Back pain

Other titles in the series

Back pain: methods for clinical investigation and assessment *edited by D. W. L. Hukins and M. A. Nelson*

Back pain: the ageing spine *edited by D. W. L. Hukins and M. A. Nelson*

Back pain

New approaches to rehabilitation and education

Edited by M. O. Roland *and* J. R. Jenner

Manchester University Press

Manchester and New York

Distributed exclusively in the USA and Canada by St Martin's Press

Published by Manchester University Press
Oxford Road, Manchester M13 9PL, UK
and Room 400, 175 Fifth Avenue,
New York, NY 10010, USA

Distributed exclusively in the USA and Canada
by St. Martin's Press, Inc.,
175 Fifth Avenue, New York, NY 10010, USA

British Library cataloguing in publication data
Back pain: new approaches to rehabilitation
and education
1. Man. Back. Backache
I. Roland, M. O. II. Jenner, J. R.
616.7'3

Library of Congress cataloging in publication data
Back pain: new approaches to rehabilitation and education/edited by
M. O. Roland and J. R. Jenner.
p. cm.
Based on papers given at a symposium held in spring 1988 at the Royal United Hospital in Bath; organized by the Society for Back Pain Research.
Includes index.
ISBN 0-7190-2789-6
1. Backache – Patients – Rehabilitation – Congresses. 2. Patient education – Congresses. I. Roland, M. O. (Martin Oliver)
II. Jenner, J. R. III. Society for Back Pain Research.
[DNLM: 1. Backache – prevention & control – congresses.
2. Backache – rehabilitation – congresses. WE 755 B126]
RD771.B217B33 1989
617'.56 – dc19
DNLM/DLC

89-2491

ISBN 0 7190 2789 6 *hardback*

Typeset in Hong Kong
by Best-set Typesetter Ltd

Printed in Great Britain
by Biddles Ltd, Guildford and King's Lynn

Contents

Preface

Few treatments for patients with back pain have been shown to be of value in scientific trials (Quebec Task Force, 1987). Education and rehabilitation are increasingly popular approaches to the management of back pain, but surprisingly little information is available on these widely used therapies. The work that has been published originates from many disciplines, including rheumatology, orthopaedic surgery, occupational medicine, general practice, osteopathy, physiotherapy, occupational therapy, ergonomics, nursing, anaesthetics and psychology; the available information is widely scattered in the literature. In an attempt to rectify this situation the Soceity for Back Pain Research organised a symposium in Spring 1988 at the Royal United Hospital in Bath, during their bicentenary anniversary celebrations, to bring together experts in these diverse disciplines. This publication is based on papers given at that meeting together with chapters from other invited authors. The result is a wide-ranging evaluation of current approaches and recent research in the fields of education and rehabilitation.

The Society felt that a fresh look at methods of prevention was essential. We have included chapters on the value of education in the form of booklets, nurse training, backschools, industrial monitoring and seating. All these important topics are given scant attention in the standard texts on the management of back pain although leaflets are frequently handed to patients, and backschools are opening in most physiotherapy departments; becoming widely available to general practitioners through 'open access' clinics.

Once a patient has developed back pain, a variety of standard treatments such as manipulation and mobilising techniques are used. These treatments are well documented and discussed in other texts, and are not included here. However, all too often treatment fails. For patients with chronic back pain three distinct methods of management are described by different authors, including an intensive in-patient programme and two out-patient appro aches – one concentrating on the physical abilities of the patient and the other utilising psychological techniques to modify the behaviour of the patient with chronic low back pain.

If progress is to be made in the evaluation of these treatments it is important that adequate methods of assessment are available. Two chapters cover this difficult area. They include discussion of the problems of assessing disability, a necessary part of the evaluation of currently available treatments.

This book should, therefore, appeal to a wide audience including the many disciplines involved in treating and trying to prevent back problems. A number of the chapters include previously unpublished approaches to treatment as well as in-depth reviews of the literature. We feel this approach of combining old and new material in each chapter provides a balanced overview of the subject matter which is not available in standard texts on the treatment of back pain.

This book will, it is hoped, serve as a cornerstone on which future services and research can be developed – at work and in the community, as well as in hospital.

M. O. Roland
J. R. Jennner

Reference

Quebec Task Force (1987). Scientific approach to the assessment and management of activity-related spinal disorders. A monograph for clinicians. Report of the Quebec Task Force on spinal disorders, *Spine*, Supplement 12, S1–S59.

Acknowledgements

The Society for Back Pain Research acknowledges with thanks the following sponsors of the meeting of Rehabilitation and Education in Back Pain: Bencard, Johnson and Johnson, Labaz, May and Baker, Ortho-Cilag and Parke Davis.

Contributors

Professor J. A. D. Anderson, MD, FFCM, Professor of Community Medicine, Guy's Hospital, London SE1.

D. J. Baker, SRN, Research Sister, Royal Orthopaedic Hospital, Birmingham B31 2AP.

A. Breen, DC, Director of Research, Anglo-European College of Chiropractic, Parkwood Road, Bournemouth BH5 2DF.

P. Buckle, PhD, FErgS, Lecturer in Ergonomics, Ergonomics Research Unit, Robens Institute of Health and Safety, University of Surrey, Guildford.

S. J. Bulstrode, MPhil, MCSP, Senior Research Physiotherapist, Royal National Hospital for Rheumatic Diseases, Bath BA1 1RL.

A. K. Burton, PhD, DO, 30 Queen Street, Huddersfield HD1 2SP.

M. D. Chard, MRCP, Senior Registrar in Rheumatology, Addenbrooke's Hospital, Cambridge CB2 2QQ.

A. K. Clarke, MRCP, Consultant in Rheumatology and Rehabilitation, Royal National Hospital for Rheumatic Diseases, Bath BA1 1RL.

C. R. Daniels, BSc, Research Assistant, ARC Occupational Health Research Unit, Guy's Hospital, London SE1.

M. Dixon, BA, Research Assistant, 125 Newmarket Road, Cambridge CB2 8HB.

C. Ellingworth, BSc, MCSP, Superintendent Physiotherapist, Doncaster Royal Infirmary, Doncaster DN2 5LT.

J. C. T. Fairbank, MD, FRCS, Director of Research, Royal Orthopaedic Hospital, Birmingham, B31 2AP.

D. C. Gardiner, BSc, Research Assistant, ARC Occupational Health Research Unit, Guy's Hospital, London SE1.

C. J. M. Getty, FRCS, Consultant Orthopaedic Surgeon, Northern General Hospital, Sheffield S5 7AU.

R. A. Harrison, MCSP, Superintendent Physiotherapist, Royal National Hospital for Rheumatic Diseases, Bath BA1 1RL.

S. Hirst, MB, Senior House Officer in Rheumatology, Addenbrooke's Hospital, Cambridge CB2 2QQ.

N. Hudson-Cook, DC, Anglo-European College of Chiropractic, Parkwood Road, Bournemouth BH5 2DF.

T. Hughes, FFARCS, Consultant Anaesthetist, Doncaster Royal Infirmary, Doncaster DN2 5LT.

J. R. Jenner, MD, MRCP, Consultant Rheumatologist, Addenbrooke's Hospital, Cambridge CB2 2QQ.

J. A. Klaber Moffett, MSc, MCSP, Research Physiotherapist, Nuffield Orthopaedic Centre, Oxford OX3 7LD.

P. Lloyd, RGN, OHNCert, RCN Advisor in Occupational Health Nursing, Royal College of Nursing, 18 Fox Street, Preston PR1 2AB.

C. J. Main, PhD, Top Grade Clinical Psychologist, Department of Clinical Psychology, Hope Hospital, Salford M6 8HD.

V. J. Markley, DipCOT, SROT, Senior Occupational Therapist, Royal East Sussex Hospital, Hastings TN34 1ER.

J. P. O'Brien, PhD, FRCS, Honorary Lecturer in Spinal Surgery, Academic Neurosurgical Unit, London Hospital, London E1 1BB.

E. Otun, BSc, MSc, Project Leader, ARC Occupational Health Research Unit, Guy's Hospital, London SE1.

H. Parker, MSc, Principal Clinical Psychologist, Department of Clinical Psychology, Hope Hospital, Salford M6 8HD.

R. W. Porter, MD, FRCS, Consultant Orthopaedic Surgeon, Doncaster Royal Infirmary, Doncaster DN2 5LT.

P. B. Pynsent, PhD, Director of Science, Royal Orthopaedic Hospital, Birmingham B31 2AP.

M. Roland, DM, MRCGP, Director of Studies in General Practice, Cambridge University School of Clinical Medicine, Addenbrooke's Hospital, Cambridge CB2 2QQ.

J. Shepperd, FRCS, Consultant Orthopaedic Surgeon, Royal East Sussex Hospital, Hastings TN34 1ER.

B. Silverman, MRCP, Registrar in Rheumatology, Addenbrooke's Hospital, Cambridge CB2 2QQ.

C. C. Spanswick, MB, ChB, FFARCS, Consultant Anaesthetist, Pain Relief Centre, Hope Hospital, Salford M6 8HD.

D. Stubbs, BEd, PhD, FErgS, Reader in Ergonomics, Ergonomics Research Unit, Robens Institute of Health and Safety, University of Surrey, Guildford.

K. Tomes-Nicholson, DC, Anglo-European College of Chiropractice, Parkwood Road, Bournemouth BH5 2DF.

F. Trailesku, MD, Senior House Officer in Orthopaedics, Doncaster Royal Infirmary, Doncaster DN2 5LT.
G. Waddell, MD, FRCS, Consultant Orthopaedic Surgeon, West of Scotland Back Pain Research Unit, Western Infirmary, Glasgow G11 6NT.

1 *G. Waddell*

A new clinical model for the treatment of low back pain*

During the past decade there has been growing concern about the present epidemic of low back disability in Western society (Cochrane Report, 1979; Nachemson, 1976; Office of Health Economics, 1985; Social Security Commission, 1986; Spitzer, 1986; Task Force on Backs, 1984). It is particularly disturbing that ever-increasing medical and health care resources are completely failing to alleviate the problem (Weber, 1986). There is a constant demand from all quarters for more research – both in basic sciences and treatment – but equally, and perhaps more fundamentally important is the question of our whole approach to low back pain. Only within the last few years has such a reappraisal really begun (Mayer *et al.*, 1985, 1986; Nachemson, 1983; Social Security Commission, 1986; Workmen's Compensation Board Symposium, 1986). This article analyses the theoretical and conceptual framework on which any real breakthrough in treatment ultimately depends.

1.1 Observations on the natural history of low back pain and disability

The following are observations about low back pain and disability:

(1) At some stage of their life, 80% of the human race will experience low back pain. Each year 2–5% of the at-risk population will seek medical attention or lose time from work because of low back problems (Benn & Wood, 1975; Cochrane Report, 1979; Horal, 1969; Hult, 1954; Kelsey & White, 1980; Office of Health Economics, 1982). As many as 60% of the normal population have

*Reprinted with permission from *Spine*.

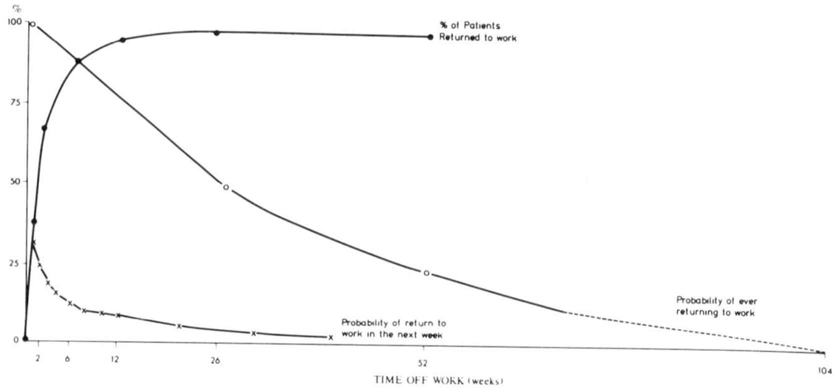

Fig 1.1 Return to work as a function of time away from work because of low back pain, showing the proportion of patients returning to work with time (Benn & Wood, 1975; Choler *et al.*, 1985; Horal, 1969; Hult, 1954; Rowe, 1969) and the diminishing probability of returning to work in the short term (Hrudey, unpublished data; Workmen's Compensation Board of British Columbia, 1986) or ever (McGill, 1968). Based mainly on data from Hrudey (unpublished data) and the Workmen's Compensation Board of British Columbia (1986)

experienced some degree of low back pain in the past year, although they will not necessarily have seen a physician or lost time from work (Consumer's Association, 1986a and b; Dunnell & Cartwright, 1972; Nuprin Pain Report, 1985; White *et al.*, 1961).

(2) A total of 80–90% of attacks of low back pain recover in about 6 weeks, irrespective of the administration or type of treatment (Figure 1.1) (Benn & Wood, 1975; Choler *et al.*, 1985; Horal, 1969; W. P. Hrudey, unpublished data; Hult, 1954; Rowe, 1969; Workmen's Compensation Board of British Columbia, 1986).

(3) Newly introduced orthopaedic services in a rapidly developing country such as Oman are inundated with patients looking for treatment for low back pain. As would be expected from the previously cited studies of Western populations, low back pain appears to be almost universal. The striking observation in Oman is that although low back pain is so common, there was very little actual disability before the introduction of Western medicine. Patients are crippled by polio, tuberculosis, or thoracolumbar fractures, but virtually no one goes to bed, stops daily life, or is permanently disabled by simple low back pain (Waddell, 1986).

(4) Low back disability has dramatically increased throughout Western society between the 1950s and 1970s (Table 1.1, Figures 1.2–1.4).

Table 1.1 United Kingdom sick certification for all forms of sickness and for back incapacities including sickness and invalidity benefit and injury benefit expressed as the annual number of spells or episodes of incapacity and as total days sick certification per 1000 persons at risk

	All incapacities				*Back incapacities*			
	Spells/1000		*Days/1000 at risk*		*Spells/1000*		*Days/1000 at risk*	
Year	*Men*	*Women*	*Men*	*Women*	*Men*	*Women*	*Men*	*Women*
1953–1954	404	406	—	—	21.7	8.0	—	—
1954–1955	432	444	14,140	17,095	22.3	8.8	506	329
1955–1956	439	444	14,107	16,807	23.8	9.5	538	352
1956–1957	410	423	13,462	16,102	25.3	9.9	545	331
1957–1958	536	574	13,736	17,596	25.3	10.2	560	365
1958–1959	479	489	14,549	16,927	27.4	11.2	595	400
1959–1960	444	459	14,005	16,177	29.1	11.9	638	438
1960–1961	488	507	14,423	16,449	29.2	12.2	630	422
1961–1962	491	526	—	—	30.5	12.9	—	—
1962–1963	494	501	15,049	15,944	31.9	13.9	720	447
1963–1964	484	497	14,999	15,919	34.9	14.5	724	530
1964–1965	505	518	15,418	16,135	37.3	15.3	761	451
1965–1966	562	565	16,562	16,487	39.1	14.9	791	423
1966–1967	512	529	16,169	15,861	41.1	16.4	863	479
1967–1968	576	600	17,704	17,237	43.8	17.3	941	491
1968–1969	582	599	17,951	16,919	43.3	18.7	976	521
1969–1970	627	631	18,780	17,365	44.1	19.0	1051	512
1970–1971	509	542	16,976	16,152	42.5	19.7	1054	547
1971–1972	504	561	17,002	16,144	41.3	20.8	1032	565
1972–1973	554	619	17,727	16,780	45.1	21.9	1097	612
1973–1974	553	621	17,895	16,630	47.3	24.1	1133	634
1974–1975	534	605	17,339	16,151	47.9	24.8	1150	642
1976–1977	535	616	18,126	15,182	51.0	29.5	1254	763
1977–1978	571	688	19,262	17,975	55.9	34.3	1432	954
1978–1979	589	752	20,210	18,307	56.9	41.3	1455	1035
1979–1980	503	705	19,337	17,966	56.1	44.6	1720	1330
1980–1981	505	690	19,314	17,433	58.2	44.7	1852	1457
1981–1982	468	655	19,859	18,171	54.6	47.7	1882	1622

No comparable figures are available from 1982 because of changes in the recording system. Back incapacities include all spinal disorders and diagnoses. Calculated from statistics supplied by the Department of Health and Social Security (DHSS).

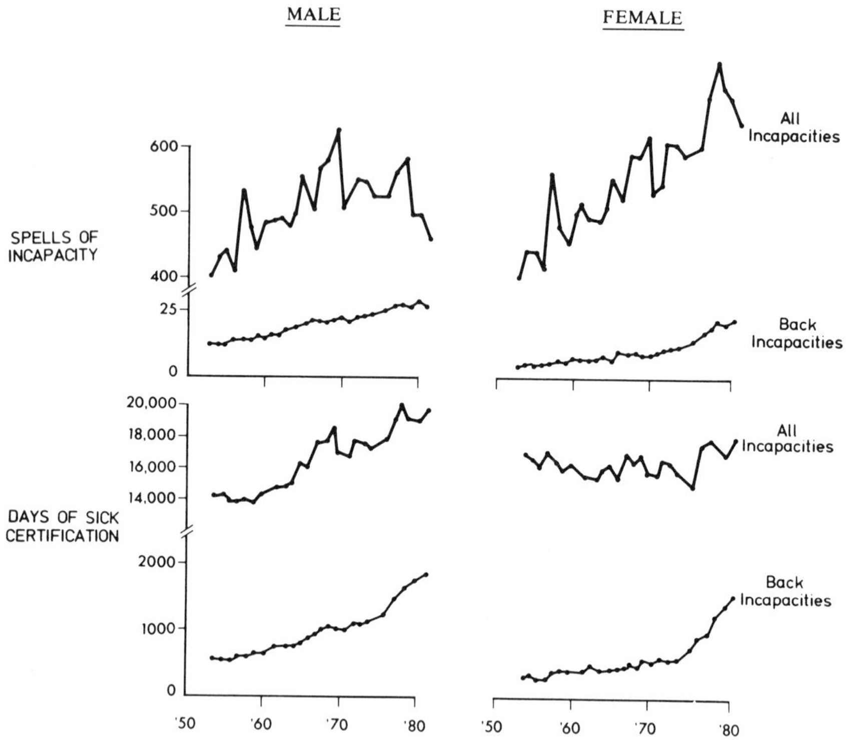

Fig 1.2 Trends of United Kingdom sick certification: annual statistics for England and Wales based on Table 1.1. Unpublished statistics supplied by the DHSS (Sample sickness and/or invalidity benefit, 1967–85)

In view of observations 1 and 5, this statement should not necessarily be interpreted as an increase in low back pain or even injuries, but more specifically as increased work loss, sick certification, compensation, and long-term disability. There may also be increased use of the diagnosis of disc prolapse (Key, 1945). However, inexorable increase in low back disability is not inevitable and some of the concepts reviewed here may already be having some impact (Figures 1.3 and 1.4).

(5) Low back pain and disability must be distinguished (American Academy of Orthopaedic Surgeons (undated); American Medical Association, 1958). Both are logically and clinically related to the underlying physical disorder or lumbar impairment, but there may be considerable disproportion in the individual patient (Figure 1.5) (Waddell, 1987; Waddell & Main, 1984). Clinical assessment of

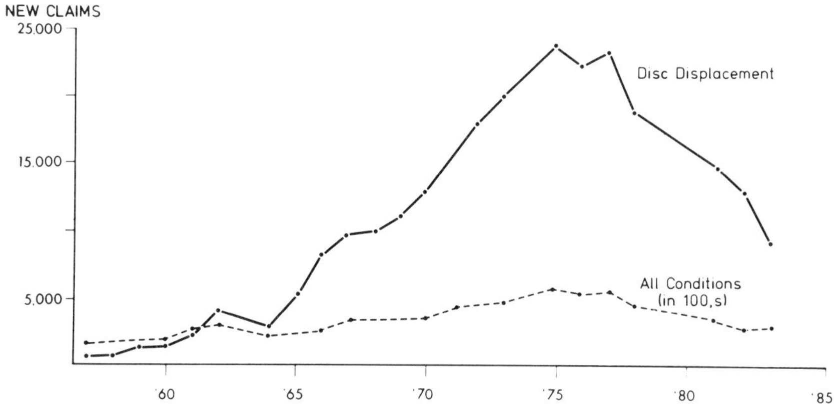

Fig 1.3 United States' Social Security Disability Insurance annual statistics of awards for permanent and total disability because of displacement of intervertebral disc, based on the Eighth Revision of the International Classification of Diseases (Social Security Bulletin, 1984–1985). During this period there was a 56% increase in the population at risk

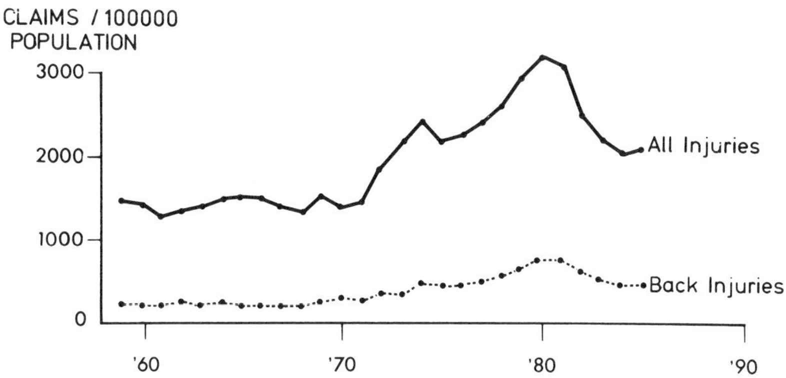

Fig 1.4 Annual statistics for Workmen's Compensation Board claims for British Columbia expressed as rates per 100 000 total population. Based on data from Hrudey (unpublished data) and the Workmen's Compensation Board of British Columbia. (1986)

pain and disability depends on the patient's subjective report, which is considerably influenced not only by the objective physical abnormality but also by the patient's attitudes and beliefs, psychological distress, and illness behaviour (Table 1.2) (Melzack, 1975; Waddell *et al.*, 1984b). The patient's report of disability based on restriction of activities of daily living may also be regarded as

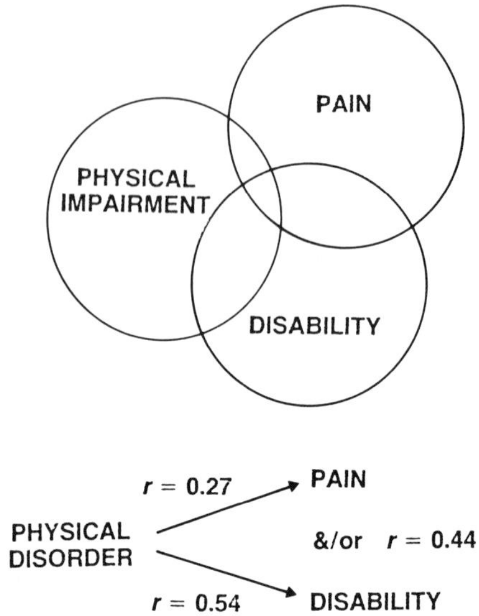

Fig 1.5 The quantitative relationship between the clinical presentation of pain, disability and objective physical impairment and the correlation coefficients (r) between them where 0 is no correlation and 1 is complete correspondence (Waddell, 1987)

avoidance learning based not only on past experience of pain but also on the patient's individual interpretation of the meaning of that pain, the assumption that pain means tissue damage and medical advice about how to react to, manage, and cope with the pain (Fordyce, 1982).

Table 1.2 Analysis of the causes of disability in chronic low back pain

Main elements of illness	*Extent to which these account for disability (%)*
Physical severity	40
Psychological distress and abnormal illness behaviour	31
Total identified[a]	71

Source: Waddell *et al.*, 1984b.
[a] Because of the inaccuracies of clinical observation, it is unusual to be able to identify such a high percentage of any biological phenomenon.

(6) Low back pain causes the greatest problem, at least as judged by health care utilisation and time away from work, in the middle working years of life with a peak age of about 40 years (Cochrane Report, 1979; Horal, 1969; Hult, 1954; Kelsey & White, 1980; Rowe, 1969). Low back pain and disability does not progressively increase with age and does not correspond to age-related changes of disc degeneration (Harris & Macnab, 1954; Urban & Maroudas, 1980). Eight controlled studies (Fullenlove & Williams, 1957; Horal, 1969; Hult, 1954; la Rocca & Macnab, 1969; Magora & Schwartz, 1976; Mensor & Duvall, 1959; Splithoff, 1953; Torgeson & Dotler, 1976) and two reviews (Nachemson, 1975; Wiltse, 1971) have shown surprisingly little relationship between clinical symptoms and radiological changes of degeneration. It is not clear why low back disability peaks in middle age.

(7) The majority of the population with low back pain and even disability cope with the problem themselves without medical treatment. Patients certainly do not go to the doctor simply because of the presence of pain or the severity of pain, and there is surprisingly little difference between patients with low back pain who see a physician and other people with low-back pain who cope with it themselves (Table 1.3) (Consumer's Association, 1986a and b; Nuprin Pain Report, 1985). Many everyday symptoms are inter-

Table 1.3 Amount and severity of back pain in people who have attended a physician and those who have received no medical attention in the past 12 months

	Medical attention in the last 12 months	
	Own physician	*None*
Duration of back pain in the last 12 months		
None	12	211
Part of the year	132	310
All or most of the year	126	79
Severity of back pain in the last 12 months on a scale of 0–10		
0–4	48	190
4–7	111	141
7–10	99	59

Calculations based on data from the Consumer's Association Back Pain Survey (1986a and b).

preted as a minor temporary nociceptive stimulus that generates little anxiety, is managed either by ignoring or resting the affected part in expectation of natural resolution, and causes little interference with life (Alonzo, 1980, 1984). Seeking health care appears to depend more on the person's perception and interpretation of the significance of the symptoms, on the availability and expectations of treatment, and on learned and cultural patterns of illness behaviour (Alonzo, 1980, 1984; Balint, 1968; Hirschfield & Behan, 1966; Mechanic, 1968, 1970, 1980; Wolff & Langley, 1968; Weinstein, 1968, 1978). The likelihood of making this decision may be increased by anxiety and emotional distress (Mechanic, 1977, 1982; Tessler *et al.*, 1976) or by life events and stress (Mechanic, 1980, 1986; Mechanic *et al.*, 1982, Mechanic & Volkart, 1960, 1961; Miller *et al.*, 1976).

(8) Once a patient reaches a physician, medical assessment and treatment is influenced more by the patient's distress and illness behaviour than by the actual physical disorder (Mechanic, 1977; Waddell *et al.*, 1984a). Medical treatment may in theory be prescribed for physical indications, but in practice both conservative (Waddell *et al.*, 1984a) and surgical (Morris *et al.*, 1986; Waddell *et al.*, 1986) treatment for a poorly understood condition such as low back pain is determined to a much greater extent than most physicians realise or would like to admit by the patient's distress and illness behaviour (Table 1.4).

(9) Despite uncontrolled personal claims for symptomatic success with particular modalities of treatment, every scientific study has shown remarkably little difference between every conceivable treatment

Table 1.4 Analysis of those elements of illness influencing how much conservative treatment patients received for low back pain

Main elements of illness	*Extent to which these account for the amount of treatment received (%)*
Duration of symptoms	14
Physical severity	11
Psychological distress	9
Abnormal illness behaviour	15
Total identified[a]	50

Source: Waddell *et al.*, 1984a.
[a] Because of the inaccuracies of clinical observation, it is unusual to be able to identify such a high percentage of any biological phenomenon.

for low back pain (Cochrane Report, 1979; Deyo, 1983; Gilbert, 1986; Nachemson, 1976b; Sackett, 1981; Weber, 1986). The few reported effects that have reached statistical significance are usually so small as to be of no practical clinical significance. It is important to distinguish between temporary or symptomatic relief and actual change in the underlying disease or natural history. It is the duty of health-care professionals to help every patient in pain. It is entirely ethical to achieve this by unscientific or even placebo means (Beecher, 1959), but this pragmatic need must be recognised for what it is and must not be confused with the demand for strict scientific proof of the effect of treatment. Viewed in this light there is no definite evidence that any treatment for low back pain is much better than a combination of natural history and placebo effect (Weber, 1986).

(10) Chronic pain becomes a completely different clinical syndrome from acute pain (Engel, 1959; Loeser & Fordyce, 1983; Sternbach, 1974, 1977; Torgeson & Dotler, 1976). Acute and chronic pain are not only different in time scale (Nachemson & Andersson, 1982) but are fundamentally different in kind. Acute and experimental pains bear a relatively straightforward relationship to peripheral stimulus, nociception, and tissue damage (International Association for the Study of Pain, 1979). There may be some understandable anxiety about the meaning and consequences of the pain (Sternbach, 1974, 1977) but acute pain, acute disability, and acute illness behaviour are generally proportionate to the physical findings. Pharmacological, physical and even surgical treatments directed to the underlying physical disorder are generally highly effective in relieving acute pain. Chronic pain, chronic disability, and chronic illness behaviour, in contrast, become increasingly dissociated from their original physical basis (Loeser & Fordyce, 1983; Philips & Jahanshahi, 1986; Wood & Main, 1985; Zarkowska & Philips, 1986) and there may, indeed, be little objective evidence of any remaining nociceptive stimulus (Fordyce *et al.*, 1981; Loeser & Fordyce, 1983; Nachemson, 1983). Instead, chronic pain and disability become increasingly associated with emotional distress, depression, failed treatment, and adoption of a sick role (Bortz, 1984; Engel, 1959; Naliboff *et al.*, 1985; Szasz, 1968; Waddell *et al.*, 1984b). Chronic pain progressively becomes a self-sustaining condition that is resistant to traditional medical management. Physical treatment directed to a supposed but unidentified and possibly nonexistent nociceptive source is not only understandably unsuccessful but may cause additional physical damage;

Table 1.5 Cause of pain in patients admitted to the Johns Hopkins Pain Clinic

Total admissions	1541
Spinal pain	1032
Low back pain with multiple surgery	826
Low back pain with no previous surgery	52

failed treatment may both reinforce and aggravate pain, distress, disability, and illness behaviour (Fordyce *et al.*, 1986; Fordyce *et al.*, 1968; Sternbach & Timmermans, 1975; Waddell *et al.*, 1979; Waddell *et al.*, 1986; Wiltse & Rocchio, 1975). Pain clinics are full of such patients who have undergone failed low back surgery (Table 1.5).

(11) Time away from work and return to work after treatment are only partly related to physical severity but appear to depend more on socioeconomic and job-related influences (Table 1.6) (Beals & Hickman, 1972; Miller, 1976; Waddell *et al.*, 1986; Weinstein, 1978). Prolonged time away from work in itself makes recovery and return to work progressively less likely (Figure 1.1) (Dworkin *et al.*, 1985; Strang, 1985). In all Western countries, however, whatever the social or medical system, work loss of more than brief duration depends on sick certification. The medical profession therefore bears the responsibility for not only sanctioning but commonly advising patients with low back pain to stay away from work.

Table 1.6 A comparison of those elements of illness influencing assessment of outcome of surgery, subjective disability, and return to work after surgery*

Patient's and surgeon's assessment of outcome of surgery (%)[a]	
Postoperative physical impairment	55
Postoperative pain	20
Total identified	75
Disability (%)[b]	
Physical impairment	40
Psychologic distress / Abnormal illness behaviour	31
Total identified	71
Return to work after surgery (%)[a]	
Postoperative disability	28
Few identified social factors†	22
Total identified	50

Sources: [a]Waddell *et al.* 1986; [b]Waddell *et al.* 1984b.

* Based on separate regression analyses of each measure.

† Very limited social information was available and this is likely to be an underestimate.

1.1.1 *Preliminary conclusions*

(1) Low back pain by its natural history appears to be a universal, benign, self-limiting condition. Indeed, low back pain may from one perspective be regarded as normal.

(2) Low back disability, as opposed to low back pain, appears to be a recent Western epidemic that is not explained by any demonstrable change in the physical disorder.

(3) Conventional medical treatment for low back pain has failed, and the role of medicine in the present epidemic must be critically examined.

1.2 **The medical model of disease**

Modern medicine traces its roots to the European Renaissance of the sixteenth and seventeenth centuries. The work of Francis Bacon (1561–1616), Galileo Galilei (1564–1642), and Isaac Newton (1642–1717) epitomised the scientific method of careful observation, systematic collection of information, and mathematical reasoning, which enabled people to unlock nature's secrets without the influence of religious revelation. Paracelsus (1493–1541), Andreas Vesalius (1514–1564), and William Harvey (1578–1657) successfully challenged the authority of Galen and applied the scientific method to the practice of medicine. Studies of human anatomy and physiology provided the basis for careful clinical observation and the application of reason to the understanding of illness. René Descartes (1596–1650), the foremost philosopher of the Renaissance, divided human existence into 'mind' and 'body' and in this dichotomy characterised pain as a simple reflex response to a physical stimulus (Descartes, 1644). Practical interpretation of pain could then be used to elucidate disease. 'A pain, an ache, a discomfort – these are the common complaint of those who seek the doctor's help. Pain issues a warning with kindly intent. She calls to action and, pointing the way, brooks no delay. And thus the ancient (sic) cycle is served, from pain to cause, to treatment to cure' (Penfield, 1969). But it was only two centuries later when Pasteur (1822–1895) discovered that infectious disease was caused by microbes (Pasteur, 1857) and Virchow (1821–1902) (Virchow, 1858) proposed the concept of cellular pathology (Virchow, 1858) that this philosophical approach could be turned into practical reality according to the following: recognise patterns of illness behaviour as symptoms and signs; infer underlying pathology for a diagnosis; relate physical therapy to underlying pathology for treatment; and expect to achieve cure with improved illness behaviour.

The industrial revolution, increasing material resources, and the explosion of technology after World War II provided the investigative and therapeutic tools that have provided for control of disease. Previous ages would regard this achievement as literally miraculous, but twentieth-century Western society has come to take it for granted. This rational physical approach to medicine reached its apogee when the mystery of life itself was unravelled in the deoxyribonucleic acid molecule (Cochrane & Crick, 1952), and it became possible to implant artificial hip joints (Charnley, 1961) and even to transplant hearts (Rider, 1975). In this mood of medical achievement and euphoria it was possible to assert confidently that the primary role of the physician was the control and, indeed, ideally the relief of all pain (Engel, 1959; World Health Organisation, 1976).

This physical approach to disease depends on the illness being due to a physical pathology, symptoms and disability being directly related to and proportionate to that physical pathology, and any psychological element being relatively unimportant or secondary to the physical disorder. Clinical recognition and diagnosis of the underlying pathology then provides the basis for rational physical treatment of the illness.

1.3 A biopsychosocial concept of illiness

Medicine has a much more ancient and richer lineage than science. Since before the time of Plato the relationship between mind and body has been held to be of fundamental importance to human existence and to medicine. Aristotle recognised that people are social animals who live and act – and become ill – in social relationships with other human beings. Hippocrates emphasised the already well-established tradition that physicians' practical roles as healers cannot be separated from their social roles of helping human beings cope with illness and suffering (Hippocrates, 1923 translation).

There is no logical reason why scientific treatment of disease should not be combined with human care of the patient (American Board of Internal Medicine, 1979). It is only because of the limitations of human nature that increased time, training, and concentration on the physical aspects of disease has led to neglect of the psychological and social aspects of illness (Flexner, 1910). All physicians agree in principle with the need to treat each patient as a human being and then in busy practice too often get on with the practicalities of treating perceived disease. Yet from Claude Bernard (Bernard, 1878) to the present day there has been a constant note of concern and criticism both from eminent members of the profession (Reiser, 1978) and independent observers (Kennedy, 1981) that too mechanistic an approach may cure many serious diseases but only deals with one half – and not necessarily the most important half – of medicine's role in society.

Application of these humanitarian principles to the daily practice of medicine has fallen behind the physical therapy of disease. Nearly a century ago Sigmund Freud (1856–1939) reaffirmed the importance of psychological factors in medicine and showed that psychoneurotic symptoms could be assessed clinically and provide insight into emotional processes (Freud, 1959). Adolf Meyer (1866–1950) originally developed the concept of 'multicausality' in psychiatry but recognised that psychosocial factors influenced the course and outcome of every illness, and that each patient must be seen and assessed as a person (Meyer, 1917). Such a holistic view of medicine has been the hallmark, inspiration and source of pre-eminence of American psychiatry (Lipowski, 1981) and it has rightly been claimed that an understanding of the psychosocial aspects of illness is one of the most important contributions that the behavioural sciences can make to medicine (Lipowski, 1969). Because mental illness has never comfortably fitted the disease model, psychiatrists have raised fundamental questions about the medical model and proposed an alternative biopsychosocial model which includes physical, psychological, and social elements. (Engel, 1977, 1982; Fabrega, 1972, 1975; Lipowski, 1969, 1981, 1983). This is very much a model of human illness rather than disease and may apply equally well to nonpsychiatric illness (Figure 1.6).

The gate control theory of pain (Melzack & Wall, 1965) provided the physiological basis for the biopsychosocial model. Pain can no longer be regarded as merely a physical sensation of noxious stimulus and disease, but conscious experience of pain may be modulated by mental, emotional, and sensory mechanisms and includes both sensory and emotional components (International Association for the Study of Pain, 1979; Mechanic, 1980; Melzack & Casey, 1968; Turk *et al.*, 1983). The major conceptual contribution of the gate control theory is that it replaces the Cartesian mind – body dichotomy and allows for the complexity of observed pain

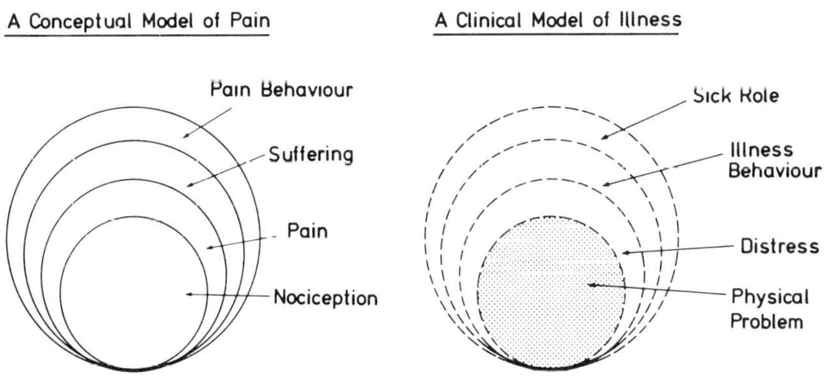

Fig 1.6 The biopsychosocial concept of illness (Engel, 1977). Loeser's conceptual model of pain (Loeser, 1982) and the Glasgow Illness Model (Waddell *et al.*, 1984a and b) – an operational model for clinical practice

phenomena. It explains how psychological and social influences may indeed modulate individual perception of and response to disease. The gate control theory has stimulated and contributed greatly to the new clinical approach to illness. However, it is important to avoid overemphasis of pain as the single most important element of human illness and even the sole aim of medical treatment (Engel, 1959; Wall, 1986). Nor must the theory be misapplied clinically merely to perpetuate the errors of the disease model in a new direction. Pain does not necessarily have to receive physical treatment independent of the ability to diagnose disease or without due consideration of non-physical factors. The gate mechanism should not be invoked simply to move failed physical treatment to a slightly higher level in the neural pathway. The true clinical application of the gate control theory lies in a fuller understanding of human pain and illness.

Several elements of the biopsychosocial model have been developed further in the behavioural sciences. Early psychological hopes that personality tests would predict individual respose to illness have not been realised (Graham, 1977; Main & Waddell, 1987) but have given birth to a number of simple psychological questionnaires mesuring distress (Beck *et al.*, 1961; Main, 1983; Zung, 1965). Medical sociology (Mechanic, 1986; Mechanic & Volkart, 1960, 1961), behavioural psychology (Fordyce, 1976; Fordyce *et al.*, 1968; Turk *et al.*, 1983) and psychiatry have combined to develop the concept of illness behaviour that has been defined clinically as 'observable and potentially measurable actions and conduct which express and communicate the individual's own perception of disturbed health' (Waddell *et al.*, 1984a). Sociologists have considered illness as a social phenomenon or sick role (Mayou, 1984; Mechanic, 1968, 1977, 1980, 1986; Mechanic *et al.*, 1982; Mechanic & Volkart, 1960, 1961; Parsons, 1951).

The whole biopsychosocial concept emphasises human illness rather than disease. This must now be applied to clinical practice (Leigh & Reiser, 1980; McWhinney, 1972).

1.4 **An analysis of success and failure in treating low back disorders**

In the past generation we have been able to a large degree to treat and even prevent many serious spinal diseases such as polio, tuberculosis, spinal deformities, and paralysis. Since the identification of the disc prolapse (Mixter & Barr, 1934) surgical relief has become routine for nerve compression that fails to resolve naturally. Disc surgery has survived the test of time for half a century because at least 70–80% of carefully selected patients obtain relief (Spangfort, 1972). Such dramatic surgical successes unfortunately only apply to approximately 1% of patients with low back disorders (Office of Health Economics, 1985). Our failure involves the remaining 99% of patients with low back pain for whom the problem has become progressively worse – despite new investigative techniques and a bewildering variety of treatments (Figures 1.2–1.4).

Diagnosis may be substantive or nominal (Zigmond, 1976). Substantive diagnoses have objective clinical features, and investigations confirm a definite pathological process, which may permit rational and successful treatment. In most patients with low back pain, however, we have neither the biomechanical nor pathological understanding to identify any definite pathological process nor even the anatomical source of pain (Nachemson, 1976a). However, human beings dislike uncertainty, fear the unknown, and search for meaning as the first stage to control (Mechanic, 1977). Preference for even a nominal diagnosis is clearly demonstrated by the vogue for the diagnosis of disc prolapse (Figure 1.3). Mixter's (Mixter & Barr, 1934) original insistence on the need for definite clinical and radiological proof before diagnosis was rapidly forgotten. By 1945 Key could state dogmatically that 99% of low back pain, apart from tumour or infection was due to 'lesions' of the intervertebral disc. Of patients coming to our clinic, 60% believe or have been told that they have a disc prolapse, although only 11% have any evidence of nerve root pain or dysfunction (Waddell, 1982). Radiological changes of degeneration are equally irresistible as a causal explanation of symptoms, ignoring their normal, age-related occurrence (see observation 6). Patients and physicians alike are much happier with even a nominal diagnosis. Unfortunately once such a nominal diagnosis has been made we forget that it was only a convenient label and treat it as if it were substantive. Not unexpectedly, the success rate of treatment based on such a nominal diagnosis is low (Spangfort, 1972). Unjustified pseudopathological diagnosis must be avoided and replaced with a clear, unambiguous term such as simple strain or non-specific low back pain (Editorial, 1979). Physical treatment, particularly potentially harmful treatment such as surgery, should be directed to objective pathological conditions that it is likely to help. A study of the indications for spinal surgery suggests that decisions to undertake surgery are frequently based on the duration and severity of the patient's pain and disability, the patient's distress and illness behaviour, and the failure of conservative treatment; completely unrelated to these factors, the outcome of surgery depends on the accuracy of diagnosis of a surgically treatable lesion (Waddell *et al.*, 1986). The patient's demand and the physician's desire to help must not confuse logical, rational decisions about physical treatment based on substantive diagnosis.

When the number of low back operations escalated after World War II it was soon realised that the failures of spinal surgery were catastrophic (De Palma & Rothman, 1970; Frymoyer & Donaghy, 1985; Greenwood *et al.*, 1952; Kelly *et al.*, 1954; Waddell *et al.*, 1979, 1986). Every study for the past 30 years has stressed the association of surgical failure with psychological disturbances (Gray *et al.*, 1984; Waddell *et al.*, 1979, 1986; Wiltse & Roccio, 1975). Wiltse and Rocchio (1975) first demonstrated that preoperative psychological tests could actually predict how patients would respond to treatment. A number of prospective studies have subsequently shown that psychological factors influence how patients respond to any form of physical treatment, whether by physiotherapy (Bergquist-Ullman & Larsson, 1977; Brown *et al.*, 1954), rehabilitation (Beals & Hickman, 1972; Flynn & Salomone, 1977), chemonucleolysis (McCulloch, 1977; Wiltse & Rocchio, 1975), surgical decompression (Dzioba & Doxey, 1984b; Oostdam *et al.*, 1981; Pheasant *et al.*, 1979), fusion (Wing *et al.*, 1973), repeat spinal surgery (Dzioba & Doxey, 1984a) or pain tract surgery (Blumetti & Modesti, 1976). The most important psychological disturbances associated with low back pain are anxiety, increased bodily awareness, and depressive symptoms; these are best interpreted clinically as psychological distress (Mechanic, 1977; Sternbach, 1974; Waddell *et al.*, 1984b, 1986). Distress is largely secondary to the physical disorder and becomes better or worse with the success or failure of treatment (Sternbach & Timmermans, 1975; Waddell *et al.*, 1986). In addition, distress arising from unrelated causes may aggravate and perpetuate physical pain.

Clinical observation should distinguish the symptoms and signs of physical disease from those of distress and illness behaviour (Ransford *et al.*, 1976; Waddell *et al.*, 1980, 1984b). This is most simply illustrated by the pain drawing (Ransford *et al.*, 1976). The way that patients draw their pain is influenced by distress, and the patient's apparently straightforward description of pain provides both physical information about the pain and psychological information about their response to it (Figure 1.7). Similarly, the adjectives that patients use to describe pain fall into two distinct patterns: those that describe the sensory qualities of pain and other adjectives that are mainly about the emotional qualities of the pain experience (Leavitt *et al.* 1978; Benn & Wood, 1975). Inappropriate descriptions of symptoms and inappropriate responses to examination have also been described in low back pain and provide a clinical measure of distress and illness behaviour (Table 1.7) (Waddell *et al.*, 1980, 1984b).

We have tested the biopsychosocial model in clinical practice by analysing the mathematical relationship between the elements of illness in chronic low back pain. We compared pain and disability and physical impairment (Figure 1.4) (Waddell, 1987). We confirmed distress as the most important psychological disturbance (Waddell *et al.*, 1984b). We examined the distinction between symptoms and signs of illness behaviour and those of physical disease (Table 1.7) (Waddell *et al.*, 1984b). Distress and illness behaviour are secondary to the physical disorder and improve or deteriorate with successful or failed treatment (Waddell *et al.*, 1986). Physical disorder, distress and illness behaviour combine to produce disability (Table 1.2)

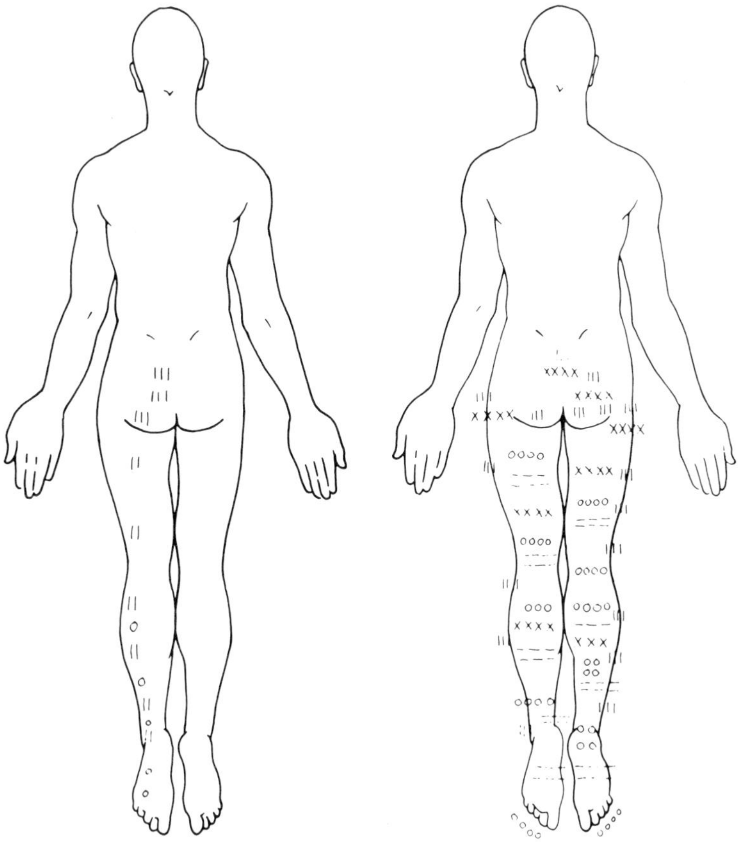

A B

Fig 1.7 The pain drawing provides clinical information about the physical and emotional characteristics of the patient's pain (Ransford *et al.*, 1976). Patient A describes the anatomical pattern of S1 pain and paraesthesia from a disc prolapse. Patient B with simple low back pain does not have cauda equina involvement but is communicating distress. Many patients do both to varying degrees: (‖) pain; (o) pins and needles; (x) ache, (=) numbness). Reproduced from Waddell *et al.*, 1984a with permission

(Waddell *et al.*, 1984b). Medical decisions about conservative (Waddell *et al.*, 1984a) and surgical (Waddell *et al.*, 1986) treatment are influenced more by distress and illness behaviour than by physical indications (Table 1.3). The interaction between physical and psychological factors determines the outcome of treatment (Waddell *et al.*, 1986). Work loss and return to work are determined more by social factors than by physical dis-

Table 1.7 A comparison of the symptoms and signs of physical disease and abnormal illness behaviour in chronic low back pain

	Physical disease/ normal illness behaviour	*Magnified or inappropriate illness behaviour*
Pain drawing[a]	Localised Neuroanatomical Proportionate	Non-anatomical Regional Magnified
Pain adjectives[b]	Sensory	Emotional
Symptoms[c]		
Pain	localised	Whole leg pain Tailbone pain
Numbness	Dermatomal	Whole leg numbness
Weakness	Myotomal	Whole leg giving way
Time pattern	Varies with time	Never free of pain
Response to treatment	Variable benefit	Intolerance of treatments Emergency admissions to hospital
Signs[d]		
Tenderness	Localised	Superficial Widespread nonanatomical
Axial loading	No lumbar pain	Lumbar pain
Simulated rotation	No lumbar pain	Lumbar pain
Straight leg raising	Limited on distraction	Improves with distraction
Sensory	Dermatomal	Regional
Motor	Myotomal	Regional, jerky, giving way
General response	Appropriate pain	Overt pain behaviour

Source: [a]Ransford *et al.*, 1976; [b]Melzack, 1975; [c]Waddell *et al.*, 1984b; [d]Waddell *et al.*, 1980.

ease (Table 1.6) (Waddell *et al.*, 1986). All these analyses confirm that the biopsychosocial concept of illness can be used as an operational clinical model (Figure 1.6B), which explains many of the observations on the natural history of low back pain and disability.

1.5 **Rest or recovery?**

Restriction of activity, rest, and even bed rest is now the treatment most commonly prescribed by physicians for low back pain (Table 1.8) apart from symptomatic analgesics. Bed rest is now unanimously taught in all standard textbooks as the first line of treatment for 'acute attacks', yet it is difficult to discover when or why it became the accepted 'conservative' treatment. One of the patients in the original description of disc prolapse

Table 1.8 Treatment for low back pain

Treatment	*One course (%)*	*> One course (%)*
Analgesics	18	69
Bed rest	21	27
Corset	14	17
Physiotherapy	10	14
Manipulation	5	5

Incidence reported by 500 patients attending orthopaedic clinics (M. Di Paola and G. Waddell, unpublished observations).

by Mixter and Barr (1934) had 'several months in absolute recumbency on a Bradford frame without relief (sic)' before surgery. As early as 1923 a standard orthopaedic text (Jones & Lovett, 1923) suggested that immediate recumbency was required for the most severe cases of back 'strains' but also cautioned against excessive bed rest and advised that 'as soon as possible, movement must be encouraged and bed forbidden'. Personal experience (R. Barnes, unpublished data), however, suggests that this was very much the exception and only employed for unusual cases before World War II. Even as late as 1966, family physicians could write that 'little discussion (of acute low back pain or its treatment)...is given in the standard textbooks of orthopaedics' (Dillane *et al.*, 1966). As bed rest of more than a few days duration is *ipso facto* associated with work loss, sick certification statistics suggest that bed rest has been widely prescribed within the last generation only.

The rationale of rest – and particularly bed rest – is not as obvious as might be imagined. It appears to be based on the clinical observation that lying down may relieve pain, although this only applies to one person in two (Table 1.9). The pathophysiological argument (Deyo, 1983; Gilbert, 1986) appears to be a combination of a nominal diagnosis of disc prolapse (Mixter & Barr, 1934) and the biomechanical observation that intradiscal pressure is lowest in the lying position (Nachemson, 1966, 1975; Nachemson

Table 1.9 Effect of activity on low back pain

	Relieves pain (%)	*No difference (%)*	*Makes pain worse (%)*
Lying down	58	30	10
Walking	16	45	36

Incidence reported by 500 patients attending orthopaedic clinics in Glasgow and the Consumer's Association Back Pain Survey (1986a and b).

Table 1.10 Most effective treatment/cure for low back pain

Type of treatment	(%)
Analgesics	35
Local heat, applications, and massage	30
Exercise, physiotherapy, and manipulation	20
Rest and lying down	14

Based on data from the Glasgow Hospital's orthopaedic outpatient clinics and the Consumers' Association Back Pain Survey (1986a and b).

& Morris, 1964), although this was certainly not intended nor interpreted in this way by the original authors. There are moreover a number of completely illogical steps in the clincial application of this argument. Symptomatic relief of pain is not necessarily associated with alteration of the natural history or cure of the pain (compare Tables 1.9 and 1.10 based on the same group of patients). Disc prolapse only constitutes a few percent of all low back pain, and treatment for disc prolapse cannot necessarily be extrapolated to all low back pain. Because of the difference between acute and chronic pain, treatment directed to the noxious stimulus of acute pain cannot simply be continued into chronic pain.

There is remarkably little scientific or clinical evidence to support the value of bed rest for low back pain or even sciatica. There are only four controlled studies of bed rest recorded in the literature (Deyo *et al.*, 1985; Gilbert *et al.*, 1985; Lidstrom & Zachrisson, 1970; Wiesel *et al.*, 1980). Only the study by Weisel *et al.* (1980) showed a clear advantage to bed rest, but this study suffered major methodological defects (Gilbert, 1986; McVeigh, 1986); it used army recruits and compared admissions to sick bay with continued, albeit modified, duties. No allowance was made for the patient's attitudes to the treatment or to training. In the particular military context there was considerable observer bias in assessing results. Yet this is the only clinical trial suggesting that bed rest is better than continued ambulation. In complete contrast, Gilbert *et al.* (1985) found no statistically significant differences between bed rest, exercise, and no treatment although the results tended to favour early mobilisation; Lidstrom & Zachrisson (1970) found little difference between exercise and rest except that exercises improved muscle strength. Deyo *et al.* (1985, 1986) showed that 2 days of bed rest was better than 7 days or, to put it the other way round, that 7 days of bed rest was proportionately more harmful than 2 days! There is no evidence whatsoever comparing bed rest in hospital with bed rest at home, which makes it difficult to justify the admission of 40–50 000 patients to hospital each year in the United Kingdom for bed rest for low back pain, permanently occupying 2000 hospital beds while other patients are kept waiting up to 3 years for the proven procedure of hip replacement for osteoarthritis (Office of Health Economics, 1982, 1985).

There is, however, little doubt about the deleterious effects of bed rest, particularly if prolonged (Bortz, 1984; Mayer *et al.*, 1985, 1986). Protracted rest leads to a catabolic state with general malaise (Bortz, 1984). There is demineralisation of bone (Sandstrom *et al.*, 1985) and 3% loss of muscle strength per day (D. Spengler, unpublished data). There is decreased physical fitness (Mayner *et al.*, 1985, 1986) and rest and inactivity may inhibit healing (Bortz, 1984). More generally, prolonged rest leads to increased psychological distress and depression, loss of the work habit, increased difficulty in starting rehabilitation, progressive loss of job opportunity, and decreasing probability of ever returning to work (Figure 1.1) (W. P. Hrudey, unpublished data; Strang, 1985). Perhaps the final test is to look at how physicians treat themselves. At a recent meeting (Workmen's Compensation Board Symposium, 1986) 60% of 230 physicians reported personal experience of low back pain. Only two had stayed in bed for as long as 2 weeks and none for longer periods. Yet physicians continue to treat their patients with prolonged periods of bed rest in a way they would never treat themselves. Some patients with simple low back pain are actually treated as if they were more seriously ill than patients with myocardial infarction who now routinely receive early ambulation (Hurst, 1975).

Conversely, there is no evidence that activity is harmful and, contrary to common belief, it does not necessarily even aggravate the pain (Table 1.9). With increasing biomechanical understanding, it is possible to avoid specific activities that increase the load on the spine (Bergquist-Ullman & Larsson, 1977; Nachemson, 1976a, 1983; Zachrisson, 1981) and several studies have demonstrated that patients with low back pain or sciatica can, despite their pain, do selected activities almost normally without increasing their pain (Berkson *et al.*, 1977; McNeill *et al.*, 1980; Nachemson & Lindh, 1965). There is, indeed, evidence that increased activity may not only promote bone and muscle strength (Bortz, 1984; Lidstrom & Zachrisson, 1970; Sandstrom *et al.*, 1985) as well as improve disc and cartilage nutrition, but may also increase systemic endorphin levels and reduce sensitivity to pain (Nachemson, 1983). There is no evidence that early return to work increases the likelihood of future recurrences. On the contrary, physically fit people have fewer and shorter attacks of low back pain and are more tolerant of pain (Biering-Soresen, 1984; Cady *et al.*, 1979; Nachemson, 1983). Fordyce and other behavioural psychologists have investigated the relationship between chronic pain and physical activity. (Fordyce *et al.*, 1981; Linton, 1985). They suggest that pain behaviours are influenced and modified by their consequences (Fordyce *et al.*, 1968, 1982). Exercise to the limit of pain tolerance is strongly influenced by conscious feedback of how much exercise has been done and, in the absence of such feedback, chronic pain patients do the same amount of exercise as normal, pain-free people (Fordyce, 1982). The exercise tolerance of chronic pain patients is markedly improved by verbal praise and reinforcement from a physiotherapist (Cairns & Pasino, 1977). Although patients with chronic low back pain almost universally report lower levels of activity, careful observation shows that subjective reports of pain are largely unrelated to actual activity levels (Fordyce *et al.*, 1981; Linton, 1985), and observed pain behaviour is actually inversely proportional to the amount of exercise done (Fordyce *et al.*, 1981). Fordyce *et al.*, (1986) compared traditional medical treatment directly with a behavioural approach to the early treatment of acute low back pain. Traditional treatment consisted of rest, analgesics, and activity prescribed as necessary; the patient was advised to 'let pain be your guide' compared with a fixed regimen of incremented activity based on tissue healing times. At 1-year follow-up, patients treated on the traditional basis reported that disability had actually increased, and patients treated on the prescribed regimen had returned to pre-onset levels of activity. Dolce *et al.* (1986) independently confirmed that a fixed exercise quota resulted in increased exercise capability, and decreased anxiety about the effects of exercise. Berntzen & Gotestam (1987) confirmed that regular analgesics gave better pain relief than medication prescribed as needed and also reduced drug dependency.

Improved understanding of the relationship between pain and activity has already been tested in clinical practice. For as long as they have existed, industrial physicians and occupational therapists have emphasised the physical, psychological, and social value of early return to work (Derebery & Tullis, 1983; Goldberg, 1982; White, 1966), although this has never been proved scientifically (Catchlove & Cohen, 1982; McVeigh, 1986). Improved spinal ergonomics combined with physiotherapy produced the 'back school' approach to patient education where improved understanding reduces fear and improves patients' ability to cope with their back problems (Hall & Iceton, 1983; White, 1979; Zachrisson, 1981). The goal of most pain management programmes is rehabilitative rather than curative and combines improvement in functional capacity with reduction of illness behaviour. Patients assume a more active role in which they can share the responsibility and begin to cope with the problem themselves (Follick *et al.*, 1985; Main, 1987; Mechanic, 1977). Mayer and colleagues (1985, 1986) have combined these principles into a sports medicine approach to the clinical rehabilitation of patients with chronic low back pain. Objective functional capacity measurements were used to guide patients on an active exercise programme, with the emphasis on improvement in disability and function rather than solely on pain. This was supplemented by psychological support and education to help patients themselves to cope better with and manage their pain. Despite some temporary increase in pain, in the long term patients not only improved their objective functional capacity but this was associated with less pain, less psychological distress, less health care utilisation, and 86% return to work. An active approach to illness can indeed be used in clinical practice to treat the whole person.

The evidence is clear. There is a fundamental antithesis between the passive and active approaches of rest or activity. There is no evidence that rest has any beneficial effect on the natural history of low back pain. On the contrary, there is strongly suggestive evidence that rest, particularly prolonged bed rest, may be the most harmful treatment ever devised and a potent cause of iatrogenic disability. There is clear evidence that, despite general belief, activity is not harmful, and active rehabilitation not only restores function but also reduces pain. It remains to be proved whether a policy of active mobilisation and early return to work can be put into widespread clinical practice (McVeigh, 1986) but the following questions can no longer be avoided: Rest or rehabilitation? Rest or restoration of function? Rest or recovery?

1.6 **Conclusions**

Low back pain is universal but low back disability is a relatively recent Western epidemic. Modern medicine can successfully treat many spinal diseases and persisting nerve compression but has completely failed to cure the vast majority of patients with simple low back pain. Overemphasis on pain alone, overdependence on a nominal diagnosis of disc prolapse, and overprescription of rest may indeed be a major cause of iatrogenic disability.

We still have a lot to learn about low back pain. We must relate improved biomechanical understanding to clinical observation in the individual patient. We must develop methods of localising the exact source of pain. We must differentiate syndromes of low back pain. And we must conduct proper, controlled trials to determine which treatments are most effective for various types of low back pain and develop a rational basis for choosing that most effective treatment for individual patients.

Equally, and fundamentally more important, we must change our whole aproach to low back disorders. We all agree in principle with the need to treat the whole person. To make this a practical reality, we must consider low back disability as an illness rather than low back pain as a disease (Table 1.11). We all recognise in theory the need to consider the physical, psychological, and social aspects of illness. In practice, we must distinguish pain from disability, distinguish the symptoms and signs of psychological distress and illness behaviour from those of physical disease, and direct treatment to restoration of function as well as relief of pain. It is unlikely that there will ever be a magic cure for all low back pain, so the physician's role as healer must be accompanied by his or her more ancient role as counsellor, helping patients to cope with their problems. The patient's role must correspondingly change from passive recipient of treatment to a more active sharing of responsibility for his or her own progress. The main theme of management must change from rest to rehabilitation and restoration of function.

This requires change in medicine, patients, and society. Some change must be at a political level. But physicians cannot escape their prime responsibility, both as the final providers of health care and for providing society with a new understanding of illness, which alone makes real change possible.

Acknowledgements

The author thanks David Allan, Michael Bond, Bill Fordyce, David Hamblen, Bill Hrudey, John Loeser, Chris Main, Alf Nachemson, Henrik Weber and Philip Wood for their ideas, information and assistance. Original data and detailed analyses were supplied by the Consumer's Association, London, the Department of Health and Social Security Headquarters Division SR8B, Newcastle-upon-Tyne, and the Workmen's Compensation Board of British Columbia.

References

Alonzo, A. A. (1980). Acute illness behaviour: A conceptual exploration and specification. *Social Science and Medicine*, **14A**, 515–26.

Alonzo, A. A. (1984). An illness behaviour paradigm: A conceptual exploration of a situational-adaptation perspective. *Social Science and Medicine*, **19**, 499–510.

American Academy of Orthopaedic Surgeons (undated). *Manual for Orthopaedic Surgeons in Evaluating Permanent Physical Impairment*, pp. 1–30. Chicago, Illinois.

American Board of Internal Medicine (1979). Clinical competence in internal medicine. *Annals Internal Medicine*, **90**, 402–11.

American Medical Association (1958). A guide to the evaluation of permanent impairment of the extremities and back, *Journal of the American Medical Association* (Suppl.), **166**, 1–122.

Balint M. (1968). *The Doctor, His Patient and the Illness*, Second edn. Pitman, London.

Beals, R. K. & Hickman, N. W. (1972). Industrial injuries of the back and extremities, *Journal of Bone and Joint Surgery*, **54A**, 1593–1611.

Beck, A. T., Ward, C. H., Mendelson, M. M., Mock, J. & Erbaugh, J. (1961). An inventory for measuring depression, *Archives of General Psychiatry*, 4, 561–71.

Beecher, H. K. (1959). *Measurement of subjective responses: Quantitative effect of drugs*. Oxford University Press, New York.

Benn, R. T. & Wood, P. H. N. (1975). Pain in the back. An attempt to estimate the size of the problem, *Rheumatology and Rehabilitation*, **14**, 121–8.
Bergquist-Ullman, M. & Larsson, U. (1977). Acute low back pain in industry, *Acta Orthopaedica Scandinavica* (Suppl.), **170**, 1–117.
Berkson, M., Schultz, A., Nachemson, A. & Andersson, G. B. J. (1977). Voluntary strengths of male adults with acute low back pain, *Clinical Orthopaedics*, **129**, 84–95.
Bernard, C. (1878). *Leçons sur les Phénomènes de la Vie Commune aux Animaux et aux Végétaux*. Baillière, Paris.
Berntzen, D. & Gotestam, K. G. (1987). Effects of on-demand or fixed interval schedules in the treatment of chronic pain with analgesia compounds: An experimental study, *Journal of Consulting and Clinical Psychology*, **55**, 213–17.
Biering-Soresen, P. (1984). Physical measurements as risk indicators for low back trouble over a one year period, *Spine*, **9**, 106–19.
Blumetti, A. E. & Modesti, L. M. (1976). Psychological predictors of success or failure of surgical intervention for intractable back pain. In: *Advances in Pain Research and Therapy*, Vol 1, ed. J. J. Bonica and D. Albe-Fessard. Raven Press, New York.
Bortz, W. M. (1984). The disuse syndrome, *Western Journal of Medicine*, **141**, 691–4.
Brown, T., Barr, J. S, Nemiah, J. C. & Barry, H. (1954). Psychological factors in low back pain, *New England Journal of Medicine*, **251**, 123–8.
Cady, L., Bischoff, D. & O'Connel, E. (1979). Strength and fitness and subsequent back injuries in firefighters, *Journal of Occupational Medicine*, **21**, 269–72.
Cairns, D. & Pasino, J. (1977). Comparison of verbal reinforcement and feedback in the operant treatment of disability due to chronic low back pain, *Behavioural Therapy*, **8**, 621–30.
Catchlove, R. & Cohen, K. (1982). Effects of a directive return to work approach in the treatment of workmen's compensation patients with chronic pain, *Pain*, **14**, 181–91.
Charnley, J. (1961). Arthroplasty of the hip: A new operation, *Lancet*, **1**, 1129–32.
Choler, U., Larsson, R. Nachemson, A. & Paterson, L-E. (1985). Ont y ryggen – farsok med vardsprogram for patienter med lumbala smattillstrand. Stockholm, *SPRI Report*, 188/85.
Cochrane Report (1979). *Working Group on Back Pain*, HMSO, London.
Cochrane, W. & Crick, F. H. C. (1952). Evidence of the Pauling-Covey α-helix in synthetic polypeptides, *Nature*, **169**, 234–5.
Consumer's Association (1986a). *Back Pain Survey*, London.
Consumer's Association (1986b). Back pain: The *Which* report, *Which?* February, 58–63.
De Palma, A. F. & Rothman, R. H. (1970). *The Intervertebral Disc*. WB Saunders Company, Philadelphia.
Derebery, W. J. & Tullis, W. H. (1983). Delayed recovery in the patient with a work compensable injury, *Journal of Occupational Medicine*, **25**, 829–33.
Descartes, R. (1644) *L'Homme*. Translated by M. Foster. Cambridge University Press, New York.
Deyo, R. A. (1983). Conservative therapy for low back pain: Distinguishing useful from useless therapy, *Journal of the American Medical Association*, **250**, 1057–62.
Deyo, R. A., Diehl, A. K. & Rosenthal, M. (1985). How much bed rest for backache? A randomised clinical trial, *Clinical Research*, **33**, 248A.

Deyo, R. A., Diehl, A. K. & Rosenthal, M. (1986). How many days of bed rest for acute low back pain? *New England Journal of Medicine*, **315**, 1064–70.
Dillane, J. B., Fry, J. & Kalton, G. (1966). Acute back syndrome – A study from general practice, *British Medical Journal*, **2**, 82–84.
Dolce, J. J., Crocker, M. F., Moletteire, C. & Doleys, D. M. (1986). Exercise quotas, anticipatory concern and self-efficacy expectancies in chronic pain: A preliminary report, *Pain*, **24**, 365–72.
Dunnell, K. & Cartwright A. (1972). *Medicine Takers, Prescribers and Hoarders*. Routledge & Kegan Paul, London.
Dworkin, R. H., Handlin, D. S., Richlin, D. M., Brand, L. & Vannucci, C. (1985). Unravelling the effects of compensation, litigation and employment on treatment response in chronic pain, *Pain*, **23**, 49–59.
Dzioba, R. B. & Doxey, N. C. (1984). *Predictors of outcome of repeat back surgery following industrial injuries*. Presented at the annual meeting of the American Academy of Orthopaedic Surgeons, 1984.
Dzioba, R. B. & Doxey, N. C. (1984b). A prospective investigation into the orthopaedic and psychologic predictors of outcome of first lumbar surgery following industrial injury, *Spine*, **9**, 614–23.
Editorial (1979). Back pain – what can we offer? *British Medical Journal*, **1**, 706.
Engel, G. L. (1959). Psychogenic pain and the pain prone patient, *American Journal of Medicine*, **26**, 899–918.
Engel, G. L. (1977). The need for a new medical model: A challenge for biomedicine, *Science*, **196**, 129–36.
Engel, G. L. (1982). The biopsychosocial model and medical education, *New England Journal of Medicine*, **306**, 802–5.
Fabrega, H. (1972). The position of psychiatry in the understanding of human disease, *Archives of General Psychiatry*, **32**, 1500–12.
Fabrega, H. (1975). The need for an ethnomedical science, *Science*, **189**, 969–75.
Flexner, A. (1910). *Medical Education in the United States and Canada*. Carnegie Foundation, New York.
Flynn, R. J. & Salomone, P. R. (1977). Performance of the MMPI in predicting rehabilitation outcome: A discriminant analysis, double-cross validation assessment, *Rehabilitation Literature*, **38**, 12–15.
Follick, M. J., Smith, T. W. & Ahern, D. K. (1985). Sickness impact profile: A global measure of disability in chronic low back pain, *Pain*, **21**, 67–76.
Fordyce, W. E. (1976). *Behavioural Methods for Chronic Pain and Illness*. CV Mosby, St Louis.
Fordyce, W. E. (1982). A behavioural perspective on chronic pain, *British Journal of Clinical Psychology*, **21**, 313–20.
Fordyce, W. E., Brockway, J. A., Bergman, J. A. & Spengler, D. (1986). Acute back pain: A control group comparison of behavioural vs. traditional management methods, *Journal of Behavioural Medicine*, **9**, 127–40.
Fordyce, W. E., Fowler, R. S., Lehmann, J. F. & DeLateur, B. J. (1968). Some implications of learning in problems of chronic pain, *Journal of the Chronic Diseases*, **21**, 179–90.
Fordyce, W. E., McMahan, R., Rainwater, G. *et al.* (1981). Pain complaint-exercise performance relationship in chronic pain, *Pain*, **10**, 311–21.
Fordyce, W. E., Roberts, A. H. & Sternbach, R. A. (1985). The behavioural management of chronic pain: A response to critics, *Pain*, **22**, 113–25.
Fordyce, W. E., Shelton, J. L. & Dundore, D. E. (1982). The modification of avoidance learning pain behaviours, *Journal of Behavioural Medicine*, **5**, 405–14.

Freud, S. (1959). *Collected Papers*. Basic Books, New York.

Frymoyer, J. W. & Donaghy, R. M. P. (1985). The ruptured intervertebral disc. Follow-up report on the first case fifty years after recognition of the syndrome and its surgical significance, *Journal of Bone and Joint Surgery*, **67A**, 1113–6.

Fullenlove, T. M. & Williams A. J. (1957). Comparative roentgen findings in symptomatic and asymptomatic backs, *Journal of the American Medical Association*, **168**, 572–4.

Gilbert, J. R. (1986). Management of low back pain in family practice: A critical review, *Canadian Family Physician*, **32**, 1855–61.

Gilbert, J. R., Taylor, D. W. & Hildebrand, A. (1985). Clinical trial of common treatments for low back pain in family practice, *British Medical Journal*, **291**, 791–4.

Goldberg, R. T. (1982). The social and vocational rehabilitation of persons with chronic pain, *Rehabilitation Literature*, **43**, 274–83.

Graham, J. R. (1977). *The MMPI: A practical guide*. Oxford University Press, New York.

Gray, I. C. M., Main, C. J. & Waddell, G. (1984). Illness behaviour and the role of psychological assessment in general orthopaedic practice, *Clinical Orthopaedics and Related Research*, **184**, 258–63.

Greenwood, J., McGuire, T. H. & Kimbell, F. (1952). A study of causes of failure in the herniated vertebral disc operation, *Journal of Neurosurg*, **9**, 15–20.

Hall, H. H. & Iceton, J. A. (1983), Back School: An overview with specific reference to the Canadian Back Education Units, *Clinical Orthopaedics and Related Research*, **179**, 10–17.

Harris, R. I. & Macnab, I. (1954). Structural changes in the intervertebral discs, *Journal of Bone and Joint Surgery*, **36B**, 304–23.

Hippocrates (1923). Translation by W. H. S. Jones. Harvard University Press, Cambridge.

Hirschfield, A. & Behan, R. C. (1963). The accident process, *Journal of the American Medical Association*, **186**, 84–90 and 193–9.

Hirschfield, A. & Behan, R. C. (1966). The accident process, *Journal of the American Medical Association*, **197**, 125–9.

Horal, J. (1969). The clinical appearance of low back pain disorders in the city of Gothenburg, Sweden, *Acta Orthopaedics Scandinavica (Suppl.)*, **118**, 1–109.

Hrudey, W. P. Workmen's Compensation Board of British Columbia. (Unpublished data)

Hult, L. (1954). The Munkfors investigation, *Acta Orthopaedica Scandinavica* (Suppl.), 16.

Hurst, J. W. (1975). Ambulation after myocardial infraction (Editorial), *New England Journal of Medicine*, **292**, 746–8.

International Association for the Study of Pain (1979). Pain terms: A list with definitions and notes on usage, *Pain*, **6**, 249–52.

Jones, R. & Lovett, R. W. (1923). *Orthopaedic Surgery*. Hodder & Stoughton, London.

Kelly, J. N., Voris, D. C., Swien, H. J. & Ghormley, R. K. (1954). Multiple operations for protruded lumbar vertebral discs, *Mayo Clinic Proceedings*, **29**, 546–50.

Kelsey, J. & White, A. A. (1980). Epidemiology and impact of low back pain, *Spine*, **6**, 133–42.

Kennedy, I. (1981). *The Unmasking of Medicine*. Allen & Unwin, London.

Key, J. A. (1945). Intervertebral disc lesions are the most common cause of low

back pain with or without sciatica, *Annals of Surgery*, **121**, 534–44.
La Rocca, H. & Macnab, I. (1969). Value of pre-employment radiographic assessment of the lumbar spine, *Canadian Medical Association Journal*, **101**, 383–8.
Leavitt, F., Garron, D. C., Whistler, W. W. & Sheinkop, M. B. (1978). Affective and sensory dimensions in back pain, *Pain*, **4**, 273–81.
Leigh, H. & Reiser, M. F. (1980). *The Patient: Biological, psychological and social dimensions of medical practice*. Plenum Press, New York.
Lidstrom, A. & Zachrisson, M. (1970). Physical therapy on low back pain and sciatica: an attempt at evaluation, *Scandinavian Journal of Rehabilitation Medicine*, **2**, 37–42.
Linton, S. J. (1985). The relationship between activity and chronic pain, *Pain*, **21**, 289–94.
Lipowski, Z. J. (1969). Psychosocial aspect of disease, *Annals of Internal Medicine*, **71**, 1197–206.
Lipowski, Z. J. (1981). Holistic-medical foundations of American psychiatry: A bicentennial, *Am J Psychiatry*, **138**, 888–95.
Lipowski Z. J. (1983). Psychosocial reactions to physical illness, *Canadian Medical Association Journal*, **128**, 1069–72.
Loeser, J. D. (1982). Concepts of Pain. In: *Chronic Low Back Pain*, ed. M. Stanton-Hicks & R. Boas. Raven Press, New York.
Loeser, J. D. & Fordyce, W. E. (1983). Chronic pain. In: *Behavioural Science in the Practice of Medicine*, ed. J. E. Carrad & H. A. Dengerink. Elsevier, New York.
McCulloch, J. A. (1977). Chemonucleolysis, *Journal of Bone and Joint Surgery*, **59B**, 45–52.
McGill, C. M. (1968). Industrial back programmes: A control program, *Journal of Occupational Medicine*, **10**, 174–78.
McNeill, T., Warwick, D., Andersson, G. B. J. & Schultz, A. (1980). Trunk strength in attempted flexion, extension and lateral bending in healthy subjects and patients with low back disorders, *Spine*, **5**, 529–33.
McVeigh, E. L. (1986). *Occupational back pain and modified work: A randomised control trial.* MSc Thesis, McMaster University.
McWhinney, I. R. (1972). Beyond diagnosis: An approach to the integration of behavioural science and clinical medicine, *New England Journal of Medicine*, **287**, 384–7.
Magora, A. & Schwartz, A. (1976). Relation between the low back pain syndrome and Xray findings, *Scandinavian Journal of Rehabilitation Medicine*, **8**, 115–25.
Main, C. J. (1983). The modified somatic perception questionnaire, *Journal of Psychosomatic Research*, **27**, 503–14.
Main, C. J. (1987). Psychological approaches to management and treatment. In: *The Lumbar Spine and Back Pain*, ed. M. I. V. Jayson. Pitman, Tunbridge Wells.
Main, C. J. & Waddell, G. (1987). Personality assessment in the management of low back pain, *Clinical Rehabilitation*, **1**, 139–42.
Mayer, T. G., Gatchel, R. J., Kishino, N. *et al.* (1985). Objective assessment of lumbar function following industrial injury, *Spine*, **10**, 482–93.
Mayer, T. G., Gatchel, R. J., Kishino, N. *et al.* (1986). A prospective short-term study of chronic low back pain patients utilising novel objective functional measurement, *Pain*, **25**, 53–68.
Mayou, R. (1984). Sick role, illness behaviour and coping, *British Journal of Psychiatry*, **144**, 320–22.
Mechanic, D. (1968). *Medical Sociology*. Free Press, New York.

Mechanic, D. (1977) Illness behaviour, social adaptation and the management of illness, *Journal of Nervous and Mental Diseases*, **165**, 79–87.
Mechanic, D. (1980). The experience and reporting of common physical complaints, *Journal of Health and Social Behaviour*, **21**, 146–55.
Mechanic, D. (1986). The concept of illness behaviour: culture, situation and personal predisposition (Editorial), *Psychological Medicine*, **16**, 1–7.
Mechanic, D., Cleary, P. D. & Greenely, J. R. (1982). Distress syndrome, illness behaviour, access to care and medical utilisation in a defined population, *Medical Care*, **20**, 361–72.
Mechanic, D. & Volkart, E. H. (1960). Illness behaviour and medical diagnosis, *Journal of Health and Human Behaviour*, **1**, 86–96.
Mechanic, D. & Volkart, E. H. (1961). Stress, illness behaviour and the sick role, *American Sociological Review*, **26**, 51–58.
Melzack, R. (1975). The McGill pain questionnaire: Major properties and scoring methods, *Pain*, **1**, 277–99.
Melzack, R. & Casey, K. L. (1968). Sensory, motivational and central control determinants of pain. In: *The Skin Senses*, ed. D. R. Kenshalo. Charles C. Thomas, Springfield, Illinois.
Melzack, R. & Wall, P. D. (1965). Pain mechanisms: A new theory, *Science*, **150**, 971–9.
Mensor, M. C. & Duvall, G. (1959). Absence of motion at the fourth and fifth lumbar interspaces, *Journal of Bone and Joint Surgery*, **41A**, 1047–54.
Meyer, A. (1917). Progress in teaching psychiatry, *Journal of the American Medical Association*, **69**, 861–3.
Miller, J. H. (1976). *Preliminary report on disability insurance*. To the Committee on Ways & Means of the US House of Representatives. US Government Printing Office, Washington, DC.
Miller, P. M. C., Ingham, J. G. & Davidson, S. (1976) Life events, symptoms and social support, *Journal of Psychosomatic Research*, **20**, 515–22.
Mixter, W. J., Barr, J. S. (1934). Rupture of the intervertebral disc with involvement of the spinal canal, *New England Journal of Medicine*, **211**, 210–15.
Morris, E. W., DiPaola, M., Vallance, R., & Waddell, G. (1986). Diagnosis and decision making in lumbar disc prolapse and nerve entrapment, *Spine*, **11**, 436–9.
Nachemson A. (1966). The load on lumbar discs in different positions of the body, *Clinical Orthopaedics and Related Research*, **45**, 107–22.
Nachemson A. (1975). Towards a better understanding of low back pain: A review of the mechanics of the lumbar disc, *Rheumatology and Rehabilitation*, **14**, 129–43.
Nachemson, A. (1976a). The lumbar spine: An orthopaedic challenge, *Spine*, **1**, 9–21.
Nachemson, A. (1976b). A critical look at conservative treatment for low back pain. In: *The Lumbar Spine and Low Back Pain*, ed. M. Jayson. Pitman, London.
Nachemson, A. (1983). Work for all, for those with low back pain as well, *Clinical Orthopaedics and Related Research*, **179**, 77–85.
Nachemson, A. (1985). Advances in low back pain, *Clinical Orthopaedics and Related Research*, **200**, 266–78.
Nachemson, A. & Andersson, G. B. J. (1982). Classification of low back pain, *Scandinavian Journal of Work and Environmental Health*, **8**, 134.
Nachemson, A. & Lindh, M. (1965). Measurement of abdominal and back muscle strength with or without low back pain, *Scandinavian Journal of Rehabilitation*

Medicine, **1**, 60.
Nachemson, A. & Morris, J. M. (1964). *In vivo* measurement of intradiscal pressure, *Journal of Bone and Joint Surgery*, **46A**, 1077–92.
Naliboff, B. D., Cohen, M. J., Swanson, G. A., Bonebakker, A. D. & McArthur, D. L. (1985). Comprehensive assessment of chronic low back pain patients and controls: Physical abilities, level of activities, psychological adjustment and pain perception, *Pain*, **23**, 121–34.
Nuprin Pain Report (1985). Louis Harris and Associates, New York.
Office of Health Economics (1982). *Hip Replacement and the NHS*. London.
Office of Health Economics (1985). *Back Pain*. London.
Oostdam, E. M., Duidenwoorden, H. J. & Pondaag, N. (1981). Predictive value of some psychological tests on the outcome of surgical intervention in low back pain patients, *Journal of Psychosomatic Research*, **25**, 227–35.
Parsons T (1951). *The Social System*. Free Press, New York.
Pasteur, M. L. (1857). Mémoire sur la fermentation appellée lactique, *Comptes Rendus de l'Académie des Sciences*, **45**, 913–16.
Penfield, W. (1969). *Pain and the neurosurgeon* (foreword). Charles C. Thomas, Springfield Illinois.
Pheasant, H., Gilbert, D., Goldfar, J. & Heron, L. (1979). The MMPI as a predictor of outcome in low back surgery, *Spine*, **4**, 78–84.
Philips, H. C. & Jahanshahi, M. (1986). The components of pain behaviour report, *Behaviour Research and Therapy*, **24**, 117–25.
Pilowsky, I. 1969. Abnormal illness behaviour, *British Journal of Medical Psychology*, **42**, 347–51.
Pilowsky, I. (1978). A general classification of abnormal illness behaviours, *British Journal of Medical Psychology*, **51**, 131–7.
Ransford, A. O., Cairns, D. & Mooney, V. (1976). The pain drawing as an aid to the psychological evaluation of patients with low back pain, *Spine*, **1**, 127–134.
Reiser, S. J. (1978). *Medicine and the Reign of Technology*. Cambridge, Cambridge University Press.
Rider, A. W. *et al.* (1975). The status of cardiac transplantation, *Circulation*, **52**, 531.
Rowe, M. L. (1969). Low back pain in industry, *Journal of Occupational Medicine*, **11**, 161–9.
Sackett, D. L. (1981). How to read clinical journals: V. To distinguish useful from useless or even harmful therapies, *Canadian Medical Association Journal*, **124**, 1156–62.
Sample sickness and/or invalidity benefit 1967–1985: DHSS Headquarters Division SR 8B, Newcastle-upon-Tyne. (Unpublished data).
Sandstrom, J., Hansson, T., Jonson, R., Roos, B. & Andersson, G. B. J. (1985). The bone mineral content of the lumbar spine in patients with chronic low back pain, *Spine*, **10**, 158–60.
Social Security Bulletin (1985). *Annual Statistical Supplement*. (1984–5) US Government Printing Office. Washington, DC.
Social Security Commission on the Evaluation of Pain (1986). *Report to US Congress*. US Government Printing Office, Washington, DC.
Spangfort, E. V. (1972). The lumbar disc herniation: A computer aided analysis of 2504 operations, *Acta Orthopaedica Scandinavica (Suppl.)*, **142**, 1–95.
Spitzer, W. O. (1986). *Rapport du groupe de travail Québécois sur les aspects cliniques des affections vertebrales chez les travailleurs*. Institut du recherche en santé et en securité du travail de Québec.
Splithoff, C. A. (1953). Lumbosacral junction: Roentographic comparison of

patients with and without backache, *Journal of the American Medical Association*, **152**, 1610–13.

Sternbach, R. A. (1974). *Pain Patients: Traits and Treatment.* New York, Academic Press.

Sternbach, R. A. (1977). Psychological aspects of chronic pain, *Clinical Orthopaedics and Related Research*, **129**, 150–55.

Sternbach, R. A. & Timmermans, G. (1975). Personality changes associated with reduction of pain, *Pain*, **1**, 177–81.

Strang, J. P. (1985). The chronic disability syndrome In: *Evaluation and Treatment of Chronic Pain*, ed. G. M. Aronoff. Urban & Schwarzenberg, Baltimore.

Szasz, T. S. (1968). The painful person, *J. Lancet*, **88**, 18–22.

Report of Task Force on Backs (1984). Ontario Council of Safety Associations. Toronto.

Tessler, R., Mechanic, D. & Dimond, M. (1976). The effect of psychological distress on physician utilisation: A prospective study, *Journal of Health and Social Behaviour*, **17**, 353–64.

Torgeson, W. R. & Dotler, W. E. (1976). Comparative roentgenographic study of the asymptomatic and symptomatic lumbar spine, *Journal of Bone and Joint Surgery*, **58A**, 850–3.

Turk D. C., Meichenbaum, D. & Genest, M. (1983). *Pain and Behavioural Medicine*, Guildford Press, New York.

Urban, J. & Maroudas, A. (1980). The chemistry of the intervertebral disc in relation to its physiological functions and requirements, *Clinics in Rheumatic Diseases*, **6**, 51–76.

Virchow, R. (1858). Die Cellular pathologie in Ihrer Begründurg auf physiologische und pathologische. A. Hirschwald, Berlin.

Waddell, G. (1982). An approach to backache, *British Journal of Hospital Medicine*, **28**, 187–219.

Waddell, G. (1986). Provision of orthopaedic services for backache in Oman, *Report to the Minister of Health.* Muscat, Sultanate of Oman.

Waddell, G. (1987). Clinical assessment of lumbar impairment, *Clinical Orthopaedics and related research*, **221**, 110–20.

Waddell, G., Bircher, M., Finlayson, D. & Main, C. J. (1984a). Symptoms and signs: Physical disease or illness behaviour? *British Medical Journal*, **289**, 739–41.

Waddell, G., Kummel, E. G., Lotto, W. N. *et al.* (1979). Failed lumbar disc surgery and repeat surgery following industrial injury. *Journal of Bone and Joint Surgery*, **61A**, 201–7.

Waddell, G., McCulloch, J. A., Kummel, E. G. & Venner, R. M. (1980). Nonorganic physical signs in low back pain, *Spine*, **5**, 117–25.

Waddell, G. & Main, C. J. (1984). Assessment of severity in low back disorders, *Spine*, **9**, 204–8.

Waddell, G., Main, C. J., Morris, E. W., DiPaola, M. & Gray, I. C. M. (1984b). Chronic low back pain, psychological distress and illness behaviour, *Spine*, **9**, 209–13.

Waddell, G., Morris, E. W., DiPaola, M., Bircher, M. & Finlayson, D. (1986). A concept of illness tested as an improved basis for surgical decisions in low back disorders, *Spine*, **11**, 712–19.

Wall, P. D. (1986). Causes of intractable pain, *Hospital Update*, **12**, 969–74.

Weber, H. (1986). *Conservative management of back pain: Critical evaluation of conservative treatment programmes*. Presented at the First European Congress on Back Pain Current Concepts and Recent Advances, Helsinki.

Weinstein, M. R. (1968). The illness process, *Journal of the American Medical Association*, **204**, 117–21.
Weinstein, M. R. (1978). The concept of the disability process, *Psychosomatics*, **19**, 94–97.
White, A. (1979). *AAOS Instructional Course Lectures. Back School*. CV Mosby, St Louis.
White, A. W. M. (1966). Low back pain in men receiving workmen's compensation, *Canadian Medical Association Journal*, **95**, 50–56.
White, K. L., Williams, F. & Greenberg, B. (1961). The ecology of medical care, *New England Journal of Medicine*, **265**, 885–92.
Wiesel, S. W., Cuckler, J. M., Deluca, F. *et al.* (1980). Acute low back pain. An objective analysis of conservative therapy, *Spine*, **5**, 324–30.
Wiltse, L. L. (1971). The effect of the common anomalies of the lumbar spine upon disc degeneration and low back pain, *Orthopaedic Clinics of North America*, **2**, 569–82.
Wiltse, L. L. & Rocchio, P. D. (1975). Pre-operative psychological tests as predictions of success of chemonucleolysis in the treatment of the low back syndrome, *Journal of Bone and Joint Surgery*, **57A**, 478–83.
Wing, P. C., Wilfling, F. J. & Kokan, P. J. (1973). Psychological, demographic and orthopaedic factors associated with prediction of outcome of spinal fusion, *Clinical Orthopaedics and Related Research*, **90**, 153–60.
Wolff, B. B. & Langley, S. (1968). Cultural Factors and the response to pain, *American Anthropologist*, **70**, 494–501.
Wood, P. L. R. & Main, C. J. (1985). *The changing influence of physical and psychological factors on subjective disability in low back pain*. Presented to the First International Congress of the International Back Pain Society, Vienna.
Workmen's Compensation Board Symposium (1986). *Low Back Pain: A multi-Disciplinary Approach*. Vancouver.
Workmen's Compensation Board of British Columbia (1986). Vancouver. (Unpublished data).
World Health Organisation (1976). *Preamble to the constitution*. Basic Documents twenty-sixth edition. Geneva, World Health Organization.
Zachrisson, M. (1981). The back school, *Spine*, **6**, 104.
Zarkowska, E. & Philips, H. C. (1986). Recent onset vs. persistent pain: Evidence for a distinction, *Pain*, **25**, 365–72.
Zigmond, D. (1976). The medical model – Its limitations and alternatives, *Hospital Update*, **2**, 424–7.
Zung, W. W. K. (1965). A self-rated depression scale, *Archives of General Psychiatry*, **32**, 63–70.

2 *J. A. Klaber Moffett*

Backschools

2.1 **Introduction**

The term 'backschool' refers to a formalised programme of back care education administered in a small group situation. Backschools are now widely used in the management of mechanical back pain problems. The concept originated in Sweden but is now used throughout Britain and similarly in Canada, USA, Australia, New Zealand and some European countries.

The principle of a backschool is to teach people who have back pain how to help themselves by giving them an insight into the problem. This approach is also used prophylactically in schools and industry, particularly in Scandinavia, to educate children and workers before they develop the problem. The emphasis is always on education but a set of exercises is often included. The professional input is usually multidisciplinary, but the sessions tend to be organised and carried out in the physiotherapy department. Apart from physiotherapists and occupational therapists, orthopaedic surgeons, psychiatrists and psychologists often contribute to the programme. In this way the patient is more likely to be presented with a comprehensive view of the problem and what can be done about it.

2.2 **Definition**

2.2.1 *Aims and objectives of backschools*

The general aims of a backschool are firstly to teach people the basic anatomy and function of the spine with special reference to the lumbar spine. This knowledge is then used to show how it is possible to minimise the stress and strain that is placed on their spines in the light of available scientific research. Close consideration is then addressed to posture of the spine throughout a 24-hour day and the individual's ergonomic environment. The overall objective is to encourage the patient to take on responsibility for looking after his own back. A positive attitude to the problem should be the major outcome and advantage gained. Patients are given a feeling of control over their problem and their quality of life is enhanced.

2.2.2 *Content and delivery*

The exact content is variable but should include:

Basic principles of anatomy of the spine
Simple applied body mechanics
Practical demonstration of correct posture during relaxation, and at work
Ergonomic advice and discussion
Relaxation/exercises.

The method of delivery is as important as the content. The success of a backshool in achieving its aims must depend on gaining the patient's interest. There is a great deal of information to get across to them and in most cases patients have little or no knowledge of how their spines are structured. They do however have many misconceptions which are nurtured by unfortunate terminology such as 'slipped disc' or 'degeneration'.

Although a reasonable level of intelligence is desirable, more important is the degree of motivation. Some backschools are run on the basis that patients are invited to attend and only those who are motivated and interested will come. In other centres patients are given an appointment to attend because it is deemed by the doctor or therapist to be beneficial for them and they are expected to attend. In this case the level of motivation at the outset will be much lower. It can be argued that it is precisely those patients who are less enthusiastic and have a negative attitude who would benefit the most. It is vital to gain their active participation in order to win them over to a more positive outlook. For this purpose a group should not consist of more than eight to ten members, in order to encourage active participation of each member. Bearing in mind that only 20% of verbal information given at a lecture is generally retained, the use of visual aids should be maximised. An overhead projector with simple colourful diagrams is ideal. A flexible life-size model of the human spine, which can be closely examined and handled by patients, is helpful if not essential.

An authoritarian approach should be avoided; a permissive attitude helps to encourage as much constructive discussion as possible. A tape-slide show may be a useful adjunct but should only form a small part of the programme, as the participants will soon take on a glazed expression of passive acceptance or even rejection! Interaction between members of the group should be encouraged, but needs to be carefully directed to make sure that one individual member does not bring down the morale of the rest of the group. The patient is more likely to be impressed by a positive statement from a fellow sufferer than by any amount of advice provided by the health professional. Members are encouraged to solve each others' ergonomic problems especially in relationship to their work situation.

2.3 The Swedish backschool

The original Swedish backshool was devised by Zachrisson-Forsell in 1970 and this now forms the basis for many backschools in this country. It is based on a slide-tape presentation to patients in small groups, aiming to teach anatomy, body mechanics and ergonomics. A position of comfort which relaxes the ilio-psoas muscle and reduces lumbar lordosis is taught. The four sessions are conducted with the members of the group in this position (Figure 2.1), to avoid exacerbating back pain with prolonged sitting. Patients are also taught to practise relaxation in this position. The overall aim of the Swedish backschool is to:

(1) help patients improve the ergonomics of their work environment;

(2) avoid inappropriate therapy;

(3) decrease the demand made on resources caused by avoidable back pain (Zachrisson-Forsell, 1980).

Berquist-Ullman and Larsson (1977) carried out a prospective study on acute back pain sufferers at the Volvo factory, in Gothenburg: 217 patients were included and were examined and assessed by an orthopaedic surgeon prior to treatment, 10 days later, and then repeatedly making a total of at least five assessments over a period of 1 year. They were randomly allocated to one of three groups:

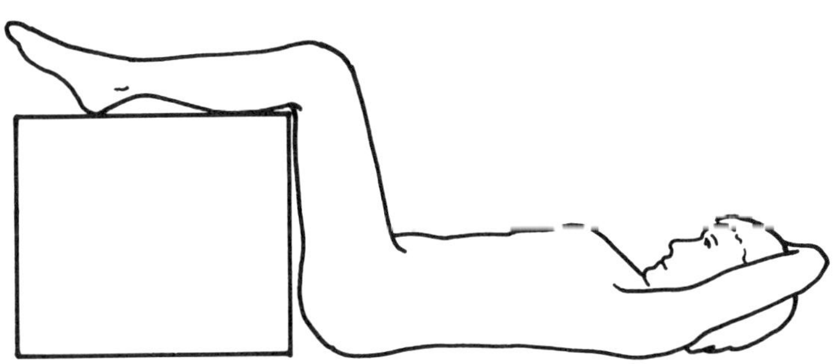

Fig 2.1 Semi-Fowler resting position to relax psoas muscle and reduce lumbar lordosis

(1) *The backschool* as described above but visits were also made to the patient's work place, with which the physiotherapist was very familiar, to evaluate their individual ergonomic problems. Where necessary, negotiations with the management were carried out to try and bring about changes in working conditions.

(2) *Manual therapy*, based on the techniques developed by Cyriax, Kaltenbourn and Lewit. The average number of treatments was four, but a maximum of ten treatments were allowed. These patients were also given instruction in posture and lifting, and exercises where the therapist felt it was appropriate.

(3) *Placebo group* consisted of short-wave diathermy applied at the lowest possible intensity which the authors remark may at the most increase bloodflow through the subcutaneous tissues. A maximum of ten treatments were given but the average was five.

The mean duration of symptoms following the first treatment was 14.8 days for the backschool and 15.8 days for the manual therapy group, which was not significantly different. But in comparison, the placebo group reported symptoms of 28.7 days duration which was significantly longer. Patients who attended the backschool went back to work significantly sooner: 20.5 days was the median duration of absence for the backschool group, but the other two groups were off work six days longer. The authors concluded that there were two economical reasons in favour of the backschool, firstly the reduction in sick-leave and secondly more economical use of therapists' time.

Lankhorst and co-workers (1983) in Holland carried out a controlled study to look at the effect of the Swedish backschool on a group of patients with chronic back pain. They allocated 48 patients in order of referral to four backschool sessions or four sessions of untuned short wave diathermy. The results were surprisingly negative.

Immediately after the treatment subjective scores such as pain and functional disability became significantly worse in the control group. However, patients in both the backschool and control groups became worse as far as objective measures (i.e. range of movement of the spine and straight leg raising) were concerned. At 1-year follow up, there was no significant effect of the backschool on objective or subjective outcome measures. The authors concluded that the negative results were due to the chronicity of back pain in their patients. They differed from the patients in Berquist-Ullman and Larsson's study, who all had a history of less than three months duration.

However their poor results could also be a reflection of the content and delivery of the programme, which is not explained in detail. In Berquist-

Ullman's study the tape-slide input formed only about a third of the total time and attention given to the group by the therapist, who then gave patients further attention individually at their work place when it was deemed necessary. If Lankhorst's programme consisted mainly of the tape-slide presentation, less attention would have been given by the therapist and other important ingredients, such as patients' active participation, would be reduced. In both studies the placebo groups are likely to have had less attention and therapist's time. Lankhorst's paper concentrated on the research methodology and the measurements, to such an extent that the treatment itself was largely ignored. Since this important factor was not apparently controlled in either of these studies it goes some way to explaining the discrepancy in their findings.

2.4 **The California backschool**

This programme was set up in 1976 and has similar aims to the Swedish backschool. It too consists of four linked sessions lasting up to 1½ hours – this is twice as long as the Swedish backschool sessions. The California backschool takes a maximum of four patients and may include either acute or chronic back problems. Patients work in pairs or are sometimes given individual training. The programme aims to evaluate the patient, help to formulate a diagnosis and provide rehabilitation for patients with 'low back dysfunction and sciatica' (Matmiller, 1980; White, 1983).

An integral part of this backschool is an obstacle course which was devised objectively to measure the performance of an individual back pain patient on a standardised form. Patients with sciatica are instructed to avoid aggravating their leg pain. Deficiencies in the use of protective body mechanics during such activities as sitting, standing, reaching, bending, kneeling, etc., are noted and used as a basis for instruction. Individual needs are assessed initially at interview and listed as biomechanical problems; a physical examination is also performed. An exercise tolerance test is carried out, taking care not to aggravate the pain for the sciatica patients. Common causes of back pain are taught in the education section. Spinal pain is explained as a position and motion-induced problem. All patients are taught how to minimise loading on the spine in sitting by using the 'contour' position aiming to support the natural curves of the spine effectively, especially the lumbar lordosis. Patients who are at work continue to review their protective body mechanics by the use of pelvic tilting and isometric abdominal bracing; this aims to reduce segmental motion and reduce loading on the lumbar spine.

A week later at the second attendance a further assessment of needs is carried out and active abdominal bracing is applied to daily living activities to help to distribute the load (Troup, 1979). The straight back or golfer's method of bending is taught where over-extended work such as reaching under the bonnet of a car is necessary, and the pelvic tilt and abdominal compression are added for further protection. A home programme of simple exercises is given. The patient is taught to maximise the strength endurance of his abdominals in the 'hook-lying' position, raising the head and shoulders but keeping the lumbar spine flat. Isometric quadriceps exercises are taught in the form of the 'human chair' with the spine pressed up against a wall and the hips and knees bent. Patients are expected to practise these exercises regularly at home and increase the length of time they hold the positions.

If the patient complains of acute pain after the second day he is sent back to the physician and may be given an epidural, or a corset to assist him to continue with the backschool programme. Alternatively the therapist may give him mobilisations, traction or heat treatment.

On the third day, that is in the third week, the aim is to get the patient back to work if he is still on sick-leave. To this end protective body mechanics in load handling are taught. This is also applied to sports activities. A special session, where appropriate, is taking the patients out for a run or a jog, with the physiotherapist observing their gait and posture, which can then be corrected with practice. A follow-up day allows the patient's condition to be evaluated again by means of the obstacle course. It is also a problem-solving day to work on the ergonomic needs of the individual. When the pain is better, a programme of McKenzie's exercises is introduced. Patients are advised to follow all flexion activities with extension. This approach will be discussed later in Chapter 3.

2.4.1 *Statistical review of the California backschool*

The review monitored 300 patients who entered the programme at intervals of one, three, and six months and after one and two years (Matmiller, 1980). The data were collected by follow-up visit, telephone interview or letter. At 2 years, information was obtained by letter or telephone. The population, which included chronic back pain sufferers, had an average duration of 60 days from the first incidence of back pain, the range extending from half a day to 8 years; 89% of the participants sought no further help after the first month of backschool training; 95% had achieved an acceptable pain level enabling them to return to normal activities after 1 month and also maintained this for the 2-year period of review. As there was no control group the results of this review must be considered with caution.

2.5 **Canadian Back Education Units**

This programme (CBEU) was developed in Toronto in 1974 (Hall, 1980; Hall & Iceton, 1983). To avoid the need for an orthopaedic surgeon repeating the same basic message to every back pain patient, two informal lectures were delivered to a group of 12 patients. This proved so popular that by 1978 the number of patients attending annually in Canada had increased to 1600. The professional services of more than 70 people are now used and a central office in Toronto co-ordinates peripheral programmes throughout Canada, and also in the USA. A full-time manager, a senior consulting physiotherapist, a business manager and a group of volunteer workers from former CBEUs run this office.

The programme is primarily aimed at chronic mechanical back problems. It does not offer diagnosis, assessment or individual treatment. The main objective is to change the patients' attitude to their pain and encourage them to accept responsibility for the management of their back problem. It aims to correct common misconceptions and emphasises the non-threatening nature of the commonest causes of back pain.

The group consists of 15 to 25 participants, a size which they claim is small enough to encourage group interaction. The first session is usually conducted by an orthopaedic surgeon and covers anatomy, physiology and pathophysiology. Non-threatening causes of back problems are explained and patients' questions are answered. The second session is led by a physiotherapist who teaches the use of correct body mechanics. The role of exercises is discussed; a 10-minute daily routine of appropriate exercises is advocated. The many different methods of obtaining temporary relief are referred to and these are compared to the methods aimed at achieving long-term control over the pain, through education and attitude modification. Session three, which is taken by a psychiatrist, introduces psychiatric aspects of pain, but patients are reassured that pain is never 'all in the mind'. The link between emotional upsets and muscle tension is pointed out. They are taught how pre-existing pain may, conversely, be magnified by chronic depression or anxiety. Session four is the last one, and is a practical demonstration which takes place outside the classroom – which is very popular with the patients. A psychologist demonstrates the principles of relaxation and the patients are taught flexion exercises and pelvic tilting.

An exercise class is not included in the programme but individual physiotherapy is provided as necessary, independently of the programme. Patients are referred by physiotherapists or doctors under whose care they remain. By the end of the course, through increased understanding of the problem, the patients co-operation with all subsequent management plans should have improved. The classes take place once a week to allow participants time to absorb the information; but for out-of-town patients a week's programme of daily lectures is also available. Low-cost accommodation is provided by the hospital. A review class takes place 6 months later. This session is led by a physiotherapist and is based on a multiple choice test to see how much information has been retained, and this is used as a basis for discussion.

2.5.1 *Statistical review of the CBEU*

Since 1978 the CBEU have employed a Research Fellow full-time to be responsible for collecting and analysing the enormous mass of data accumulating from patients' questionnaires. Information is obtained initially on their first visit and again at their 6-month follow-up. Subjective evaluation of patients' pain and functional disability is recorded. Also, a multiple choice examination is given prior to starting the course, at the end of the series, and again at 6 months, to see how much information is retained. This facilitates evaluation of the effects of the patient education programme and allows demographic data relevant to back pain to be studied, over a 6-month period.

A statistical review of 6418 participants who completed the initial programme obtained a 38% response rate on follow-up at 6 months (Hall & Iceton, 1983). The average age was 45 years but there was a surprisingly high incidence of women between the ages of 55 and 59. The ratio of males to females was 4: 6. Most were largely sedentary in their life-style and occupation. Their limitations were mainly due to pain during lifting, carrying and sports activities. Comparing the data for height and weight with the 1975 Canadian census, men included in the CBEU were between 6.3 and 7.6 cm taller than average and 2.7 kg heavier. Women were between 3.8 and 5.0 cm taller and weighed less than the Canadian average. The extra height of course might increase the amount of stooping an individual is likely to do. The weight difference could be explained in terms of reduced activity for the men; alternatively, it may be due to the fact that larger-than-average men, because of their size, may more frequently be expected by others to help out with heavy tasks.

At the follow-up class the number of patients who said that their condition was deteriorating dropped from 27 to 6%. Most of the participants said that their condition had improved. The number of patients seeking help from other services decreased markedly in the month after attendance at the programme. While, prior to the programme, 38% had consulted three or more different health professionals patients, only 2% of them consulted this number of professionals in the month after the course.

Those patient who could not give a specific diagnosis did significantly worse compared with the whole group ($p = 0.004$) whereas those who said that the pain was due to a pulled muscle ($p = 0.06$), wear in the discs ($p = 0.02$), or facet joint problems ($p = 0.0001$) had significantly better results. This underlines the need to emphasise the non-threatening nature of most back problems. The meaning of the pain is very important to the patient and fear of the unknown, which leads to unnecessary suffering, can be reduced through education.

The patients who claimed they did regular exercise fared better (p = 0.007) and so did those who practised routine back care (p = 0.04); whereas patients who restricted or avoided activities, or used a spinal corset or regular traction as a means of pain control were significantly worse.

Analysis of the questionnaires also showed that patients who had high-school education and recognised the emotional component of the problem gained the best results. Patients who believed their pain was due to an accident fared less well. Also patients who were claiming from the Workmen's Compensation Board did less well. Those who had pain persistently below the knee did not do so well.

It is interesting to note that a positive correlation was found between the subjective improvement that patients reported and the amount of information that they could recall. This provides further evidence for the role of education in the management of back problems. This uncontrolled review demonstrates the importance of different factors associated with individuals response to back pain.

2.6 **Backschools in Britain**

Backschools are now commonly found throughout Britain. They tend to be organised on a less formal basis, since the facilities and resources available are usually quite limited compared with the North American programmes. They vary greatly in their content, especially as far as emphasis on exercise is concerned. In Derbyshire, substantial emphasis is put on exercises (Haynes, 1984). Patients selected for this backschool attend each working day for 2 weeks. Each session lasts for 1 hour and they have hydrotherapy twice a week. On the other 3 days of the week, 25 minutes is devoted to an exercise class in the gymnasium, prior to a session on back-care education.

Many other backschools in this country follow more closely the pattern of the Swedish Backschool where education is the main aim. One example of such a programme is that in Oxford which has been running at the Nuffield Orthopaedic Centre since 1979.

2.6.1 *The Oxford backschool*

Patients are referred mainly from the orthopaedic and rheumatology out-patient clinics and tend to have a long history of back pain, with or without referred leg pain. They are drawn from a cross-section of the population, which in Oxford includes factory workers, housewives, students and academics. Many have already had a variety of different forms of physiotherapy and/or other forms of treatment. They are examined and assessed individually by a physiotherapist and, according to the findings, taught a set of suitable home exercises. They are then given an appointment to attend the four linked sessions which comprise the Oxford backschool. An overhead projector, transparencies and a model of the spine are used to teach simple anatomy, biomechanics of the spine and common causes of back pain. The content is similar to the Swedish back school, although the tape-slide programme is not used. The third session is led by an occupational therapist and consists of a practical demonstration, discussion and practice of daily living activities, especially household activities, taking into account all that has been taught. This session is the last one of the three in the first week.

If it is successful, each member of the group should be making an active contribution including those who at the outset may have been passive and perhaps negative in their attitude. At this stage it is often possible to observe a marked change in attitude and motivation. Much of this is gained from the influence of other more positive minded members of the group, and also from the realisation that many other people are coping with similar pain problems. A follow-up session takes place 3 weeks later where patients fill in a short quiz to test how much they have remembered. This is used as a basis for discussion which is directed towards particular problems which people have encountered at work. Members are encouraged to try and solve each others' problems. The American video called 'Backfire' is shown, which not only adds a touch of both drama and humour but also helps to reinforce information that they have already been taught.

2.6.2 *Evaluation of the Oxford backschool*

A controlled study was carried out at the Nuffield Orthopaedic Centre to evaluate the effectiveness of this backschool compared with an exercise-only regimen (Klaber Moffett *et al.*, 1986). In this trial patients with a history of more than 6 months' back pain were randomly allocated to attend three linked sessions of either the backschool described above or an exercise-only class. Both groups were taught four simple Lumbar Isometric Flexion Exercises (LIFE) which were considered safe for all types of chronic back pain patients who might attend. No more than six to eight people were included in any one group. The exercise-only group acted as a control and were not taught any backcare, but for ethical reasons they were given a handout which gave them some guidelines. Patients were assessed by a physiotherapist and a rheumatologist on three occasions, prior to attending the sessions, at 6 weeks and at 4 months after entering the study. The assessors were blind to which group each patient had attended. Results showed a mean decrease in pain and functional disability scores at 6 weeks for both treatment groups. However at 4 months there was a significant difference between the two groups; the backschool patients had continued to improve whereas the exercise-only patients had regressed.

The mean duration of history of back pain was 7.5 years and 46% of the patients had a history extending over more than 10 years. The only difference in treatment between the two groups was the education package offered in the backschool. It seems that this engendered a more positive attitude on the patients' part so that they felt more able to cope.

2.7 A follow-up study of the Oxford Backschool evaluation

Approximately 5 years after entering the trial described above, the same group of patients was followed up by means of a postal questionnaire, to try and discover whether any of the apparent benefits of the backschool over the exercise-only class were still quantifiable.

2.7.1 *Method*

Questionnaires were sent out to 92 patients who had entered the original study, 5 years before: 70 completed questionnaires were returned, after a reminder and a phone call where necessary. The remaining patients could not be contacted because no current address could be traced. Considering the large time interval, the 76% return was unexpectedly high.

All patients were sent a copy of the Oswestry Low Back Pain Questionnaire (Fairbank *et al.*, 1980) to measure their current level of functional disability. They were also sent a questionnaire, designed to elicit:

(1) whether they still had back pain problems;

(2) how they were managing their back pain;

(3) how it was effecting their lifestyle.

2.2.2 *Results*

Analysis of the Oswestry Back Pain Questionnaire for Functional Disability scores showed no significant difference at the 5-year follow-up between the backschool and exercise-only groups but inspection of Figure 2.2 shows that the backschool group still tend to function slightly better than the exercise-only group. However comparing the two groups, there was no significant difference in the changes in functional disability scores from the third assessment to the 5-year follow-up, or in the changes from the pretreatment assessment to the 5-year follow-up. A greater number of patients in the backschool group claimed to have no functional disability and this was significant at the 5% level (Table 2.1).

The responses of patients to questions in the second questionnaire, which was sent to both groups, is shown in Table 2.2.

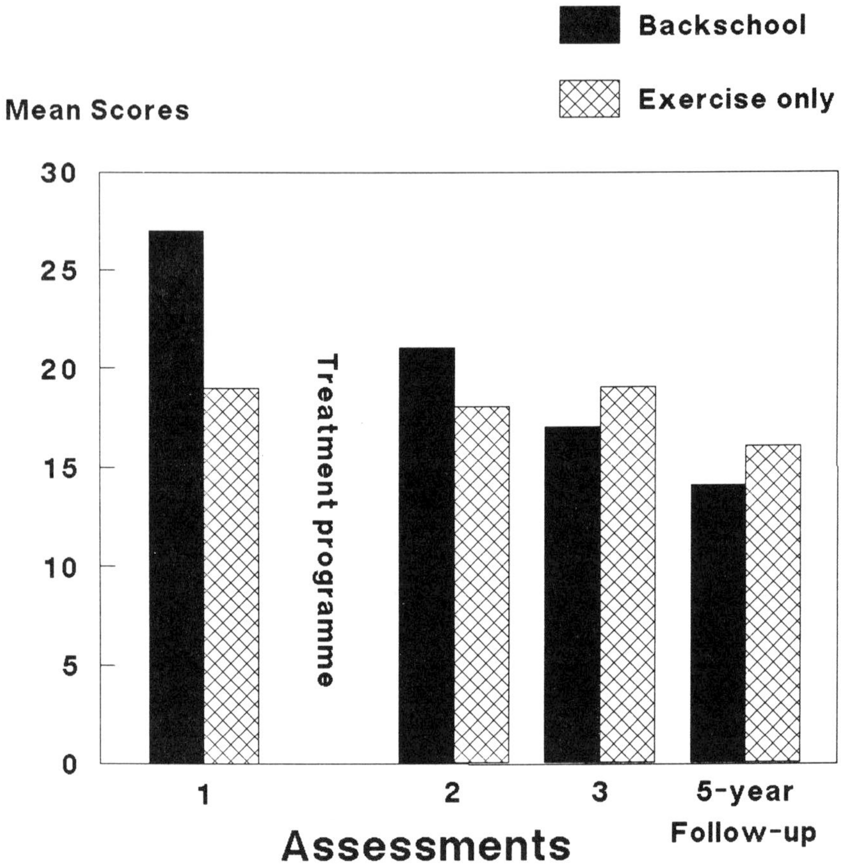

Fig 2.2 Comparison of functional disability scores: solid columns, backschool; cross-hatched, exercise only

Table 2.1 Number of patients in each group at the 5-year follow-up who claimed to be free of any functional disability

Treatment group	*No functional disability*	*Some functional disability*	*Total*
Backschool	9 (27%)	24 (73%)	33
Exercise only	2 (5%)	35 (95%)	37
	11	59	70

$\chi_1^2 = 4.754$ (with Yates correction); $p < 0.05$.

Table 2.2 History of back trouble in preceding 12 months, 5 years after entry to back school trial

	Backschool (n = 33)	*Exercise only (n = 37)*
Able to minimise it by looking after your back?	27	34
Any back and/or leg pain in the last 12 months?	23	29
Consulted GP?	11	9
Consulted hospital specialist?	7	2
Saw a physiotherapist?	4	4
Saw a chiropractor or osteopath?	3	5
Other form of treatment?	4	3
Time off work? None	16	27
1–6 days	7	4
1–2 weeks	2	0
2–4 weeks	3	2
1–3 months	1	1
Over 3 months	2	2

Table 2.3 shows that there was no significant difference between the two groups in numbers of patients who had seen a hospital specialist in the past 12 months or in the percentage of patients in each group who took time off work (Figure 2.3). 29% of backschool patients and 27% of exercise-only patients stated that they had changed their jobs during the past 5 years for a variety of reasons. When questioned about the extent to which they were still doing their exercises, 55% of the backschool claimed that they did them daily, compared to 62% of the exercise-only patients.

Patients who attended the backschool were sent a third questionnaire to find out if they had made any changes in their lifestyle since they had attended 5 years previously. 65% reported that they had made changes in

Table 2.3 Number of patients who has consulted a hospital specialist in the preceding 12 months, 5 years after entry to the backschool trial

Treatment group	*Consulted hospital specialist*	*Did not consult hospital specialist*	*Total*
Backschool	7 (23%)	20 (77%)	27
Exercise only	2 (5%)	29 (95%)	31
	9	49	58

$\chi_1^2 = 2.8$ (not significant).

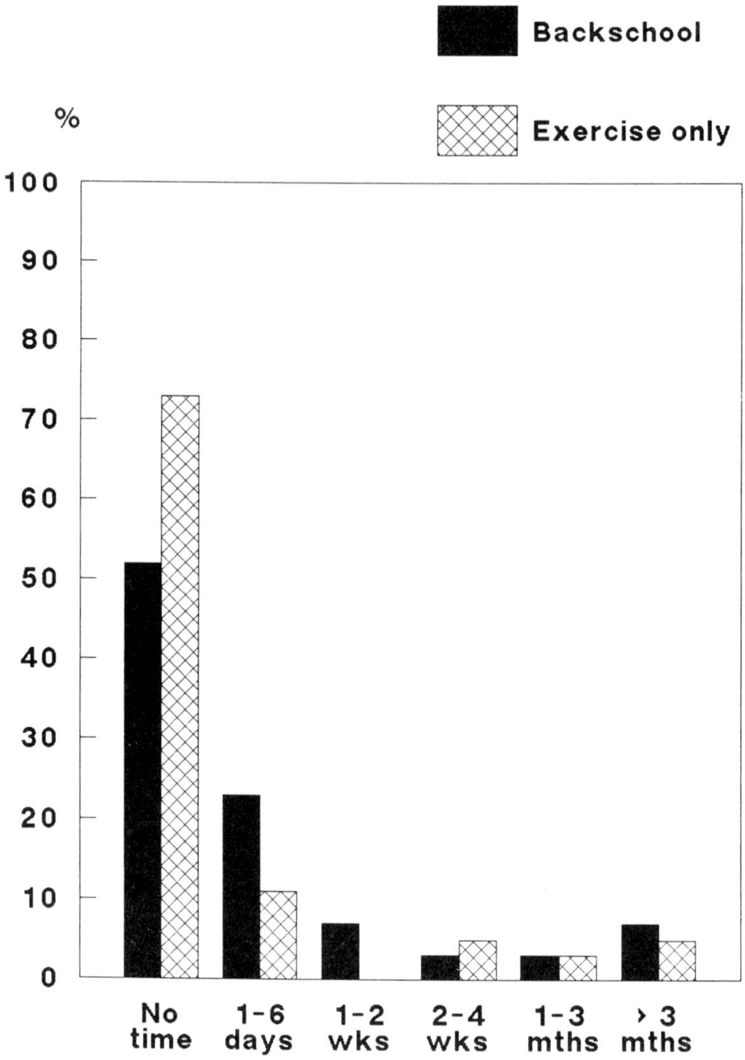

Fig 2.3 Time off work: solid columns, backschool; cross-hatched, exercise only

their home but only 52% said they had done this in their workplace. Only 16% said that they had taken up a new hobby, and 10% that they had taken up a new sport.

2.7.3 *Discussion*

It may perhaps be over-optimistic to expect to see any significant differences between the two groups 5 years after they had attended the backschool. It is interesting that a larger number of backschool patients still reported no functional disabilty. But the otherwise negative results do underline the need to emphasise to patients the non-threatening nature of the problem. Possibly too much emphasis was put on the need to rest if the pain was acute and to avoid excessive activity in the presence of pain (Waddell, 1987). This could explain the unexpectedly dependent and over-cautious attitude of the backschool patients 5 years later, as shown by their attendance to a hospital specialist and time taken off work.

These results contrast with the findings of the Canadian and Californian backschools, which both report a significant reduction of patients seeking further help from health professionals. However the North American figures relate only to immediate follow-up at 1 month, compared to the very long time interval of 5 years for the Oxford study. Also the patients in the Oxford study had a much longer history of back pain.

The Oxford backschool has been reviewed and developed since the original study was carried out and is currently being updated again taking into account these recent findings.

It is worth noting that patients were less likely to make alterations in their workplace than in their home. Frequently they said that however much they would like to make changes in the work environment to make it more ergonomically acceptable it would not be possible. They did not have control over this and they did not expect their managers to be enthusiastic about changes which might potentially imply capital outlay. It is therefore vital that professionals in this area should became more involved. There is a need to convince company managers that it is not only their obligation to make the environment at the workplace fit the individual worker but also to understand that any extra capital outlay may actually lead to greater productivity. If the worker is free of pain or discomfort then he can be expected to work more efficiently and he is also less likely to need sick leave. Physiotherapists and ergonomists need to play a greater part in planning industrial design. Trade unions could also play a more active role in promoting an ergonomically satisfactory environment at work where the worker's back is not put at risk.

Every effort should be made to return the patient to work as soon as possible. Long periods off work are undoubtedly detrimental to the well-being of an individual and if someone is off work for more than 6 months the chances of ever getting back to work are reduced to only 30% (Nachemson, 1983). Use of leisure time is also important and there is a danger that a back pain patient will be afraid of producing pain by particular activities; this fear may have been reinforced by the doctor or the therapist. He may conclude that it is 'safer' not to do any of the hobbies or sports that he would like to do and give up all the activities which he previously enjoyed. This should not happen and the clinicians must do everything they can to encourage the person to continue with the same activities or to try and find some other alternative activity or interest which they enjoy.

2.8 **Conclusions**

To conclude, there is evidence to suggest that the backschool as a concept has an important role to play in the management of back pain. The programme, however, needs to be structured with great care to make sure that a positive attitude is engendered in the individual, and that a return to normal function is encouraged as far as possible, and as soon as possible, in spite of pain. Patients should be taught how to reorganise their environment to reduce loading the spine and to modify the way certain activities are carried out, but need to be given maximum encouragement to be as active as possible.

References

Berquist-Ullman, M. & Larsson, U. (1977). Acute low back pain in industry, *Acta Orthopaedica Scandinavica* (Suppl.), 170.

Fairbank, J. C. T., Couper, J., Davies, J. B. & O'Brien, J. P. (1980). The Oswestry low back pain disability questionnaire, *Physiotherapy*, **66**, 271–3.

Hall, H. (1980). The Canadian Back Education Units, *Physiotherapy*, 66, 115–7.

Hall, H. & Iceton, J. (1983). Backschool, *Clinical Orthopaedics and Related Research*, **179**, 10–17.

Haynes, C. R. (1984). Back schools and total back-care programmes – a review, *Physiotherapy*, **70**, 14–17.

Klaber Moffett, J. A., Chase, S. M., Portek, I. & Ennis, J. R. (1986). A controlled, prospective study to evaluate the effectiveness of a Back school in the relief of chronic low back pain, *Spine*, **11**, 120–22.

Lankhorst, G. J., Van de Stadt, R. J., Vogelaar, T. W., Van der Korst, J. K. & Prevo, A. J. H. (1983). The effect of the Swedish back school in chronic idiopathic low back pain. *Scandinavian Journal of Rehabilitation and Medicine*, **15**, 141–5.

Mattmiller, A. W. (1980). The California back school, *Physiotherapy*, **66**, 118–22.

Nachemson, A. L. (1983). Work for all, *Clinical Orthopaedics and Related Research*, **179**, 77–85.

Troup, J. D. G. (1979). Biomechanics of the vertebral column, *Physiotherapy*, **65**, 238–44.

Waddell, G. (1987). A new clinical model for the treatment of low back pain, *Spine*, **12**, 632–44.

White, A. H. (1983). *Back school and other conservative approaches to low back pain*. The C. V. Mosby Company, St Louis.

Zachrisson-Forsell, M. (1980). The Swedish back school, *Physiotherapy*, **66**, 112–14.

Discussion

Troup (Liverpool): How far does your education extend – does it extend to the family or to the GP?

Moffett: We would certainly like to get at the families though we don't do so at present. We would like to get at these problems early, before they become chronic.

Carter (St Mary's): Did you make any attempt to correlate the type of condition with your success? I would also be interested to know about radiological findings.

Moffett: I agree that would be interesting but the problems of diagnosis are so fraught that we didn't actually get involved with that area at all. We included all patients with mechanical back pain problems.

Nelson (Leeds): It is a question which always comes up in a study like this. Are you satisfied that doing something is better than doing nothing? Have you been able to find a group which you could call a control group? How do we know what happens to these people when untreated for 5 years. Do you have any information on that?

Moffett: I think the simple answer is no. Obviously it would be good if one could have a control group, but the group would have to be exactly the same type of patient and the same type of patient is obviously going to have had some form of treatment.

Morrison (Swindon): I think we want to encourage this type of research rather than denigrate it. It's all very easy when someone produces a paper to get up and ask, 'Have you had enough controls?', or, 'have you had this or that which is statistically significant?' I would suggest that it would be incredibly difficult to find a group of patients that went for 5 years with back pain and hadn't had any treatment from anybody and indeed one might even suggest it was unethical to deny them that treatment.

3 *J. A. Klaber Moffett*

Exercises for back pain

3.1 **Flexion and extension exercises for back pain**

Exercises are commonly assumed to be of benefit for back pain. Although various different types of exercises for back pain have been recommended over the past decades, their effects have not been sufficiently researched. Active extension exercises have been widely used for at least 30 years and indeed are still often prescribed. Their purpose is to strengthen the spinal extensor muscles, to afford a greater protection to the spine. Some evidence of weakness of these muscles in back pain patients is reported in the literature (Addison and Schultz, 1980; McNeill, *et al.* 1980) but it seems likely that these findings could be confounded by the patient's willingness to tolerate pain during the testing procedures. Extension exercises are often carried out in a prone lying position in order to work the muscles against gravity, and the arms and legs are used to provide a variable length lever to grade the difficulty of the exercise (Figure 3.1). In this position the extensors are worked in their inner range which would rarely be the case in work or daily living activities. The well-researched and documented subject of specificity of muscle training (see, for example, Rasch *et al.*, 1957; Coyle *et al.*, 1981) tends not to be taken into account in rehabilitation. Another problem with this exercise is that the intradiscal pressure is greatly raised (Nachemson, 1976); this is undesirable if there is disc involvement. In practice, it is often found that these exercises exacerbate signs and symptoms of back pain. If a need to strengthen the spinal extensors is apparent the exercise may be more safely and beneficially carried out from a starting position of about 45° flexion through to the neutral position (Figure 3.2).

Flexion exercises are also frequently prescribed in the form described by Williams (1965) but Jackson and Brown (1983) found little scientific evidence to support their use. Blackburn and Portney (1981) carried out an EMG study of the paraspinal muscles during Williams' flexion exercises

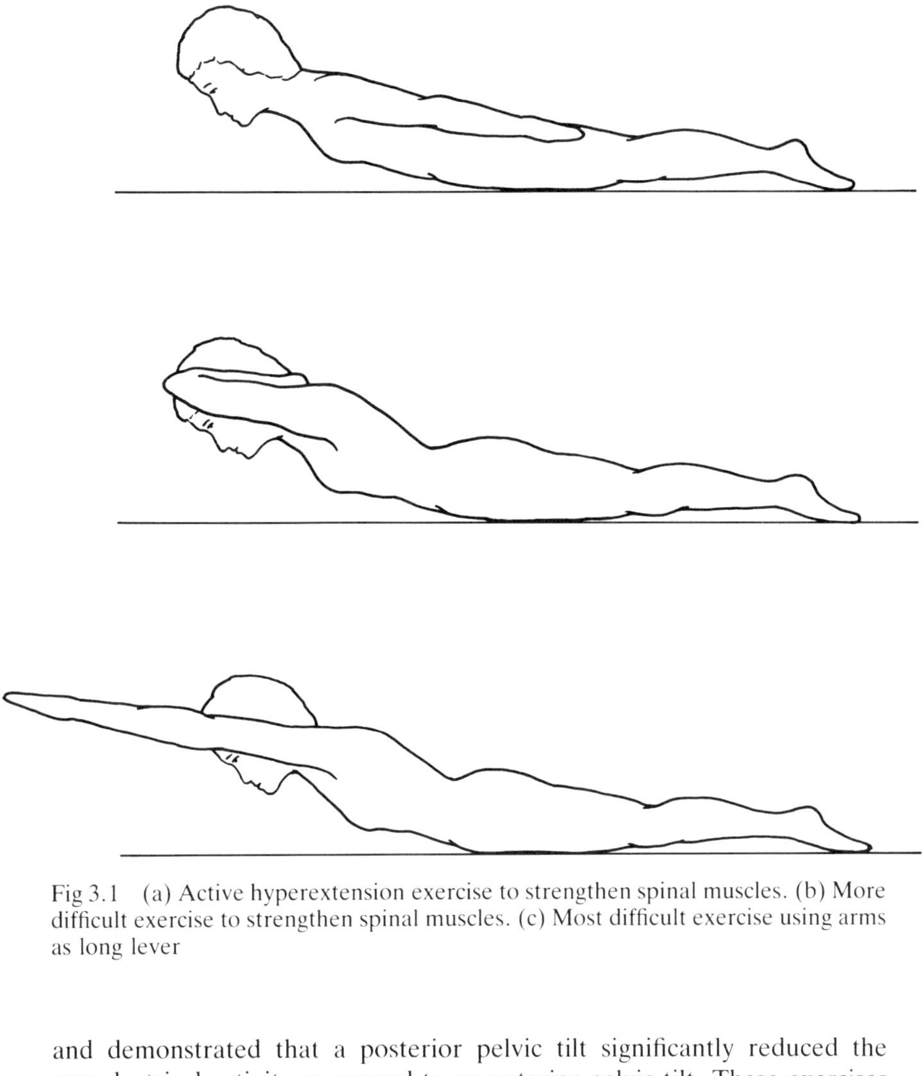

Fig 3.1 (a) Active hyperextension exercise to strengthen spinal muscles. (b) More difficult exercise to strengthen spinal muscles. (c) Most difficult exercise using arms as long lever

and demonstrated that a posterior pelvic tilt significantly reduced the myoelectrical activity compared to an anterior pelvic tilt. These exercises are sometimes referred to as mobilising exercises, which is a misleading term as the regimen described by Williams includes exercises which aim:

(1) to relieve pressure on the nerve root by opening the intervertebral foramen;

(2) to stretch the hip flexors and back extensors;

(3) to strengthen the abdominal and gluteal muscles with exercises, including sit-ups or partial sit-ups.

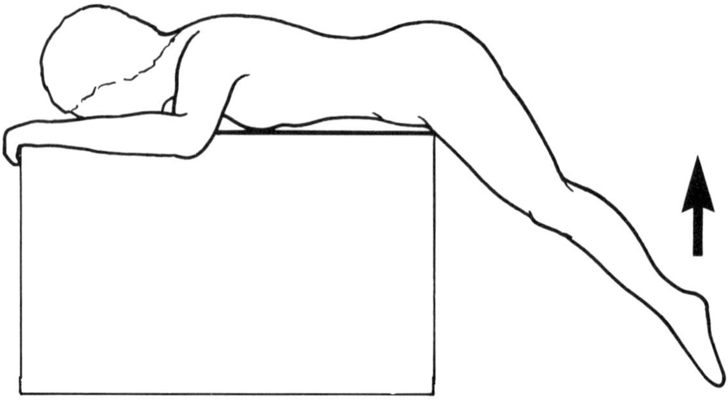

Fig 3.2 Exercise to strengthen spinal extensor muscles (from 45° flexion)

The latter should be used cautiously due to the great increase in intradiscal pressure produced by this manoeuvre (Nachemson, 1976) and are contraindicated if the back pain is caused by a bulging disc or disc protusion. The last two exercises are particularly aimed at patients who are found to have lax abdominal muscles and an exaggerated lumbar lordosis.

By combining static abdominal contractions with static gluteal contractions the patients are taught how to eliminate their lumbar lordosis (Figure 3.3). The ability to alter the pelvic tilt and therefore the degree of lumbar lordosis is useful for many patients who have this postural problem, and can sometimes provide immediate pain relief.

Advocates of the flexion regimen such as Williams (1965), Hume Kendall and Jenkins (1968b), and Caillet (1981), also claim that it is beneficial for back pain patients to maintain a slightly flexed lumbar spine at all times. They even suggest that back pain patients should sit slightly forwards in a chair to allow the lumbar spine to flex and so make sure that the lordosis is obliterated. This advice is very controversial and the opposite view is submitted below.

Hume Kendall and Jenkins (1968b) developed a programme of Lumbar Isometric Flexion Exercises (LIFE) which can be more safely recommended to the majority of back pain patients without risking an exacerbation of their problem. They conducted a double-blind controlled trial (1968a) in which they compared:

(1) the LIFE programme;

(2) twelve exercises designed (a) to mobilise the spine and (b) to

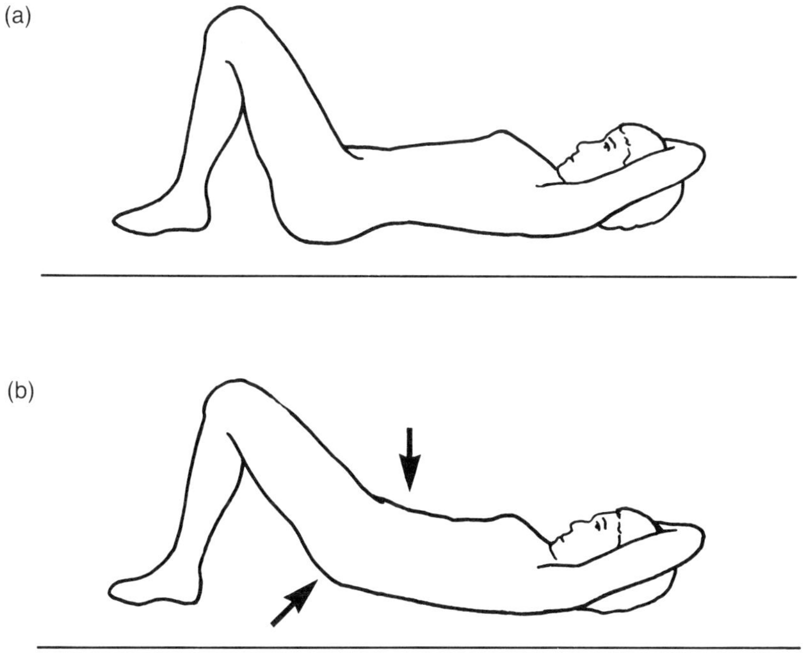

Fig 3.3 Pelvic tilting exercise: (a) forward tilt; (b) backward tilt

strengthen the muscles of the spine, both including flexion and extension;

(3) five exercises to strengthen the spinal extensor muscles, three of which were carried out in hyperextension.

At the end of a 3-month period of doing these exercises, of the 47 patients included in this study: 11 patients were symptom-free, seven of these from the LIFE group; 14 patients improved with the treatment; five patients withdrew from the study; five were made worse by the extension exercises (group 3); and two by the combined mobilizing exercises (group 1). No information was supplied as to the patients' diagnosis, symptomatology (e.g. whether any referred leg pain or neurological symptoms were present), age, sex or duration of history. It is also not known if any other forms of treatment were carried out. The most notable finding appears to be that LIFE exercises are less likely than the other two types of exercise programmes to exacerbate symptoms. This is not surprising as the other programmes were much more demanding.

In a rather better designed, more recent study, Davies *et al.* (1979)

attempted to reproduce these results by studying the effects on back pain patients, of the following three treatment groups:

(1) short-wave diathermy, as a control group;

(2) short-wave diathermy and back extension exercises;

(3) short-wave diathermy and LIFE exercises.

Their population consisted of patients of any age whose back pain was interfering with their sport and they included patients with a duration of symptoms ranging from 3 weeks to 6 months. Their findings showed that there were more cases of complete remission of symptoms with extension exercises (group 2), compared to the two other groups although the results were not statistically significant. This difference in results compared to those of Hume Kendall and Jenkins' trial may be due to a difference in population studied.

It has been widely assumed that abdominal muscles play an important role in supporting the spine, because of the relationship between their activity (particularly the oblique abdominals) and the intra-abdominal pressure. This in turn is directly related to the intradiscal pressure both of which increase when the spine is loaded (Andersson, 1977). However Hemborg and co-workers (1985) carried out a study in which they reported that increased strength in the abdominal muscles was not related to an increase in EMG readings or an increase in intra-abdominal pressure during various lifting procedures. Twenty male patients with chronic back pain undertook a rigorous exercise programme designed to increase the strength of the oblique abdominals. Interestingly, although the abdominal muscles were demonstrably stronger, they found that there was a significant decrease in EMG activity and no change in the intra-abdominal pressure during all the lifting procedures after training. One explanation is that the training was not specific enough in relationship to the task performance measured which, as mentioned above in relationship to strengthening the extensors, is an important consideration. But since the EMG readings were consistently reduced, the authors conclude that, rather than taking advantage of their ability to recruit more motor units, the subjects apparently utilised the metabolic effects of the strengthening exercise in some other way.

Abdominal bracing does seem to reduce loading on the spine in some way but the mechanism of the abdominal muscles is not yet understood. One theory is that they act on the spine through their attachment to the very strong lumbodorsal fascia, which provide an extensor moment and /or a hydraulic amplifier mechanism (Gracovetsky *et al.*, 1981).

There is some doubt as to whether the exercise programmes discussed above do actually produce the physiological effects such as strengthening or mobilising which they purport to achieve. In a very carefully designed study, Martin *et al.* (1986) allocated patients with a history of back pain of more than 6 weeks, most of whom had a long history of chronic back pain, to one of three treatment groups:

(1) mobilizing exercises;

(2) LIFE exercises;

(3) attention-control-placebo group: dummy ultrasound and dummy short-wave diathermy.

They found no significant improvement in strength or mobility resulting from the exercises. One way of explaining these results is in terms of the specificity of muscle strength training, referred to above. Interestingly there was no significant difference in outcome of pain or functional disability when comparing the three groups. The exercise groups did no better than the attention-placebo-control group.

3.2 **The McKenzie approach**

McKenzie (1981) advocates a totally different and innovative approach to the management of back pain. He maintains that back pain is so prevalent because of the amount of time spent with the lumbar spine in a flexed position. This is substantiated by epidemiological studies which show a high incidence of herniated disc problems in a sedentary population (Kelsey, 1977) and biomechanical studies which demonstrate an increase of 30% in intra-abdominal pressure readings when sitting compared to standing (Nachemson, 1976). McKenzie describes three factors which are primarily responsible for precipitating episodes of back pain:

Prolonged sitting
Prolonged or repeated stooping
Decreased range of lumbar extension.

He emphasises the importance of maintaining the lumbar lordosis at all times. This principle fits in very well with a new model of the spine in which the spine is described as an arch (Aspden, 1987). The lumbar lordosis is central to the theory and in its presence the intra-abdominal pressure can provide a stabilising mechanism for the spine. McKenzie stresses the importance of maintaining a lordosis especially during relaxed sitting when it decreases on average by 38 degrees (Andersson *et al.*, 1979). This can be restored by the use of a lumbar roll of adequate thickness.

The exercises, which are based on his initial findings from the history and examination, are very simple and easily performed. They are based on the mechanical properties of the intervertebral disc and other soft structures of the spine. Experimental work has shown that the position of the nucleus within the intervertebral disc is influenced by movements of the spine so that flexion tends to move the nucleus posteriorly and extension shifts it anteriorly (Shah *et al.*, 1978). McKenzie is prepared to treat any patient with a mechanical back pain problem except those with unremitting, constant nerve-root pain and neurological signs. In this group of patients it is likely that the nuclear material has been extruded through a breach in the annular wall and in this situation it is not possible to influence derangement.

McKenzie believes that it is possible, on the basis of the examination and the history, to categorise mechanical back pain into three distinct syndromes:

(1) *Postural:* the pain is caused by a prolonged posture, e.g. stooping which puts the richly innervated ligaments on a constant stretch. It is immediately relieved by altering the posture. No pathology is present.

(2) *Dysfunction:* adaptive shortening of the periarticular structures has occurred and so pain is produced as soon as these tissues are put on a stretch, which is likely to result from particular postures and movements.

(3) *Derangement:* pain may be constant or intermittent, due to the alteration in position of the fluid nucleus pulposus. There is disturbance of the normal resting position of the two adjacent vertebrae, which often results in a kyphosis or scoliosis. On testing lumbar spine movements, peripheral pain is reduced by certain movements and the pain is produced more centrally. For example in posterolateral protusions the nuclear material can be shifted away from the nerve by repeated extension. The programme recommended for such patients is therefore repeated passive extension (see Figure 3.4). The compressional forces on the spine are reduced if the spinal extensors are inactive, so patients have to learn to perform the exercise without using these muscles. All the strain must be taken on the arms and the pelvis must not be raised. These exercises are therefore not comparable with the programme of active extension exercises described above and illustrated in Figure 3.1.

There is a need for this approach to be thoroughly evaluated. Meanwhile McKenzie's approach is a particularly useful one and frequently appears to provide rapid improvement. The great advantage is that the patient recognises that if recovery is made it is due to his own efforts and so prophylaxis and self-reliance are encouraged.

Some evidence of the usefulness of this approach is afforded by a retro-

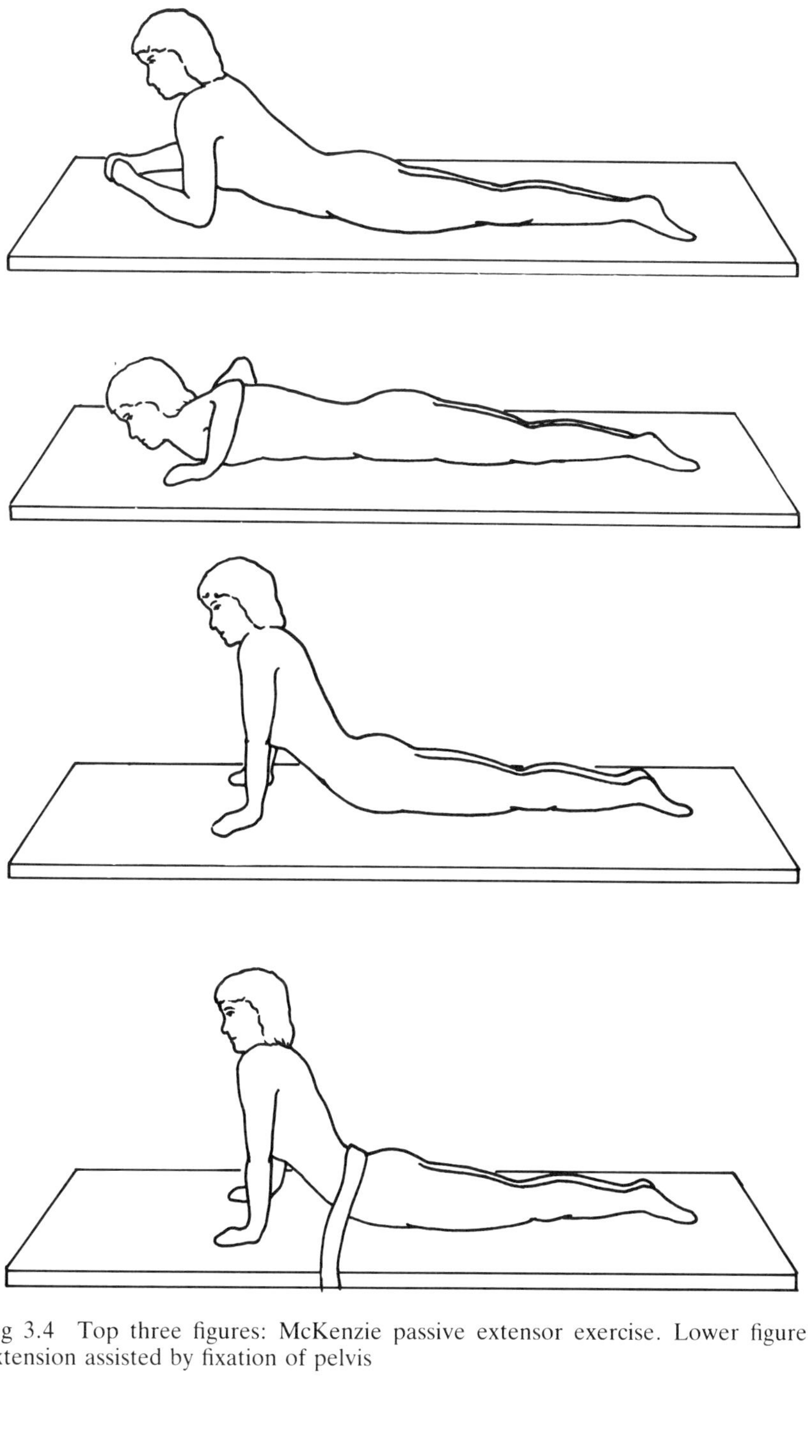

Fig 3.4 Top three figures: McKenzie passive extensor exercise. Lower figure: extension assisted by fixation of pelvis

spective study of patients admitted as probable acute herniated lumbar discs (Kopp *et al.*, 1986). Out of 67 patients, 35 responded to conservative treatment and all but one achieved normal lumbar extension within 5 days. Of the other 32 patients requiring surgery, 75% were found to have free fragments of disc material or nerve root displacement. Only two of the surgical cases had been able to achieve 30 degrees of extension prior to their operation. The authors suggest that this could be a useful test to ascertain which patients are going to require surgery.

3.3 General fitness exercises

There is a definite argument in favour of a general fitness programme being included in the routine management of back pain patients. Cady and co-workers (1979), in a study of firefighters, demonstrated that the least fit were ten times more likely to have subsequent back injuries. The type of exercise programme will depend on the patient population, the requirements for a group of young men engaged in strenuous physical activities obviously differing greatly from a group of chronically debilitated back pain patients.

A general fitness programme is especially important in chronic back pain patients where deconditioning through inactivity may lead to a major disability. Fear and avoidance of pain which are common features of a back pain problem (Lethem *et al.*, 1983) need to be recognised and countered, as soon as possible. Otherwise exaggerated illness behaviour and the increasing avoidance of activity is likely to be perpetuated. This learned pattern of behaviour is often reinforced not only socially but also in the clinical setting.

Exercise quotas have been shown not only to increase levels of activity but also to reduce exaggerated fear of pain anticipated on movement (Dolce *et al.*, 1986). In this system the patient is set a quota of exercise or specified activity, and is rewarded for attainment of the quota which is gradually increased. The patient is encouraged to work through the pain or discomfort and pain complaints are not rewarded by attention. This is an example of how the principle of operant conditioning described by Fordyce (1978) can improve function and reduce pain behaviour.

Thomas and co-workers (1980), at Rancho Los Amigos Center in California, carried out a study on 15 subjects with chronic back pain who took part in a gradually progressive activity programme. They demonstrated that those patients who had measurably reduced levels of physical fitness and functional ability had, by the end of the programme, improved their energy cost during exercise and were able to walk significantly further although not always faster. These results were achieved without an operant-conditioning programme, simply by gradually increasing the amount of daily walking or bicycling undertaken.

Multidisciplinary programmes may include exercise quotas, operant conditioning, biofeedback, relaxation, vocational and recreational rehabilitation. Such comprehensive programmes which are usually run on an in-patient basis are expensive and are not readily available at present in Britain. Success rates, which are much higher than one would expect from a very chronic population of back pain patients who have already had a great deal of unsuccessful treatment often including surgery, are reported in several studies of a variety of different multidisciplinary programmes (e.g. Cairns *et al.*, 1976; Keefe *et al.*, 1981; Gottlieb *et al.*, 1982).

In an evaluative study of a comprehensive treatment programme Mayer and colleagues (1985) at the Productive Rehabilitation Institute of Dallas for Ergonomics (PRIDE) included 111 patients with back pain: 73 of the patients took part in the treatment programme having authorisation from their insurance company, whilst the other patients acted as a control group. The programme aimed to restore range of movement and strength of muscles as well as increase cardiovascular fitness and simulate working situations. They found that return to work was related to increase in range of motion, muscle strength and functional capacity. Mayer suggests that these factors could be useful predictors of the ability for returning to work, rather than the more subjective report of pain.

It is likely that all back pain patients would benefit from some form of general fitness activity but they may require considerable encouragement and need to be convinced of the positive benefit in the face of pain. Patients with chronic back pain have been shown to have reduced levels of endorphins which is likely to increase their sensitivity to pain (Johansson *et al.*, 1980) but it is possible to raise these endorphin levels through exercise (Puig *et al.*, 1982). Also chronic back pain patients may exhibit demineralisation of the axial skeletal (Hansson *et al.*, 1980), presumably due to inactivity which could be prevented, if not reversed, by exercise. One more argument in favour of exercise is to counter the effect of depression which is often associated with chronic back pain. Aerobic exercise can have a specific effect on depression as shown in a controlled study carried out by Martinsen and co-workers (1985).

3.4 **Conclusion**

The role of exercise in the management of back pain is still controversial. The type of exercise administered must depend on the needs of the individual patient and they may be aimed at any of the following problems:

Pain
Posture
Loss of range of movement
Muscle weakness

Loss of confidence in the spine
Loss of general fitness.

It is the physiotherapist's responsibility to examine and assess the patient and devise a set of exercises aimed at reducing the patient's particular problem. For this reason exercises given in a group situation are of limited value as the suitability of the exercise will always depend on the individual. Classes are however useful for general fitness exercises, so long as the competitive spirit is carefully monitored and controlled. It is essential that patients should pace themselves in a manner appropriate to their condition, in order to avoid disappointing setbacks.

One of the greatest problems for the patient (and also the therapist) is to know how hard to push themself especially in the presence of pain and its attendant threatening implications. However, not only the possibility of a recurrence of an acute episode must be taken into account, but also the thought that if normal movement and activity are not encouraged soon after the onset of an acute attack there is a real danger that the patient will continue to protect their spine for fear of an exacerbation and pain. In this way the chronic back pain patient, with all his accompanying disability, comes into being.

Since conservative treatment to date offers no magic cure, it seems that the simplest, least costly and most effective methods available should be used.

An exercise programme may be an important adjunct to a backschool, especially in the form of a graded general fitness class where the competitive spirit can be used for patients to strive to beat their own records on each station of a circuit. They should be able to use this as a goal-oriented model of how to pace themselves, and to develop their activities at home by setting targets for themselves and, as far as possible, to return to a normal active life.

References

Addison, R. & Schultz, A. (1980). Trunk strengths in patients seeking hospitalization for chronic low back disorders, *Spine*, **5**, 539–44.

Andersson, G, B. J., Murphy, R. W., Ortegren, R. & Nachemson, A. L. (1979). The influence of backrest inclination and lumbar support on lumbar lordosis, *Spine*, **4**, 52–58.

Aspden, R. M. (1987). Intra-abdominal pressure and its role in spinal mechanics, *Clinical Biomechanics*, **2**, 168–74.

Blackburn, S. E. & Portney, L. G. (1981). Electromyographic activity of back musculature during Williams' flexion exercises, *Physical Therapy*, **61**, 878–85.

Cady, L. D., Bischoff, D. P., O'Connell, E. R., Thomas, P. C. & Allan, J. K. (1979). Strength and fitness and subsequent back injuries in firefighters, *Journal of Occupational Medicine*, **21**, 269.

Caillet, R. (1976) *Low back pain* (3rd Edn.). F. A. Davis Co., Philadelphia.

Cairns, D., Thomas, L., Mooney, V. & Pace, J. B. (1976). A comprehensive treatment approach to chronic low back pain, *Pain*, **2**, 301–8.

Coyle, E. F., Feiring, D. C., Rotkis, T. C., *et al.* (1981). Specificity of power improvements through slow and fast isokinetic training, *Journal of Applied Physiology*, **51**, 1437–42.

Davies, J. E., Gibson, T. & Tester, L. (1979). The value of exercises in the treatment of low back pain, *Rheumatology and and Rehabilitation*, **18**, 243–7.

Dolce, J. J., Crocker, M. F., Molletteire, C. & Doleys, D. M. (1986). Exercise quotas, anticipatory concern and self-efficacy expectancies in chronic pain, *Pain*, **24**, 365–72.

Fordyce, W. F. (1978). Learning processes in pain. In: *Psychology of Pain*, ed. R. A. Sternbach. Raven Press, New York.

Gottlieb, H. J., Koller, R. & Alperson, B. L. (1982). Low back pain comprehensive rehabilitation program: a follow-up, *Archives of Physical Medicine and Rehabilitation*, **63**, 458–60.

Gracovetsky, S., Farfan, H. F. & Lamy, C. (1981). The mechanism of the lumbar spine, *Spine*, **6**, 249–61.

Hansson, T., Sandstrom, J., Roos, B., Jonson, R. & Andersson, G. B. J. (1985). The bone mineral content of the lumbar spine in patients with chronic low back pain, *Spine*, **10**, 158–60.

Hemborg, B. Moritz, U., Hamberg, J., Holmstrom, E., Lowing, H. & Akesson, I. (1985). Intra-abdominal pressure and trunk muscle activity during lifting, *Scandinavian Journal of Rehabilitation and Medicine*, **17**, 15–24.

Hume Kendall, P. & Jenkins, J. M. (1968a). Exercises for backache: A double blind controlled trial, *Physiotherapy*, **54**, 154–7.

Hume Kendall, P. & Jenkins, J. M. (1968b). Lumbar isometric flexion exercises, *Physiotherapy*, **54**, 158–63.

Jackson, C. P. & Brown, M. D. (1983a). Is there a role for exercise in the treatment of patients with low back pain? *Clinical Orthopaedics and related research*, **179**, 39–45.

Jackson, C. P. & Brown, M. D. (1983b). Analysis of current approaches and a practical guide to prescription of exercises, *Clinical Orthopaedics and related research*, **179**, 46–55.

Johansson, F., Almay, B. G. L., Von Knorring, L & Terenius, L. (1980). Predictors for the outcome to treatment with high frequency transcutaneous electrical stimulation in patients with chronic pain, *Pain*, **9**, 55–61.

Keefe, F. J., Block, A. R., Williams, R. B. & Surwit, R. S. (1981). Behavioral treatment of chronic low back pain: clinical outcome and individual differences in pain relief, *Pain*, **11**, 221–31.

Kelsey, J. L. (1975). An epidemiological study of acute herniated lumbar intervertebral discs, *Rheumatology and rehabilitation*, **14**, 144–5.

Klaber Moffett, J. A., Chase, S. M., Portek, I. & Ennis, J. R. (1986). A controlled, prospective study to evaluate the effectiveness of a back school in the relief of chronic low back pain, *Spine*, **11**, 120–22.

Kopp, J. R., Alexander, A. H., Turocy, R. H., Levrini, M. G. & Lichtman, D. M. (1986). The use of lumbar extension in the evaluation an treatment of patients with acute herniated nucleus pulposus, *Clinical Orthopaedics and Related Research*, **202**, 211–18.

Lethem, J., Slade, P. D., Troup, J. D. G. & Bentley, G. (1983). Outline of a fear-avoidance model of exaggerated pain perception-1, *Behavioural Research*

Therapy, **21**, 401–8.

McKenzie, R. A. (1981). *The Lumbar Spine*. Spinal Publications Ltd., New Zealand.

McNeill, T., Warwick, D., Andersson, G. & Schultz, A. (1980). Trunk strengths in attempted flexion, extension and lateral bending in healthy subjects and patients with low back disorders, *Spine*, **5**, 529–38.

Martinsen, E. W., Medhus, A. & Sandvik, L. (1985). Effects of aerobic exercise on depression: a controlled study, *British Medical Journal*, **29**, 109.

Mayer, T. G., Gatchel, R. J., Kishino, N. *et al.* (1986). Objective assessment of lumbar function following industrial injury, *Spine*, **12**, 482–93.

Martin, P. R., Rose, M. J., Nichols, P. J. R., Russell, P. L. & Hughes G. I. (1986). Physiotherapy exercises for low back pain: process and clinical outcome, *International Rehabilitation Medicine*, **8**, 34–38.

Nachemson, A. L. (1976). The lumbar spine: an orthopaedic challenge, *Spine*, **1**, 59.

Puig, M. M., Laorden, M. L., Miralles, F. S. & Olaso, M. J. (1982). Endorphin levels in cerebrospinal fluid of patients with postoperative and chronic pain, *Anesthesiology*, **57**, 1.

Rasch, P. J. & Morehouse, L. E. (1957). Effect of static and dynamic exercises, *Journal of Applied Physiology*, **11**, 29–54.

Shah, J. S., Hampson, W. G. J. & Jayson, M. I. V. (1978). The distribution of surface strain in the cadaveric lumbar spine, *Journal of Bone and Joint Surgery*, **60B**, 246–51.

Thomas, L. K., Hislop, H. J., & Waters, R. L. (1980). Physiological work performance in chronic low back disability, *Physical Therapy*, **60**, 407–11.

Williams, P. C. (1965). *The Lumbosacral Spine, Emphasising Conservative Management*. McGraw-Hill, New York.

4 *P. Buckle and D. Stubbs*

Ergonomic aspects of back pain rehabilitation

4.1 Introduction

This chapter has been divided into three sections: Section 4.2 outlines what ergonomics is and examines its role within the health care setting. The benefits of ergonomics and the role of education of teams working towards rehabilitation and primary prevention of back pain are considered. In section 4.3 the role which ergonomics plays in existing rehabilitation programmes is the examined in the light of a review of studies undertaken both in the United Kingdom and elsewhere. In addition, areas have been identified where additional ergonomic inputs might be beneficial and methods for implementing these have been advanced. A number of case studies are presented in the final section 4.4 which illustrate the ways in which ergonomics can help and the dangers of inappropriate or delayed interventions.

4.2 What is ergonomics?

Both the study and the application of ergonomics attempt to optimise the fit between an individual and the task that the individual is undertaking. In order to ensure that the operation of the task is safe and efficient, and that the individual is comfortable and not at risk of ill-health, the ergonomist must rely on the body of scientific knowledge which is available for both physical and behavioural capabilities and limitations. This requires knowledge of the four main pure scientific disciplines: anatomy, biomechanics, physiology and psychology, which together with a knowledge of engineering design, form the basis of ergonomics (Oborne, 1982; Grandjean, 1980; Pheasant, 1984; Chaffin & Andersson, 1984; Tichauer, 1978; Warr, 1978; McCormick, 1978).

Ergonomics is concerned with the practical application of these disciplines, often within specialist areas, e.g. environmental aspects, workspace design, interface design and work organisation.

In spite of the range of specialist areas, a general principle runs through the study of ergonomics problems in complex work environments. The best way to approach a satisfactory solution is to consider the whole problem in terms of a systems approach. This takes into account the fact that each part of the work system may have an effect on another, i.e. that changes or problems in one area may have an influence on another. Such an approach involves consideration of people, tasks, equipment and environments all of which interact in the work system. It is only through understanding the complex nature of the work system, and the interactions between physical and behavioural demands that one can develop work practices and work places that are safe, healthy, efficient and comfortable.

It is perhaps not surprising, therefore, that the majority of ergonomists in this country have been trained at postgraduate level and that many come to such courses with a first degree of a scientific nature.

Increasingly the ergonomist is involved in either information technology and the role of human factors in designing systems or remains in the more traditional areas of job and equipment design. This polarisation has, to some extent, limited the number of ergonomists who are available to work within a health care setting (Stubbs & Buckle, 1984) and it is frequently left to other professional groups to provide what ergonomic input they can. Whilst it is true that physiotherapists, occupational therapists, general practitioners and other occupational health personnel may have some knowledge in the area (Stubbs, 1987), it is unlikely that many will have received professional training.

Where professional training in ergonomics is provided, its variety can be vast, as noted at a recent meeting hosted by the Commission of the European Community. Training courses included those for ergonomic technicians from Belgium (60 hours), physiotherapists and occupational therapists from Denmark (10 weeks), occupational physicians from the Netherlands (10 hours), occupational physicians from France (2 years) as well as undergraduate and postgraduate degrees from the United Kingdom (4 years and 1 year respectively). The meeting concluded that it is unlikely that many will have received professional training in ergonomics.

If we move away from the health care setting and consider those responsible for job design or redesign, it is evident that even here the human operator in the system is frequently not considered by the design engineers. Similarly there are some groups (e.g. industrial physiotherapists) who have some responsibilities in this area but for whom such matters are of secondary concern. Others within industry who might be considered as possible sources of ergonomic knowledge include occupational hygienists, occupational health nurses, safety officers and, to a lesser extent, some areas of personnel. The knowledge and awareness base in the general public is even more disappointing, although those who have suffered as a result of some mismatch, and this inlcudes many back pain sufferers, may have sought out information in an attempt to remedy their problems.

It is also probably true to say that, historically, ergonomists within this country have been more involved in primary prevention with respect to ill health issues than in rehabilitation.

In order to consider the role of ergonomics in rehabilitation one has to look primarily outside the United Kingdom to, for example, Scandinavia where many rehabilitation programmes in industry have involved ergonomics. It should be pointed out that this knowledge has not usually been provided by ergonomics experts. However, some form of team approach to rehabilitation involving ergonomics similar to that outlined recently for Occupational Health Services (International Labour Office, 1985) does seem to be a useful model and its success will be considered in section 4.3. The different roles required for a team approach to Occupational Health Services (including rehabilitation) and their respective training needs require further consideration. It will not, for example, usually be possible to have access to specialist knowledge at all times. It will be important therefore to generate criteria for seeking such advice (e.g. when the problem is very complex or when there are no previous studies of the problem available).

4.3 **The role of ergonomics in the rehabilitation of back pain sufferers**

4.3.1 *Current rehabilitation programmes*

A recent monograph (Spine, 1987) has considered the approaches to the assessment and management of activity-related spinal disorders. The report by the Quebec Task Force on spinal disorders endorsed only that which had been established through valid scientific study. This led them to call for further research as the treatment of activity-related spinal pain has infrequently been studied on a scientific basis. The extent of this limitation becomes obvious when therapeutic modalities for lumbar spinal disorders are reviewed. The vast majority of treatments have not been validated in randomised controlled trials, nor indeed in non-randomised controlled studies. The use of treatment modalities is usually based on common practice without support of scientific evidence. There is also an increasing trend towards the uptake of uncommon practice methods which similarly lack scientific support. The Quebec Task Force concluded that, in general, symptoms of acute pain tend to resolve spontaneously and that bed rest for low back pain (without significant radiation) should not usually be necessary. If required, it should not normally exceed 2 days.

4.3.2 *What then of ergonomics and ergonomic advice?*

The Quebec Task Force review indicated that a number of modalities which related to ergonomics, or where a knowledge of ergonomic issues was imparted, were of importance. These included the provision of postural information, the use of functional training, the provision of backschools and the modification of the work environment through ergonomic intervention. All these approaches have been shown to be useful in non-randomised controlled trials for at least some categories of low back pain patients, and backschools have also been found to be effective in randomised controlled trials.

It would seem therefore that, given the admitted limitations of most therapeutic modalities currently advanced, ergonomics can play an important role.

What is perhaps more difficult to establish is the extent to which ergonomic education is, or can be, provided. Similarly, consideration must be given to those who should be providing this education. At a practical level, ergonomic advice may be required in terms of temporary or permanent modification of the work environment. The same considerations then apply as to who could, should, or does have the expertise.

What then are the types of ergonomic input currently found in rehabilitation programmes both in the United Kingdom and around the world?

The major source of information transferral seems to occur within some of the backshool programmes. These frequently provide general information on the spine, its structure and function, and how the role of posture and physical activities may load this structure. Aspects of prevention and exercises for the back are frequently incorporated.

Other areas where ergonomic information forms an integral aspect of rehabilitation are in the provision of postural advice, in the use of functional training (Mayer *et al.*, 1985), and in the ergonomic intervention of occupational aspects.

It is not clear to what extent all or any of these aspects are present in rehabilitation programmes within this country, or the extent to which resources have been allocated to consider, implement or evaluate this approach.

A number of studies carried out in the United Kingdom in recent years have incorporated aspects of ergonomic advice in their backschool rehabilitation programmes. Klaber-Moffett *et al.* (1986) concluded that the backschool approach seemed to be more effective than an exercise-only regime, especially in the longer term outcomes, which in this study represented a period of 16 weeks. The ergonomic input to this programme included: anatomical and biomechanical aspects of the spine, ergonomic aspects of manual handling of loads, postural stress and practical methods for carrying out activities with minimal strain on the spinal structures (see Chapter 2).

Such an input was limited in time and would also be considered to be insufficient to deal with the topic as outlined above.

4.3.3 *When should ergonomic advice be provided?*
It would perhaps be of benefit to all sufferers (and non-sufferers) at least to have an awareness of ergonomic principles. To this extent perhaps such topics should be introduced as part of a national school syllabus! Failing this, and restricting our appraisal to rehabilitation of sufferers, it is perhaps useful to consider the pattern of return to work of back pain sufferers. The Quebec Task Force (Spine, 1987) observed that approximately 75% of workers reporting activity-related spinal disorders will be returned to work within 1 month. On the strength of this, they do not consider that advice on ergonomic aspects, other than some postural counselling from the treating physician, is required at this stage. Indeed, it is not until the patient has not resumed work for at least 3 months that any ergonomic assessment is considered. The percentage of all sufferers who reach this stage is estimated to be approximately 12%.

It would appear at first sight, therefore, that as the large majority of sufferers return to work within 1 month there is little purpose in using valuable resources on ergonomic input at this early stage. In contrast however, Lankhorst *et al.* (1983) found that backschools were of little help to chronic back pain patients, but argued the need to prevent the chronicity of back pain and that this could best be achieved by backschools in the early phase of idiopathic low back pain. Waddell (1987) also provides further insight into active rehabilitation that not only restores function but also reduces pain. If, in addition, the available information on repeat sufferers and multiple attacks of pain are considered, it becomes apparent that there may in fact be considerable justification for providing ergonomic awareness to sufferers at the earliest possible stage in order to minimise the risk of repeat attacks which may be triggered through, for example, occupational activities (see section 4.4). Table 4.1 illustrates that, within a nursing population, 43% of all those nurses who had had back pain reported that they had experienced at least seven episodes (Stubbs *et al.*, 1986b). It is therefore a matter of some conjecture as to how many of these repeats might have been prevented if more attention had been paid at an earlier stage to the work environment and the tasks the sufferers were being asked to undertake. Similarly, in a study of department store staff and of supermarket store staff (Buckle *et al.*, 1986) it was found that of those with some history of back pain, 54 and 53%, respectively, had suffered at least five attacks. Whilst it is not known how many of these repeat attacks required treatment it seems probable that they represent a significant proportion of the overall problem.

Further supportive data appear in the most recent set of statistics produced by the Royal College of General Practitioners *et al.* (1986). Approxi-

Table 4.1 Number of separate episodes reported by nurses with back pain (from Stubbs *et al.*, 1986b)

No of episodes	*No of respondents (%)*
1	327 (15.3)
2	316 (14.8)
3	282 (13.2)
4	181 (8.5)
5	72 (3.4)
6	40 (1.9)
7 or more	924 (43.1)

mately one in four of the back pain episodes experienced by individuals in the working age group, and seen by general practitioners, are not the first episode suffered by that patient.

Evidence from a controlled study of the effectiveness of back schools, containing some ergonomic input, compared with combined physical therapy and a placebo group has been presented by Bergquist-Ullman & Larsson (1977). Whilst the type of treatment did not seem to have a significant effect on the number of patients who had recurrences during the follow-up period of 1 year, the analysis was confounded by the very large percentage who changed jobs during that period (over 50%).

This study was of particular interest as it provided an opportunity for the working conditions to be inspected by a physiotherapist. It is unclear to what extent the working environment and tasks were, or could be, modified to conform with ergonomic principles.

It is on such topics that the backschool philosophy and ergonomic approach seem to come adrift. In this country it would seem that many of the backschool programmes in operation have some educational input on specific topics appertaining to ergonomics (e.g. biomechanics of the spine, lifting loads, and chair lumbar supports) but do not perhaps place them in their real context or show that ergonomics is about the design of work and work systems to fit the capabilities of the user or operator. Perhaps there is a greater need to encourage physiotherapists and occupational therapists to pursue courses in ergonomics and thus improve the quality of advice and education in this area that they can provide.

The role of the occupational physician in the rehabilitation of the back patient is also vital. There is perhaps a tendency to accept the return to work recommendation of the patient's own general practitioner, who has usually never seen the patient's place of work, rather than to investigate what might need to be done with respect to job or workplace redesign (see section 4.4).

Some complications with respect to these aspects are known to arise where a legal claim is being pursued and work-place changes may be seen as an admission of guilt.

4.4 **Extending rehabilitation after a return to work**

4.4.1 *When should the sufferer return to work?*

There are many good reasons why a sufferer should return to work at the earliest opportunity following an episode of back pain. Mayer *et al* (1985), Waddell (1987) and the Quebec Task Force (*Spine*, 1987) have produced a number of recommendations concerning the demands of the workplace, establishing restrictions on work activity, return to light work or part-time work, alternative jobs and use of a multidisciplinary rehabilitation team (including an ergonomist). Against this background the following case studies illustrate the diversity of current practice with respect to rehabilitation after a return to work.

The first of these case studies illustrates the possible effects of early intervention, the second the effects of late intervention, and the final study considers the effects of no intervention.

4.4.2 *Early ergonomic intervention*

A 45-year-old male office worker presented with acute low back pain. He had a previous history (three episodes) all of which had improved with conservative treatment. At his presentation to the occupational physician, nothing abnormal was found. The case was subsequently discussed with the industrial physiotherapist who then saw the patient and determined the nature and extent of his work task, work station, etc. This was followed, upon his return to work 1 week later, by an assessment of his working conditions. This revealed potential mismatches which included the desk height and the office chair. Conservative treatment was given twice weekly, during which time the physiotherapist also talked about the importance of ergonomics, e.g. the avoidance of static postures, postural variety. Improvements were made to his work station and a new chair was selected by an industrial physiotherapist using ergonomic criteria and which was tried and tested before being purchased for him by the company, where he is still working today.

4.4.3 *Late ergonomic intervention*

A 45-year-old male office clerk had suffered for 2 years with chronic low back pain. He had frequent appointments with the occupational physician and had received physiotherapy treatment. He was given a new chair a year ago, chosen by the company, but still suffered from back pain, particularly when seated, and had considerable time off work. An ergonomist was called in by the company to try and 'solve' the problem. The work station presented as an ergonomic disaster area: range of height adjustments were incorrect; armrests were too long to enable a close proximity to the desk; and lumbar support was inadequate. Several adjustments were made to the work station and a number of different chairs were given trials. In addition the importance of changing postures, e.g. stand/sit variations, were emphasised. Within 2 weeks of the ergonomist's visit this patient was medically retired due to his back pain.

4.4.4 *Inadequate ergonomic intervention*

As part of a major investigation of back pain in the nursing profession (Stubbs *et al.*, 1984), the circumstances surrounding 40 episodes of back pain were examined. Twelve nurses were reporting their first attack, whilst 28 were presenting with a repeat episode. For 32 of the nurses the onset of pain had been sudden with most occurring whilst on duty. Twenty cases were associated with handling a patient and 12 with other activities. Of the latter, five involved the movement of equipment.

The patient-handling tasks associated with the onset of pain were found to place considerable postural and load-handling demands on the nurse. Onset of pain frequently accompanied 'taking the weight' either in an awkward posture (e.g. combinations of bending, reaching and twisting) or in an emergency (e.g. when a patient collapsed). During transfer procedures (e.g. moving a patient from a bed to a chair) there was evidence of mismatched and inappropriate equipment increasing the problems.

The analysis suggest that the provision of suitable physical work environments, including the design of appropriate equipment and space, has not kept pace with the demands placed on the nurse by the greater emphasis on rehabilitation and maintenance of mobility in highly-dependent patients in both the hospital and the community (Stubbs *et al.*, 1984).

The High Court case of More *v*. Norfolk Area Health Authority (Manos, 1986) illustrates the consequences of such an incident. A nurse, after two previous episodes of back pain associated with lifting, suffered a final incident and left nursing, as many other nurses do (Stubbs *et al.*, 1986a). Her only consolation was the judgement against the Health Authority. Despite the large amount of research data now available, no guidance has been forthcoming from National Health Service management boards concerning either primary or secondary prevention or rehabilitation.

4.4.5 *Ergonomic consideration of the workplace*

The National Board of Occupational Safety and Health (1987) have estimated that of the 22 390 occupational diseases reported to the authorities in Sweden in 1983, 11 918 (55.7%) were attributable to factors amenable to ergonomic intervention. Some 20% of these cases were directly related to the back. It seems probable that the situation in other countries will be similar.

Many workplace factors have been shown to be associated with back pain (Andersson, 1982; Buckle, 1984). These include: heavy physical work, static work postures, frequent bending and twisting, lifting and forceful movements, repetitive work, vibration and psychological work factors. In a recent study of the nursing profession a combination of high static and moderate dynamic postural loading was considered to be the main contributory factor associated with the high incidence of back pain experienced by this group. The preventive approach proposed identified a need to reduce the overall postural loading of nurses and that this could best be achieved by proper consideration of the work system, that is, optimising the fit between nurses and their tasks, equipments and working environments (Stubbs *et al.*, 1986b). The full extent to which this and other strategies that have included ergonomics (e.g. Westgaard & Aaras, 1984, 1985; Stubbs, 1987; Troup & Rauhala, 1987) are effective in primary prevention or in the rehabilitation field is unclear, but the inclusion of ergonomics seems to hold more promise than other conventional approaches such as training or personnel selection (Snook *et al.*, 1978).

The extent to which the ergonomic approach may be effective in reducing these problems has been illustrated in a number of studies (Westgaard & Aaras, 1984, 1985; Spilling *et al.*, 1986) of musculoskeletal illness carried out at a major STK telephone plant in Norway over the period 1967–1982. The researchers undertook a quantitative study of the occurrence of musculoskeletal illness (i.e. sick leave with a relevant medical diagnosis) among workers in situations demanding high static muscle loads. Between 1967 and 1974 all workstations were fixed height. The scientists showed that this created excessive muscular load due to the need to adopt awkward postures at work. In 1975, an extensive ergonomic redesign of all workstations was undertaken which gave each operator greater flexibility for altering working postures. In particular, adjustments were sufficient to allow work to be carried out either standing or sitting.

The average musculoskeletal sick leave (expressed as the percentage of possible working time each year) for the period 1975–1982 was 3.1%, as opposed to 5.3% between 1967 and 1974. The effect was far greater when the figures were compared directly before and after ergonomic intervention. In addition, there were significant reductions in labour turnover from 30.1% (1967–1974) to 7.6% (1975–1982). This shows a clear positive effect of ergonomic intervention for both improved musculoskeletal health in the workplace as well as significant cost benefits to the organisation with respect to labour turnover, training, and sickness benefits. It has been estimated that the cost of the intervention, relative to the savings was of the order 1:10.

4.5 **Conclusions**

In reviewing this topic it has become apparent that there are many views as to what ergonomics is and what role it might have to play in the rehabilitation of back pain patients. We have attempted to put forward our view of ergonomics and the principles which underly good ergonomic design and practice. In so doing we realise that a number of dilemmas have been raised. For example, some would argue that hard physical activity at work keeps you fit and that active rehabilitation through work is beneficial. Our point of view on these two issues is, however, somewhat different. One of the major problems with heavy physical jobs is that they often leads to employment discrimination of groups in the working population (e.g. againt many elderly workers). In addition, such work is well established in the literature (Andersson, 1982; Buckle, 1984) as being associated with an increased risk for back disorders. Most ergonomists would argue that the job can, and should, be redesigned to be within the capacity of as many individuals as is reasonably possible. Whilst workers without a history of back pain will benefit from such an approach, the needs of back pain patients or ex-sufferers is less clear. It would seem that the application of ergonomic principles should be a minimum requirement it any event and that active rehabilitation should be encouraged within such constraints. More vigorous exertions should, one would argue, be undertaken only under controlled situations (e.g. during physiotherapy). Some have argued (Mayer *et al.*, 1985) that victims of low back pain should confront their pain and resume active bending and heavy work as soon as possible. Views on such issues vary widely (Troup *et al.*, 1987) but what is required is a research programme designed to obtain objective data on the capabilities and the capacities of sufferers and non-sufferers alike. Data are equally urgently required to span the temporal changes in abilities as patients recover from an episode.

It has been estimated that some 80% of the population will suffer from back pain at some time in their lives and in many occupational groups this figure will be higher. One is therefore forced to consider how many jobs have been designed bearing this fact in mind? Similarly, how many patients are being sent back to the very tasks and stresses which initiated their problem without any help in identifying or changing those aspects of their work? Between 1971 and 1981 (Royal College of General Practitioners *et al.*, 1986) the back pain episodes incidence rate increased by 30%. If the chain of events is to be broken, work-place intervention of an ergonomic nature must surely be a key place to start.

References

Andersson, G. B. J. (1982). Occupational aspects of low back pain. In: *Proceedings of the International Symposium, Low Back Pain and Industrial and Social Disablement*, ed. M. Nelson, pp. 45–51. Back Pain Association, London.

Bergquist-Ullman, M. & Larsson, U. (1977). Acute low back pain in industry: a controlled prospective study with special reference to therapy and confounding factors, *Acta Orthopaedica Scandinavica*, Suppl. **170**, 1–117.

Buckle, P. W. (1984). Ergonomic needs in epidemiological studies of low back pain. In: *Occupational Aspects of Back Disorders*, ed. J. Brothwood, pp. 24–33. Proceedings of the Society of Occupational Medicine, London.

Buckle, P. W., Stubbs, D. A. & Baty, D. (1986). Musculoskeletal disorders (and discomfort) and associated work factors. In: *Ergonomics of Working Postures*, eds. N. Corlett, J. Wilson & I. Manenica, pp. 19–30. Taylor and Francis Ltd., London.

Chaffin, D. B. & Andersson, G. B. J. (1984). *Occupational Biomechanics*. John Wiley, New York.

Grandjean, E. (1980). *Fitting the Task to the Man: An ergonomic approach*. Taylor and Francis Ltd., London.

International Labour Office (1985). *Convention 161 and Recommendation 171*. Occupational Health Service, ILO, Geneva.

Klaber-Moffett, J. A., Chase, S. M. Portek, I. & Ennis, J. R. (1986). A controlled, prospective study to evaluate the effectiveness of a back school in the relief of chronic low back pain, *Spine*, **11**, 120–22.

Lankhorst, G. J., Van de Stadt, R. J., Vogelaar, T. W., Van der Korst, J. K. & Prevo, J. H. (1983). The effect of the Swedish Back School in chronic idiopathic low back pain, *Scandinavian Journal of Rehabilitation Medicine*, **15**, 141–5.

Manos, J. (1986). Legal liability for back injury, *Occupational Health Review*, August/September, 7–10.

Mayer, T. G., Gatchel, R. J., Kishino, N., Keeley, J., Capra, P., Mayer, H., Barnett, J. & Mooney, V. (1985). Objective assessment or spine function following industrial injury. A prospective study with comparison group and one year follow-up, *Spine*, **10**, 482–93.

McCormick, E. J. (1978). *Human Factors in Engineering and Design*. McGraw-Hill, New York.

National Board of Occupational Safety and Health (1987). *Occupational Injuries in Sweden, 1983*, National Board of Occupational Safety and Health, Stockholm, Sweden.

Oborne, D. J. (1982). *Ergonomics at Work*. John Wiley, New York.

Pheasant, S. T. (1984). *Anthropometrics: An introduction for schools and colleges*. PP 7310, British Standards Institution, London.

Royal College of General Practitioners, Office of Population Censuses and Surveys, Department of Health and Social Security (1986). *Morbidity Statistics from General Practice 1981–1982*. HMSO, London.

Snook, S. H., Campanelli, R. A. & Hart, J. W. (1978). A study of three preventive approaches to low back injury, *Journal of Occupational Medicine*, **20**, 478–81.

Spilling, S., Eitrheim, J. & Aaras, A. (1986). Cost benefit analysis of work environment investment at STK's telephone plant at Kongsvinger. In: *The Ergonomics of Working Postures*, eds. N. Corlett, J. Wilson, and I. Manenica, pp. 380–97. Taylor and Francis Led, London.

Spine (1987). Scientific approach to the assessment and management of activity-related spinal disorders: a monograph for clinicians. Report of the Quebec Task

Force on Spinal Disorders, *Spine*, **12**, 7, Supplement.

Stubbs, D. A. (1987). Ergonomics in nursing: introduction. *International Journal of Nursing Studies*, **24**, 285–9.

Stubbs, D. A. & Buckle, P. W. (1984) Health care and ergonomics – a review paper. In: *Proceedings of the 1984 International Conference on Occupational Ergonomics. 2*, eds. M. Matthews & R. Webb, pp. 154–61. Human Factors Association of Canada, Ontario Canada.

Stubbs, D. A., Buckle, P. W., Baty, D., Fernandes, A., Hudson, M. & Rivers, P. (1984). *Patient handling and back pain in nurses*. DHSS Report No. JR/125/120, London.

Stubbs, D. A., Buckle, P. W., Hudson, M. P., Rivers, P. M. & Baty, D. (1986a). Backing out: nurse wastage associated with back pain, *International Journal of Nursing Studies*, **23**, 325–36.

Stubbs, D. A., Baty, D., Buckle, P. W., Fernandes, A., Hudson, M., Rivers, P., Worringham, C. J. & Barlow, C. (1986b), *Back pain in nurses: summary and recommendations*. Robens Institute, University of Surrey, Guildford.

Tichauer, E. R. (1978). *The Biomechanical Basis of Ergonomics*. John Wiley, New York.

Troup, J. D. G. & Rauhala, H. H. (1987). Ergonomics and training, *International Journal of Nursing Studies*, **24**, 325–30.

Troup, J. D. G., Foreman, T. K., Baxter, C. E. & Brown, D. (1987). The perception of back pain and the role of psychophysical tests of lifting capacity. *Spine*, **12**, 645–57.

Warr, P. B. (1978). *Psychology at Work*, 2nd Edn. Penguin Books, London.

Waddell, G. (1987). A new clinical model for the treatment of low back pain, *Spine*, **12**, 632–44.

Westgaard, R. & Aaras, A. (1984). Postural muscle strain as a causal factor in the development of musculoskeletal illnesses, *Applied Ergonomics*, **15**, 162–74.

Westgaard, R. & Aaras, A. (1985). The effect of improved workplace design on the development of work-related musculoskeletal illnesses, *Applied Ergonomics*, **16**, 91–97.

Discussion

Loebl (London): You haven't mentioned whether in ergonomics there are significant results in randomised trials as yet or whether they are in the pipe-line?

Buckle: There are some good studies which indicate that ergonomic intervention has long term effects in terms of general musculoskeletal disorders, not specifically back pain but including shoulder pain and so on, where you modify the whole work process.

5 *P. Lloyd*

Recent educational initiatives in the nursing profession for back pain avoidance

5.1 Introduction

The problem of back pain and its disabling effects remains despite the extensive efforts made to research the causes and prevention of this symptom. It is a problem familiar to large numbers of people in all walks of life and in all sorts of occupations. In varying degrees, it can adversely affect peoples lives, sometimes dramatically, yet it is a condition which evokes little sympathy or concern as far as the general public is concerned, probably because it is not seen as a life-threatening condition. Clearly if the more serious conditions can be prevented then many people will be freed from a lifetime of misery and restriction. Therefore every effort must be directed into researching the causes and prevention of this condition especially when it occurs as a result of occupation.

Despite the conclusions of some researchers that conventional instruction to promote correct lifting techniques has been shown to be of little value (Simpson, 1984), the emphasis on training as a preventive approach must not be diminished in favour of the ergonomic approach however attractive that may be. The two must run side by side. Where research points the way to a preventive strategy then it is imperative that every effort is made to find practical means of reducing and ultimately eliminating the problems of back pain by harnessing research results. Ergonomic design, staff selection and safety training are generally accepted as the three main preventive approaches.

5.2 Training programmes

In this chapter only the training aspect will be considered. If a training strategy is to succeed, it is first necessary to raise the level of awareness of the problem among the target group and emphasise the risks they run of a disabling back injury if they ignore the principles and systems of work prescribed. Secondly, it is necessary to give individuals a framework or point of reference upon which they can hang their behavioural modifications. If the training programme fails to achieve changes in behaviour, the purpose and end result will not have been achieved.

5.2.1 *Training children to avoid back pain*

The obvious starting point is to direct the training and educational effort towards the child whilst still in a formative stage of development. The Educational committee of the National Back Pain Association has drawn together a number of experts in this subject who are currently working towards producing a manual for school teachers both in primary and secondary schools. Many difficulties surround this initiative, one of which is to find the right choice of narrative which both inspires and interests the reader without making the subject either too complicated to understand, on the one hand, nor too elementary on the other.

The members of the committee are convinced that it is important to teach children how to look after their backs whilst they are still at school so that good postural and lifting habits can be instilled. The appeal of the manual will be further enhanced by line drawings and photographs to get the message across. If the working party succeeds in alerting teachers to the problem and this topic becomes an integral part of the health promotion syllabus in the school curriculum, a great step forward will have been taken.

5.3 **The nursing profession and back pain**

As an occupational group, nurses have a high incidence of back pain. Various studies indicate that nurses show relatively high prevalence rates when compared to other occupations. Stubbs *et al.* (1983) have estimated the size of the problem in a retrospective survey of back pain among 3912 nurses in the NHS as:

Annual prevalence – 431 per 1000 at risk
Point prevalence – 170 per 1000 at risk
Annual incidence – 77 per 1000 at risk.

These figures should not lead to complacency on the part of the nursing profession itself, nor of the employers of nurses, whether in the NHS or the private sector, for the problem is a serious one. This is not surprising given the combination of various adverse factors which conspire to cause the maximum amount of damage to nurses' backs. Poor work place design, lack of space, unco-operative patients, excessive weights to be moved, lack of adequate training, inadequate resources, and too few staff to look after too many patients, are just some of the reasons.

5.3.1 *Preventive approach to nurses' back pain – training and education*

A preventive strategy has long been adopted by employers in the form of training, although in early nursing textbooks produced in the fifties, sixties and early seventies the subject was hardly given a mention. Increasing attention was, however, given to training in the late seventies and the current editions of most nursing textbooks are much more forthcoming about lifting and handling techniques for nurses.

The Chartered Society of Physiotherapists produced a short illustrated booklet *Lifting patients in hospital* in 1962 which seems to have been the only standard advice available to nurses at that time. The illustrations show young women in one-piece swimming costumes lifting other similarly dressed young women. The whole thrust of such training was to show nurses three basic lifting methods: namely, the three-person lift, used to transfer a patient from bed to trolley; the shoulder lift; and the orthodox lift to move a patient up a bed.

Any practical training was usually accompanied by visual aids which dealt with the principles of manual lifting. These visual aids usually showed the subject picking up a box from the floor, or similar activities. Unfortunately such approaches took little account of many other factors which made the outcome of the lift unpredictable, not the least of which was the behaviour of the patient being lifted (RCN, 1979; Stubbs *et al*; 1980).

A further complicating factor was the question of maximum safe weight limits. The instructors' approach in health care services was to ignore this aspect, an approach which led nurse students into believing that provided they followed the particular lifting technique to the letter they would avoid back injury, irrespective of how heavy a patient was. There are no maximum weight limits laid down for nurses, and an attempt by the Health and Safety Commission to define manual weight limits for workers by regulation failed to get past the first round of consultation (HSC, 1984).

The approach to the training of nurses and other health care workers who had to lift and move patients was too simplistic, considering that the subject was fraught with many difficulties. The changes in the treatment pattern of patients in hospital and the community has also been a significant factor over the past 20 years. Patients are no longer allowed to stagnate in bed even if death is not far away. The emphasis was, and still is, on getting all patients, including the very elderly and infirm, out of bed, rehabilitated as far as possible, and mobilised.

There are good medical reasons for this because the movement of the patient helps to improve blood flow and restore lost function, with the laudable objective of improving the quality of the patient's life. However, the consequences of these changes have resulted in nurses having to handle and lift more and more patients and having to cope with patients who collapse suddenly. Nurses just have to hold them up and injure themselves doing so.

A report of a working party (RCN, 1979) identifying these problems was published. The aim was to persuade the nursing profession that back injury should not be seen as an inevitable consequence of nursing practice. Given the right attitude to change, the authors hoped to point the profession in the right direction to encourage the adoption of a more positive preventive strategy through a problem-solving approach.

The report highlighted the wide variations in approach in schools of nursing to the question of training. Teaching in-patient manual lifting techniques was the only preventive measure in most cases. It was concluded that, on average, learner nurses received one hour's instruction and one hour's practice in the subject of manual handling and hardly any training in the use of hoists or mechanical lifting aids.

Although questions were asked about hoists, almost no training school had a hoist of its own and nurses in training were simply not taught to use such equipment as an alternative to lifting manually.

The problem was perceived to be self-perpetuating because trained ward sisters and managerial grade nurses relied on their own inadequate training which did not encourage innovation nor reappraisal of poor techniques.

A recent research study (Troup *et al.*, 1987) makes the point that the skills in handling which instructors teach are sometimes inadequately used in practice because the senior nurses in charge of the wards have not received similar instruction. Consequently, the students are not able to practise their skills under competent supervision. To overcome this problem it was recommended (RCN, 1983) that training programmes should begin with the senior managers responsible for nursing care.

Attitudes to training are now changing. This process has been helped not only by the work of the Royal College of Nursing but also by the report produced by the Health and Safety Commission Health Services Advisory Committee *The Lifting of Patients in the Health Services* (Health and Safety Commission, 1984). This report recommended that each health authority should develop a patient-handling policy which also defined safe handling procedures at all appropriate levels, with emphasis placed on the use of hoists with a hoist co-ordinator appointed to act as an information resource. Most importantly, a positive policy on education and training in patient handling was recommended for all health service workers involved in handling patients. This report revealed that porters and nursing auxiliaries who did most of the lifting received least training if any at all.

Innovative educational approaches to the avoidance of back injury among nurses are now being developed. Greater emphasis is being placed

Table 5.1 Instructor's syllabus for handling and moving patients (RCN, 1988)

Unit 1	Legal and Professional Responsibilities (2 hours)
Unit 2	Biomechanics Basic Theory (1 hour) The Practical Aspects of Biomechanics (2 hours)
Unit 3	Elimination of Postural Stress and back injury (2 hours)
Unit 4	Assessment and principles of patient handling needs (half an hour plus a minimum of 3 hours practice)
Unit 5	Hoists and lifting equipment (minimum of 5 hours practice)
Unit 6	Problem solving situations (4 hours practice)
Unit 7	Body awareness and trust exercises (1½ hours practice)
Unit 8	Principles of teaching/handling (5 hours theory plus teaching practice)

on supervised practice in the actual patient-care situation. Also greater efforts are being made to relate training to the reality of the situations in which nurses are expected to lift patients. Training is no longer seen as a 2-hour lecture and demonstration of a few manual lifts with practice on fellow learners, but as an ongoing exercise with emphasis on refresher training at stated intervals.

Greater attention is now being focussed on the need to find solutions to problem cases on a team basis with the ward-based practical lifting and handling co-ordinator taking responsibility. The tendency in the past has been to leave the problem to junior nurses to solve; if they made a wrong judgement and become injured they are then castigated for it.

A new instructor's syllabus for handling and moving patients has now been published (RCN, 1988). This syllabus is the result of the initiative taken by the Royal College of Nursing's advisory panel on back pain in nurses when it ran a pilot course in the University Hospital in Nottingham intended for senior handling instructors from health authorities who were invited to participate in a week-long residential course. As a result of the course evaluation, the syllabus was produced by colleagues on the panel led by Cynthia Attwell, Duncan Troup and Brian Fletcher.

The syllabus is divided up into units and each unit can be taught as a separate entity in any order. A time limit is suggested for all the units which if taken together would be 26 hours plus teaching practice (see Table 5.1).

5.4 Case studies

Another innovation is the use of case studies, as accompaniments to the new syllabus for handling and nursing patients (RCN, 1988).

There are an increasing number of nurses' back injury cases coming before the courts; the plaintiffs seek damages against their employers for their injuries. Each case is different and liability hinges on the particular circumstances of each incident because of all the factors involved. There is increasing success in this direction with some nurses winning large damages for back injuries where it has been shown that employers failed to take reasonable care of an employee when it was forseeable that a back injury could occur. These cases have served to heighten awareness of the problem and have forced employers to look much more carefully at their responsibilities for providing a safe and healthy working environment.

The case study is therefore turned to the advantage of both nurses and employers by analysing the factors involved and then providing a preventive strategy for coping with the difficulties that emerge. Thus the case studies, although all different in detail, conform to the same format, i.e. venue, patient, staff, situation, accident, causes and prevention.

The Royal College of Nursing's strategy has been to make the best possible use of research by attempting to educate the nursing profession about the dangers of back injury and by providing instruction, training, and up-to-date advice. Its advisory panel on back pain in nurses consists not only of officers of the Royal College of Nursing, who have an interest and expertise in the subject, but also practising nurse educators, an occupational therapist, an occupational physician and a professor of ergonomics. The panel members act as expert witnesses in court cases. *The Guide for Nurses* (National Back Pain Association, 1987) has been produced with an expanded text and many more line drawings. The authors have attempted to cover many of the situations which create the greatest difficulties for nurses when lifting or handling patients. These include lifting children, toiletting the elderly semi-dependent person, and mobilising the patient liable to fall.

The Advisory Panel concentrates on education as the primary preventive approach because the state of affairs in the health service does not at present lead one to believe that there will be any dramatic overnight solutions to the ergonomic problems which exist. Any major reduction in work-related back injury can only be brought about when this aspect is adequately dealt with.

For this reason the next most important task facing the Royal College of Nursing's back pain panel is to tackle the problem of poor work-place and equipment design by offering nurses practical solutions to the problems they face when handling patients. The advisory panel hopes to produce a guide to practical ergonomics for nurses and others in health care establishments. The panel welcomes every opportunity to preview new patient lifting and handling devices as well as new visual aids concerned with patient handling directed towards nurses. They aim to ensure that redundant techniques such as the orthodox lift are perpetuated.

5.5 Use of mechanical aids

The manufacturers of hoist and transfer equipment are also playing their part. Two new lifting aids by Mechanaids deserve mention, namely the Dextra and the Stella. The Dextra is an extra-light mobile hoist which is very comfortable because it has an all-enveloping sling with very good head support and, most importantly, it lifts in half the time because of its simplicity and mobility. The Stella is an elegent name for a most inelegent looking piece of apparatus. Quite simply it is used to pluck a dependent patient out of a chair, support the patient whilst the nurse removes the lower clothing and then deposits the patient onto a toilet, thus avoiding all the bending and twisting a nurse has to do while she is trying to hold up a patient who at any moment might collapse on her.

These innovations are just what is needed. Nurses are reluctant to use mechanical aids to lift patients because they perceive them as being slow and cumbersome (Bell, 1984). Some of them are. Some patients are apprehensive about being lifted by a mechanical device and sometimes need considerable reassurance before they accept the need.

The time is right, however, for manufacturers to put their minds to harnessing the latest technology and providing electricially-operated hoists instead of pumping and winding mechanisms. In the future nurses might be replaced by robots programmed to do the heavy lifting tasks. The need for human contact and a reassuring touch will remain paramount but not at the expense of a back injury.

References

Bell, F. (1984). *Patient-lifting devices in hospitals*. Croom Helm, London.

Health and Safety Commission (1982). *Manual Handling of Loads. A Consultative Document*. Health and Safety Commission, London.

Health and Safety Commission Health Services Advisory Committee (1984). *The Lifting of Patients in the Health Services*. Health and Safety Commission, London.

National Back Pain Association in Collaboration with the Royal College of Nursing (1987). *The Handling of Patients. A Guide for Nurses*, 2nd Edn. National Back Pain Association, Teddington, Middlesex.

RCN Advisory Panel on Back Pain in Nurses (1983). *Guidance on the Handling of patients in Hospital and the community*. Royal College of Nursing, London.

RCN Advisory Panel on Back Pain in Nurses (1988). *An Instructor's Syllabus for Handling and Moving Patients*. Royal College of Nursing, London.

RCN Working Party Report (1979). *Avoiding Low Back Injury Among Nurses*. Royal College of Nursing, London.

Simpson, G. (1984). Ergonomic problems and solutions. In: *Proceedings of the Society of Occupational Medicine Back Pain Symposium*, ed. J. Brothwood. Society of Occupational Medicine.

Stubbs. D. A. Buckle. P. W. Hudson. M. P. Rivers. P. M. & Worringham. C. J.

(1983). Back pain in the nursing profession. Part 1. Epidemiology and pilot methodology, *Ergonomics*, **26**, 755–65.

Stubbs, D. A. Hudson. M. P. Rivers P. M. & Worringham. C. J. (1980). *Patient Handling and Truncal stress in nursing, Conference Proceedings*, Conference organised by the Nursing Practice Research Unit, Northwick Park Hospital , Back Pain Association and the DHSS, 26 September, 1980, pp. 14–22.

Troup. J. D. G. & Rauhala H. H. (1987). Ergonomics and training, *International Journal of Nursing Studies*, **24**, 325–30.

Discussion

Troup (Liverpool): I would like to refer to something I said in the *Nursing Mirror* about the want of evidence on the value of training. Perhaps I could now bring that a little up to date. We have developed in Helsinki a 40-hour training programme for student nurses. We have shown that the effect of that training programme is to increase patient-handling skills. We also have done a follow-up on the patient-handling skills on graduation as a nurse, and virtually all the nurses who had reported injury in their first year of work thereafter had had or poor handling skills but none of the excellents had any back injuries at all. So we are now being very much more positive about the value of training.

Mulholland (Nottingham): In the face of that excellent presentation it is perhaps daring of me to question the entire role of trauma in producing significant back disability. We all know that major back injury in terms of people breaking their spine or being run over by cars, etc., is not an enormous problem in terms of producing chronic back pain. We also know that an injury is an activity that an individual has done many times before without any trouble and it is an activity which other members of the staff have equally done. For example, patients are collapsing on the ward frequently, they are often picked up. Only one nurse in 20 will experience back pain. Surely our third difficulty is that we constantly speak with forked tongue when we emphasise that injury is the cause of back pain by asking, 'When did you injure your back?'. The patient will recall that the last time their back 'went' was when they bent down to pick up a matchbox or when they turned to the left to pick up something. The patient then logically thinks, 'My back went, doctor, I must have injured it'. The emphasis on injury constantly undermines any attempt to get people who are frightened of their backs back to normal activity.

Lloyd: Well, I won't argue about the medical issues involved in that question because I do not feel qualified to do so. Certainly from the point of view of compensation unfortunately the way the cards are stacked in this country you have to show that an untoward event occurred whilst carrying out an activity, such as lifting, moving, handling. If you can't show that, it is extremely difficult to persuade the courts that an accident did indeed occur. We did win a court case, for instance against a Lancaster Health Authority, on the argument of cumulative strain, of heavy repeated lifting throughout a whole night's duty on an intensive care unit, understaffed, with heavy patients. Nothing untoward occurred, no particular incident occurred, but nevertheless the judge accepted the argument and I think that was encouraging. So we have to look to all these factors, the weight of the patient, the frequency of lifting, and so on, and perhaps the quicker we move in this country to no fault compensation for health service workers the better.

Loebl (London): You didn't mention anything about medical screening of student nurses before they start their training to see whether they might have some pre-existing spine problems. Is in fact this being done or encouraged?

Lloyd: Well, I deliberately didn't mention pre-employment screening because I was talking about training and pre-employment screening is another issue. I believe there are no predictive tests which have any value. I know Richard Porter has done a lot of work on spinal canal diameters and whether the Occupational Health departments in this country are in a position to use his techniques routinely I am not in a position to say, but my suspicion would be that they are not. The equipment is expensive and you need specially trained technicians to use it. So the only significant evaluation one could ask is whether there had been any pre-existing back pain and exclude on that basis.

6 *M. Roland and M. Dixon*

The role of an educational booklet in managing patients presenting with back pain in primary care

6.1 Introduction

Back pain is a common symptom in the population. In one community survey in Great Britain, back pain was the fifth commonest reported symptom and 21% of the sample said that they had experienced back pain in the previous 2 weeks (Dunnell & Cartwright, 1972). Most patients with back pain do not seek medical advice. In a study of young women in South London, it was estimated that only one episode of back pain in 52 was presented to the patient's general practitioner (Morrell & Wale, 1976). Nevertheless, back pain is the seventh commonest symptom seen in general practice, and a general practitioner with an average list size can expect to see between 80 and 125 new episodes of back pain in his patients each year.

The management of back pain in general practice is unsatisfactory because diagnosis is usually imprecise, and effective methods of treatment are not available. Of patients who present to general practitioners with back pain, only about 5% have a prolapsed intervertebral disc with clear signs of nerve root compression, serious systemic disease is very uncommon, and the great majority have non-specific mechanical low back pain (Morrell, 1972; Barton *et al.*, 1976).

Most patients with non-specific low back pain will get better on their own. The general practitioner's role is often limited to general advice, support, and prescription of analgesics. This advice may include a period of bed rest, but even this is controversial as, of the three controlled studies which have been done on the place of bed rest in acute low back pain, two suggested that bed rest delayed recovery (Gilbert *et al.*, 1983; Deyo *et al.*, 1986), and only one suggested benefit from initial bed rest (Wiesel *et al.*, 1980). General practitioners sometimes prescribe non-steroidal anti-inflammatory agents, though there is little evidence that they are more effective than simple analgesics (Deyo, 1983). They may also use skeletal muscle relaxants: there is some theoretical basis for the use of these drugs, but little evidence that they actually work (Roland, 1986).

Some general practitioners have access to a physiotherapist, and some may provide educational material to help patients to look after their own backs. Access to such resources may reduce the sense to nihilism with which the general practitioner faces his patient, but there is little evidence that they help. Indeed in the only randomised controlled trial of physiotherapy and education for acute back pain in primary care, patients allocated to physiotherapy (isometric abdominal exercises) and education (tape–slide presentation and leaflet) appeared to fare slightly worse than patients receiving no attention at all (Gilbert *et al.*, 1983).

This result contrasts with the use of educational methods in specialist clinics and in industry, where 'back-schools' are becoming increasingly popular, with some evidence that they may be effective (Bergquist-Ullman & Larsson, 1977; Klaber Moffatt *et al.*, 1986). The backschool approach is probably not appropriate in general practice, partly because such resources are not widely available, and partly because many patients will get better spontaneously within a few days. However, it may be valuable for the general practitioner to give general advice about the prevention and self-care of back pain. It is difficult to give such advice verbally in a consultation because of shortage of time and because patients are only able to retain limited amounts of information in the course of one consultation. It may be, therefore, that such information would be provided more effectively in the form of an educational booklet.

The study described in this chapter is a randomised controlled trial of an educational booklet for patients presenting with back pain in primary care. The hypotheses tested were that, when compared to a control group, patients receiving the booklet would:

(1) consult their doctor less frequently with back pain over the following year;

(2) have less sickness absence due to back pain in the following year;

(3) be referred to hospital less frequently;

(4) have improved knowledge of back problems.

6.2 **Method**

The sample consisted of all patients presenting to five British general practices with a complaint of low back pain between September 1985 and September 1986. Back pain had to be the main reason for the consultation, but all patients with back pain, whether acute or chronic, were included. Patients were included if they were between 16 and 64 years old. The practices were group practices, each with between four and seven general practitioners, and they were situated in Cambridge and in London.

Low back pain was defined as pain in an area bounded by the lowest palpable ribs, the buttock creases, and the posterior axillary lines. Certain patients were excluded from the study. These included pregnant patients, patients with flu-like illnesses and patients known to be illiterate. In addition, patients who moved away from the practice during the study year were excluded so that the period of follow-up would be the same for all patients in the study.

Patients were randomised into two groups according to their day of birth. Patients whose day of birth was an odd number (e.g. 7 August 1952) formed the intervention group and were given the booklet, while those whose day of birth was an even number (e.g. 8 August 1952) formed the control group. This method of randomisation can be used as births are randomly distributed on odd and even days of the year, and it has the advantage of permitting randomisation without disruption of the consultation. Randomisation was therefore made by the doctor at the initial consultation.

Information was extracted from the patients' medical records 1 year after entry into the study. This included the number of consultatons for back pain recorded in the 2 years prior to entry into the study and consultations for back pain during the 1-year study period. Information about consultations in the first few weeks of the study year was collected separately from that in the later part of the year, as it was thought that a high proportion of consultations in the initial period would be doctor-initiated or related to certification and might therefore not be affected by the booklet. In addition to information on consultations, the amount of certified sickness absence for back pain during the study period was recorded. In Great Britain a doctor's certificate is generally required for more than 1 week's absence from work due to illness. A referral to hospital was recorded if there was a copy of the referral letter or a reply from a hospital department in the medical records.

A questionnaire was sent by post to patients 1 year after they entered the study. The questionnaire was designed to test knowledge about back pain and included 15 questions which could have been answered on the basis of information contained in the booklet. These questions all required the response 'Yes' or 'No' to statements in the form: 'Knees should be bent when lifting', or, 'Tummy muscles help support your back'. Questions were also asked concerning the patients' perceived general health, how much time they had had off work because of back problems during the preceding year, and age leaving full-time education. Patients in the booklet group were asked additional questions about the acceptability of the booklet.

6.3 **Results**

1096 patients were entered into the study. Of these, 114 moved away from the practice with which they were registered during the study year, 31 patients were found to have been entered into the study incorrectly, and the notes of 15 patients could not be found. Data on 936 patients were therefore available for analysis: booklet group 483 (51.6%); control group 453 (48.4%). The mean age of the sample at entry into the study was 38 years.

At the end of the study year 83% of patients returned the questionnaire. Of patients in the booklet group who returned their questionnaire, 94% said that they had read the *Back Book*: 84% said that they found it useful and 68% said they still had their copy. At the time of filling in the questionnaire, which was 1 year after they had received it 58% of patients said that they could still find the booklet.

As anticipated, the effect of the booklet on consulting behaviour varied in different parts of the study year. There was no significant effect of the booklet on consultations in the first 2 weeks after entry to the study. However, excluding the first 2 weeks of the study, there was a significant reduction (Table 6.1) in the proportion of patients in the booklet group who consulted with back pain in the rest of the study year (35.6% of patients in the booklet group compared to 42.2% of patients in the control group; $p < 0.05$). This effect was particularly marked in patients who had no consultations for back pain recorded in the 2 years prior to entry into the study (Table 6.2) and in patients who had left full-time education after the age of 20 (Table 6.3). There were no significant effects of the booklet on certified absence from work due to back pain.

Comparing the booklet group to the control group, there were reductions in the proportion of patients referred to physiotherapy, referred to hospital, admitted to hospital, and undergoing laminectomy (Table 6.4). These differences reached statistical significance at the 10% level for combined referrals to hospital and physiotherapy, and for laminectomies.

When patients' knowledge about back pain was tested in the question-

Table 6.1 Number of patients consulting with back pain (excluding first 2 weeks of study period)

	Number of patients who did not consult with back pain	*Number of patients with one or more back pain consultations*	*Total number of patients*
Booklet	311 (64.4%)	172 (35.6%)	483 (100%)
Control	262 (57.8%)	191 (42.2%)	453 (100%)

$\chi^2_1 = 4.2$; $p < 0.05$.

Table 6.2 Effect of booklet on number of patients consulting GP with back pain, controlling for past history of consultations with GP for back pain

	Number of patients (%) consulting with back pain during study year (excluding first 2 weeks)	
	Booklet group	*Control group*
No consultations for back pain in previous 2 years	88 (28.8%)	108 (36.4%)
One or more consultations for back pain in previous 2 years	84 (47.5%)	82 (52.2%)

naire sent 1 year after entry into the study, patients in the booklet group had significantly higher scores than patients in the control group. The median knowledge score in the booklet group was 12, compared to 11 in the control group (Mann-Whitney test: $z = 4.1$, $p < 0.001$). The difference in knowledge scores between the groups was mainly due to the higher proportion of patients in the booklet group with a score of 12 or more out of a maximum possible score of 15 (53% of the booklet group compared with 41% of the control group).

6.4 **Discussion**

The purpose of the booklet written for this study was to provide information about back pain in a way that would be acceptable both to general practitioners and to patients, and to encourage patients to look after their own episodes of back pain without recourse to medical advice. The outcome measures used were designed to measure changes in both knowledge and behaviour.

No formal analysis was carried out of the acceptability of the booklet

Table 6.3 Effect of booklet on number of patients consulting GP with back pain, controlling for educational status

	Number of patients (%) consulting with back pain during study year (excluding first 2 weeks)	
Age left full-time education	*Booklet group*	*Control group*
15–16 yrs	90 (38.6%)	108 (41.9%)
12–20 yrs	20 (33.9%)	18 (36%)
21–25 yrs	6 (18.2%)	11 (40.7%)

Table 6.4 Effect of the booklet on referral to hospital and physiotherapy

	Booklet group	*Control group*
Referred to physiotherapy	50 (10.4%)	61 (13.5%)
Referred to hospital	46 (9.5%)	51 (11.3%)
Referred to hospital or physiotherapy	96 (19.9%)*	112 (24.7%)
Admitted to hospital	11 (2.3%)	19 (4.2%)
Laminectomy	2 (0.4%)*	8 (1.8%)

* Difference significant at the 10% level.

to the general practitioners in the study, but comments were almost universally favourable. Doctors often feel that they have little to offer patients with back pain. When talking about the *Back Book*, one doctor commented, 'You actually felt you were doing something useful'. Others commented that it was easier and sometimes quicker to end the consultation if the patient was in the booklet group as time spent giving advice to the patient could be restricted – another comment from a participating doctor was, 'With the booklet, you didn't have to turn on the record all over again.'

The booklet appeared to be very acceptable to patients, as well over three quarters of patients claimed to have found it useful and two thirds still had their booklet 1 year after they had received it. The questionnaire was sent with an accompanying letter from the patient's own doctor, so some patients may have been over-complimentary about the booklet. Nevertheless patient acceptability appeared very high and, of many additional comments written on the questionnaire by patients, only one was directly critical of the booklet.

It was remarkable that the booklet was retained for a year by such a high proportion of patients. Patients clearly valued a booklet given to them by their doctor when they consulted with back pain.

Receipt of the *Back Book* was associated with significant changes in both knowledge and behaviour. When consultations with the GP for back pain were analysed, the booklet had a different effect in different parts of the study year. In the first 2 weeks after receiving the booklet, the booklet had no significant effect on consultations for back pain. However, once the first 2 weeks of the study year were excluded, receipt of the booklet was associated with a reduction in the proportion of patients consulting with back pain, an effect which was maintained throughout the remainder of the study year.

There are a number of possible explanations for the booklet having different effects in different parts of the study. In the first 2 weeks after entry to the study, some patients may have been asked by the doctor to return in order, for example, to assess their progress or the effect of a treatment. Consultations later in the study year will for many patients have been related to a separate episode of back pain. The decision about whether to consult for a new episode of pain rested to a greater extent with the patient, and it was at these times that the booklet had a greater effect on consulting behaviour.

The booklet was particularly effective in reducing the proportion of patients consulting in two groups of patients. These were patients who had not consulted with back pain in the 2 years prior to entry into the study and patients with higher education. Patients with a previous history of back pain may either already have known what there was to be learned from the booklet or already have established a pattern of consulting when they had back pain in order, for example, to get a medical certificate. The greater effect of the booklet in patients with higher education could not be explained on the basis of increased knowledge scores in this group. Perhaps these patients were more able than the rest of the study population to act on the implicit message in the book that back pain can often be managed without recourse to the general practitioner.

The booklet had no effect on absence from work due to back pain. However, there were fewer referrals to physiotherapy and hospital, fewer admissions, and fewer laminectomies in the booklet group. Some of these differences almost achieved statistical significance despite the small number of patients referred and admitted to hospital. There are a number of ways in which the booklet could have affected referral and admission rates. Reassurance about the natural history of back pain coupled with clear instructions on pain management may make patients less demanding of their general practitioners. General practitioners know that there is often little benefit from a hospital or physiotherapy referral and such referrals are often made under pressure from the patient. Information contained within the booklet could have reduced the demands of some patients that 'something must be done'. Equally, except in emergency situations, a decision about laminectomy is often influenced by pressure from the patient. The long-term outlook of conservative management of prolapsed discs is good, but patients are often unwilling to accept slow natural resolution of problems. The information in the booklet could have enhanced patients' perception of back pain as a symptom which they were able to manage without professional help.

In the case of back pain, it is very uncommon for episodes of back pain presenting to general practitioners to be caused by serious or life-threatening disease. It is therefore appropriate to use educational material to encourage patients to learn more about back problems and to look after themselves during episodes of pain. In these respects, the booklet written for this study was modestly successful and would encourage the view that the provision of educational material on back pain is of value and may encourage appropriate health seeking behaviour. In addition, the provision of an educational booklet was a method of providing information which was appreciated by both patients and doctors.

Acknowledgements

This study received financial support from the East Anglian Regional Health Authority and the Health Education Council.

References

Barton, J. E., Haigh, R. O., Marsland, D. W. & Temple, T. E. (1976). Low back pain in the primary care setting, *Journal of Family Practice*, **3**, 363–6.

Bergquist-Ullman, M. & Larsson, U. (1977). Acute low back pain in industry, *Acta Orthopaedica Scandanavica*, Suppl. **170**, 1–117.

Deyo, R. A. (1983). Conservative therapy for low back pain. Distinguishing useful from useless therapy, *Journal of the American Medical Association*, **250**, 1057–62.

Deyo, R. A., Diehl, A. K. & Rosenthal, M. (1986). How many days of bed rest for acute low back pain? A randomised controlled trial, *New England Journal of Medicine*, **315**, 1064–70.

Dunnell, K. & Cartwright, A. (1972). *Medicine Takers, Prescribers and Hoarders*. Routledge and Kegan Paul, London.

Gilbert, J. R., Taylor, D. W., Hildebrand, A. *et al.* (1985). Clinical trial of common treatments for low back pain in family practice, *British Medical Journal*, **291**, 791–5.

Klaber Moffatt, J. A., Chase, S. M., Portek, I. & Ennis, J. (1986). A controlled prospective study to evaluate the effectiveness of a back school in the relief of chronic low back pain, *Spine*, **11**, 120–22.

Morrell, D. C. (1972). Symptom interpretation in general practice, *Journal of the Royal College of General Practitioners*, **22**, 297–309.

Morrell, D. C. & Wale, C. J. (1976). Symptoms perceived and recorded by patients, *Journal of the Royal College of General Practitioners*, **280**, 769–71.

Roland, M. O. (1986). A critical review of the pain–spasm–pain cycle in spinal disorders, *Clinical Biomechanics*, **1**, 102–9.

Wiesel, S. W., Cuckler, J. M., Deluca, F. *et al.* (1980). Acute low back pain: an objective analysis of conservative treatment, *Spine*, **5**, 324–30.

Discussion

Clarke (Bath): One of the problems we found with booklets is educational attainment. In particular we as professionals often put things into books which we think important but which patients think entirely irrevelant and we often miss out things that patients feel are important but we don't. How much actual field testing of your booklet did you do to arrive at the final version you have presented?

Roland: We tried to write it with no words greater than three syllables but we did look at the effect of educational level on response to the booklet which in fact was quite interesting. As you might expect the score of knowledge about back pain was greater in patients who had greater educational achievements but when we looked at the effect on consultations this effect was particularly marked on patients with higher education but was independent of their knowledge scores. So we suspect that patients with higher education don't perhaps have greater knowledge about back pain but they perhaps have greater capacity to respond to this sort of educational message which in essence says, 'You can look after your own back pain.'

Maddocks (Birmingham): Did you select who should have the booklet in fact? The reason I ask this is that I find there are very generally two types of back patient. There is the type who responds to the extension exercises and the type who responds to flexion exercises. Clearly if you were going to have a booklet like that it would not be suitable for every type of patient.

Roland: Indeed there was a problem in deciding what exercises to put into the book. We chose lumbar isometric flexion exercises rather than extension exercises because of the evidence that probably they don't do any patients any harm, whereas I think there is some evidence that some patients may be harmed by doing extension exercises. We have no information whether the patients did any of the exercises or not.

Fairbank (Birmingham): I think you have quite a well-educated population in Cambridge but in Birmingham the IQ is lower. I believe the consultation rate does vary quite a lot for all conditions in terms of educational achievement and maybe you are having an impact on more educated people.

Roland: The study was conducted in two practices in Cambridge and three practices in South London. All the South London practices were fairly strongly working-class though in fact we were surprised what a small percentage of our Cambridge patients had higher education and in fact the differences between the London and the Cambridge practices were not significant. The effects that we demonstrated in the booklet were independent of whether the patient came from Cambridge or London, so it might work in Birmingham.

Jenner (Cambridge): Do you have any idea which bit of the book the patients found most important and the most influential?

Roland: No. We didn't ask them that.

7 *M. D. Chard, B. Silverman, J. R. Jenner and S. Hirst*

The in-patient rehabilitation of chronic back pain patients – a retrospective review of an intensive treatment programme

7.1 Introduction

The value of intensive rehabilitation in the treatment of chronic low back pain remains controversial. The relative merits of exercises, education and the more recently developed concept of the 'backschool' are reviewed in Chapters 2 and 3. Despite these and other therapeutic measures, such as manipulation, local injections, traction, electrical therapy, surgery and corsetry, there is a group of patients who remain chronically disabled by their low back pain. This group is often referred to in the American literature as the 'low back losers' (Mayer, 1983).

7.2 The diagnosis of chronic back pain

The cause of persistent low back pain is frequently difficult to establish. A careful history and examination together with plain X-rays, a blood count, an ESR and a biochemical screen will usually exclude any sinister underlying pathology such as metabolic bone disease. A bone scan may be helpful in revealing secondary bone metastases and tissue typing may prove helpful in identifying patients suffering from previously undiagnosed ankylosing spondylitis. A radiculogram will show any mechanical cause for the pain which would be amenable to surgery. Finally further investigations such as computerised tomography scanning (CT) or magnetic resonance imaging (MRI) are carried out. Often these reveal only minor abnormalities of the lumbar discs or apophyseal joints which are probably of little clinical significance. A frequent finding is evidence of fibrosis around the nerve root especially in the post-surgical patient. Jayson (1987) has postulated that patients with chronic low back pain have abnormalities of fibrinolysis resulting in profuse or abnormal fibrous tissue being laid down around the nerve root which may be the cause of the chronic pain, but this theory remains controversial. Other possibilities suggested as the cause of the persistent pain are that it is coming from structures in the spine which cannot be clearly visualised, such as the spinal ligaments, or that the pain may be reflexly perpetuated in an ill-understood way. However an accurate diagnosis of the pain source is all too often impossible. Despairing of a diagnosis and having exhausted all forms of out-patient treatment, the therapeutically destitute doctor may finally recommend a period of intensive in-patient rehabilitation. These programmes have been available for many years but have rarely been subjected to critical analysis.

7.3 **Early in-patient rehabilitation**

In 1825, Jacques Malthieu Delpech, a French surgeon, founded an orthopaedic institute in Montpellier for the treatment of spinal deformities due to non-tuberculous conditions. The institute was palatial, covering 3½ acres, and included an enclosed gymnasium (Figure 7.1). Treatment placed considerable emphasis on exercise consisting primarily of balancing and climbing (Figure 7.2). Patients remained as residents in the Institute for 1 to 2 years. Unfortunately Delpech was assassinated by a deranged patient (whose hydrocoele he had treated) before he could publish his results, so we have no records of the outcome (Delpech, 1828; Peltier, 1983). In England back rehabilitation developed more slowly. A number of rehabilitation units were opened in the early 1950s and an inpatient rehabilitation programme for the treatment of back pain was well established by 1962 in Garston Manor (Mattingly, 1971).

7.4 **Assessment of in-patient rehabilitation**

The earliest studies of in-patient rehabilitation were performed in America. Gottlieb *et al.* (1982) have developed and reported on a comprehensive in-patient rehabilitation programme. Their patients were treated with a wide variety of methods including bio-feedback to improve relaxation, physical therapy, back education, psychological counselling, vocational rehabilitation and a self-regulated reduction in medication. They studied 78 patients with chronic low back pain, only 8% of whom were employed on entry to the programme: 68% of the patients had undergone at least one surgical operation and they had been disabled for an average of 5 years, with 64% being involved in litigation. Follow-up at 6 months and 1 year showed an encouraging 42 and 44%, respectively, were working. Patients who stayed in the programme for 4 weeks or more also did better than those who undertook a short period of treatment. These findings are encouraging but were both uncontrolled and retrospective.

More recently Aberg (1984), working in Sweden, conducted a pro-

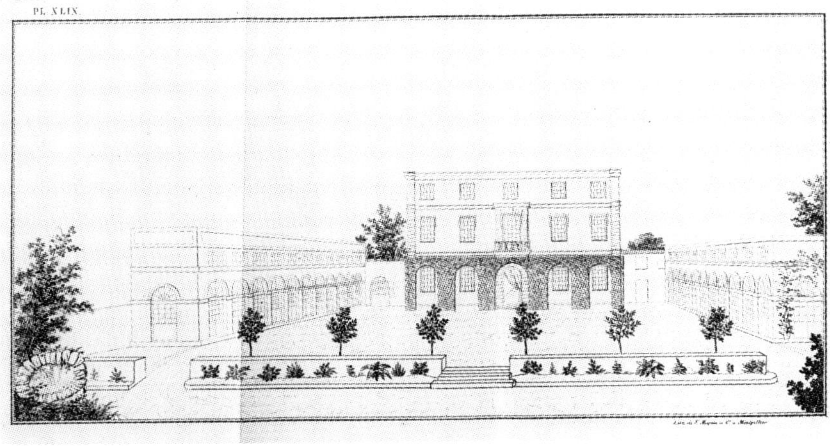

Fig 7.1 The Orthopaedic Institute in Montpellier

spective randomised controlled trial of a 6-week intensive in-patient rehabilitation programme for patients with chronic low back pain *versus* a control group who were patients on the waiting list. All his patients had been off work for at least 1 year and the majority were blue-collar workers. No mention is made of previous surgery. His findings were disappointing. Despite large groups, 164 treated and 189 control patients, the only positive finding at 4 months was that the treated group was earning more. At a year the only difference in the two groups was that the treated group had a more positive attitude to their back. This study does, however, suffer from being conducted as a questionnaire survey with a high level of non-responders (55 in the treated and 23 in the control group), although this is said by the author not to affect the conclusions.

No controlled studies have been performed in Britain, but a prospective study of 101 patients with chronic back pain undergoing an intensive rehabilitation programme using a multidisciplinary approach has recently been reported from the Royal National Orthopaedic Hospital (Wynn Parry & Girgis, 1988): 72% of patients had received surgery; the average duration of symptoms was 10 years; 58% of the patients improved and were living useful and fulfilling lives at a 2-year follow-up. They found that transcutaneous nerve stimulation and exercises were the two most beneficial items in their programme. Patients considered to have 'non-organic' symptoms and signs were also helped by this programme.

7.4.1 *Patient selection*

One of the major problems with all studies of back pain rehabilitation, including Aberg's controlled study, is the problem of selecting patients

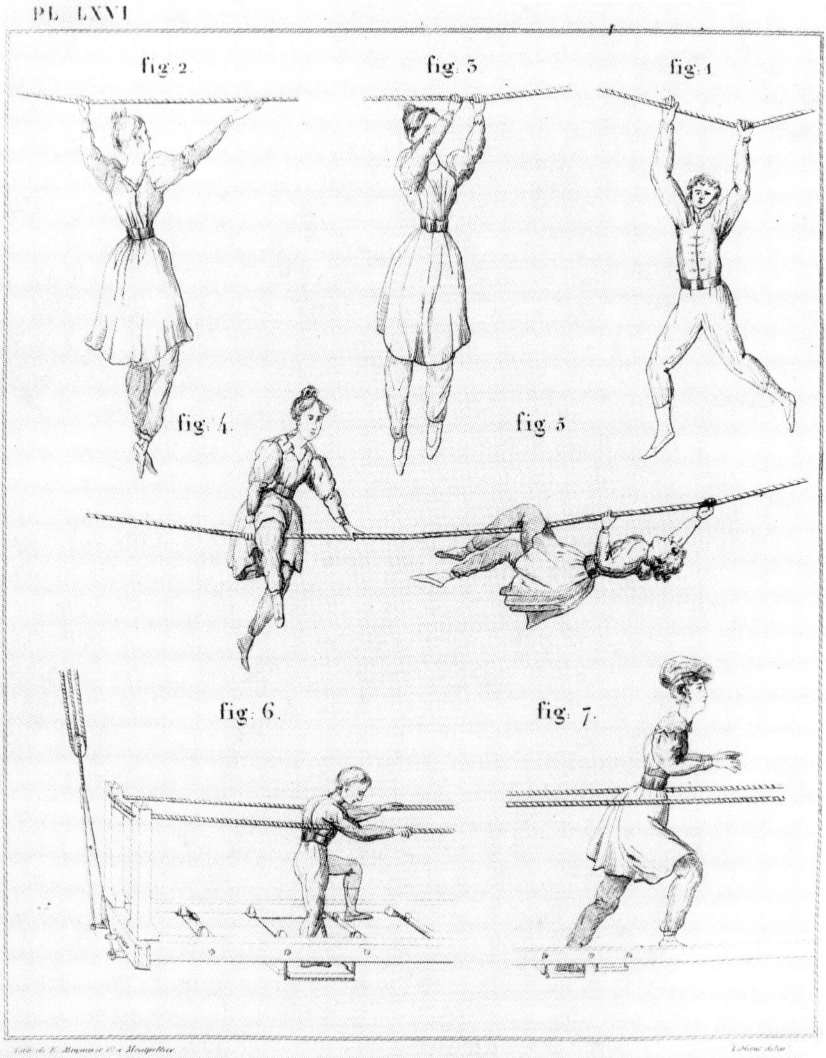

Fig 7.2 Balancing and climbing exercises

likely to benefit from such programmes. As mentioned previously, it is usually not possible to make an accurate diagnosis as to the cause of pain so other methods of selection must be sought. Sandstrom (1986) analysed the results of 52 patients who underwent a rehabilitation programme in Goteborg and found that a high analgesic intake, a negative attitude and widespread pain prior to rehabilitation indicated a bad prognosis. Interestingly, the length of sickness absence prior to rehabilitation only seemed to indicate a bad prognosis in patients in an older age group (over 41 years). None of these patients had undergone spinal surgery.

Cairns *et al.* (1984), working in California, compared a group undergoing in-patient rehabilitation at Rancho Los Amigos Hospital with a group undergoing out-patient treatment at the Downey Community Hospital. Direct comparisons between these groups was not possible as the in-patient group was older, had a longer duration of symptoms, and had a higher incidence of post-surgical patients. They used the results to develop a complex formula combining a number of features including the patient's age, sex, time off work, length of symptoms and the Minnesota Multiphasic Personality Inventory (MMPI). The results suggested that it was possible to select those who were likely to return to work in approximately 70% of patients (using different formulae for in-patients and out-patients). The authors felt that predictive formulae could possibly be developed further.

7.4.2 *Outcome measures*

Studies of rehabilitation also suffer from difficulties in establishing successful outcome. Return to work is used as the gold standard but is often not appropriate (e.g. for housewives) and some patients may improve considerably with treatment but not obtain re-employment, particularly in areas of high unemployment. McArthur *et al.* (1987) have looked at a variety of outcome measures in the short-term follow-up of 702 patients and long-term follow-up of 210 of these patients, all of whom underwent an intensive multidisciplinary rehabilitation programme of at least 4 weeks duration. The programme was dominated by married, middle-aged, middle-class Caucasians suffering from chronic low back pain of more than 4 years duration. A third had undergone previous surgery and only 6% were thought to be employable on admission. Visual analogue measurements were made of pain. Function was measured on a 4-point scale for exertion measures (walking, strength, flexibility) and non-exertion measures (sitting tolerance, muscle tension). Psychological assessments (pain behaviour, assertiveness, comprehension of programme goals) were also measured on a 4-point scale as well as performing the MMPI and the Wechsler Adult Intelligence Scale.

They found that although improvements were found in response to treatment the outcome measures changed independently of each other, except for the two psychological profiles which improved together.

The assessments in this and other studies have been made by self-reported questionnaire. The inadequacy of this form of assessment alone was considered by Trief (1983) who suggested that a tripartite model of outcome, including self-reports, physical measures and objective indices of success (return to work or goal achievement), was needed to monitor the effectiveness of a treatment programme.

With the acceptance that medical intervention is often unhelpful in patients with chronic back pain, much interest has developed in understanding and treating the psychological aspects of pain and indeed these form a large part of most American programmes, usually being the aspects that are most closely measured and reported. In recent years, however, an alternative approach has developed in at least one centre, the so-called 'Dallas programme'.

The method used by Mayer *et al.* (1985) is a physical training approach to treatment aiming to increase back strength and endurance with little direct attention to pain. In doing this they have developed a number of tests to assess spine mobility, trunk strength, endurance, co-ordination and dynamic lifting capacity. Associated with improvement in these tests, a reduction in pain was achieved with an 82% return to work in a previously 92% unemployed group of 66 patients. These objective tests would appear encouraging; objective and reproducible methods of assessment that correlate with improvement in function are vital if in-patient rehabilitation programmes are to be properly assessed. Such programmes are both time-consuming and expensive and the data supporting their efficacy sparse. There seems little doubt, however, that some individuals, even a few with seemingly intractable problems, can be helped by such treatments. The difficulties with patient selection continue to make worthwhile trials difficult to construct; if only a small percentage of those selected actually benefit, a controlled study will have to be large to show the effect.

7.5 The present study and its aims

A 3- to 4-week in-patient rehabilitation programme for chronic low back sufferers has been in operation for almost 10 years at the Rehabilitation Unit at Addenbrookes Hospital, Cambridge. It differs from other programmes in that the patients are referred through two main channels. The neurosurgeons and orthopaedic surgeons refer a post-surgical group who have failed to mobilise satisfactorily after surgery, while the rheumatologists and general practitioners refer a mainly non-surgical group who have failed to respond to conventional out-patient measures and are not candidates for surgery. Both of these groups can be divided into patients with either a relatively short history (less than 1 year) or those with a more chronic problem (greater than 1 year). With such relatively clear-cut groups of patients, it was felt that it would be useful to perform a retrospective study of patients entering the programme in order to establish if any one of these groups fared better or worse than another – in the hope that this may improve the selection of patients for the programme in the future.

7.5.1 *Patients and methods*

The patients selected for inclusion in the in-patient treatment programme suffer with chronic low back pain, with or without associated leg pain. Symptoms have been present for more than 6 months unresponsive to out-patient conservative therapy or have failed to mobilise satisfactorily after lumbar surgery, usually discectomy.

They are medically assessed prior to inclusion into the programme in order to exclude sinister underlying pathology. Relevant further investigations are carried out such as CT scanning, bone scans, or electromyography.

All those selected are made fully aware of the nature of the programme that they are offered. Patients with compensation claims outstanding are not excluded. Most have conditions related to disc disease or non-specific mechanical and soft-tissue low back pain. A few patients with ankylosing spondylitis requiring very active treatment are included.

7.5.2 *The rehabilitation unit*

Admission is undertaken in groups of six into the 27-bed general Rehabilitation Unit. This enables group therapy and support in a general rehabilitation environment. It also helps patients to change their perspective of their problems in the light of the disabled people around them. Admitting patients helps to develop the group feeling and a suitable therapeutic milieu. It stops some patients having to travel long distances for daily treatment and also removes patients from their home where unidentified physical and psychological factors could all potentially aggravate their pain. The rehabilitation team consists of rheumatologists, nurses, physiotherapists and occupational therapists.

7.5.3 *The philosophy of the programme*

The programme does not set out to 'cure' the patient's back pain problem but rather the aim is to improve function with a reduction in pain. The patient is told that the philosophy behind the treatment is to 'do more for less pain'. Improvement in function of the spine and body in general is the prime goal, suppressing pain as needed. It is then envisaged that this improved function will subsequently reduce the pain. Patients are aware that success is not guaranteed.

7.5.4 *Assessment*

In addition to the out-patient pre-admission assessment, the patients are reassessed medically on entry to the programme as are their X-rays and investigations to ensure nothing specifically treatable has been missed. The

Table 7.1 Assessments undertaken on chronic back pain patients

Pain (visual analogue)	Lumbar movement (fingertips to floor)
Posture	Physical tolerance (standing, sitting, walking, driving)
Gait	Functional assessment
Neurological	
Straight leg raise (goniometer)	

majority will have had a CT scan of the lumbar spine or a radiculogram. They are then extensively assessed by the therapist staff (Table 7.1). The functional assessment includes self-care and daily living activities plus ability to undertake workshop tasks and, where relevant, those related to occupation; these activities are scored for performance. A note is made of the pre-admission activities level as well as of the patient's perceived affect, social factors and goals. Suitable individual aims are identified.

7.5.5 *The treatment programme*

Although essentially carried out by physiotherapists and occupational therapists, the treatment programme has additional input and reinforcement from the unit's medical and nursing staff. The emphasis of the programme is on physical approaches to treatment. There is no specific clinical psychologist input but all staff encourage positive attitudes and suppress negative ones.

The therapists work together to provide an integrated programme with overlaps to reinforce particular aspects especially education. There is a full multifaceted treatment regime each weekday with rest and personal exercises at weekends (Table 7.2).

Treatment days consist of an initial warm-up period and then the day is split into four 1-hour sessions. Hydrotherapy is a constant element and the

Table 7.2 Facets of the treatment programme

Warm-up exercises	Education (anatomy and back care)
Hydrotherapy	ADL (advice and equipment)
Pain relief (e.g. TENS)	Work preparation
Mobilisations	Activities to increase physical tolerance
Relaxation	Ergonomics
Exercises (isometric and isotonic)	Strengthening (workshop activities)

rest of the time is spent undertaking either physiotherapy or occupational therapy. Where appropriate, group sessions, such as back education, relaxation classes, anatomy and back-care, are undertaken.

The time and content of other parts of the treatment programme are individually tailored to the patient's particular problems. The exercises used are a combination of isometric flexion and the McKenzie extension type. All are attempted initially and pain-inducing exercises are excluded in that particular patient, although progressing to more difficult exercises is often possible during the treatment period. Persistent pain and stiffness is treated individually with a variety of techniques, including Maitland Mobilisation, Transcutaneous Nerve Stimulation (TENS) and analgesia. Patients are encouraged to keep analgesic intake to a minimum.

As well as the activities undertaken in the occupational therapy department, suitable gadgets, appliances and chairs can be assessed and arranged there. Where necessary vocational guidance is given and liaison undertaken with the Disablement Resettlement Officer and Manpower Services Commission.

7.5.6 *Reassessment and follow-up*

At the end of the 3-week course patients are reassessed by the same therapists on the parameters used on admission plus a medical review. An appropriate change of at least 10% in a particular parameter is generally considered significant. More importantly, the patient's reduction in pain and attainment of their individual goals is considered.

If there has been no benefit at the end of treatment the patient is considered for any further investigation or other avenues of treatment such as attendance at the pain clinic or the use of a rigid polythene jacket. Occasionally a patient may be encouraged to stay for a further week of therapy.

Patients having at least some benefit have subsequently been followed until full domestic activities or return to work have been achieved and reviewed again as necessary. Others having lesser benefit have been followed until stable or until other treatment has been given as indicated above.

7.6 **Results**

The 78 patients treated during the course of 1 year have been separated into the four groups outlined above, based on chronicity and the presence or absence of previous lumbar surgery (Table 7.3). Nearly three quarters of the patients had had pain for more than 1 year with over 45% having had previous lumbar surgery.

A profile of the patients in each group in terms of age, sex and percentage with abnormal neurological signs is given in Table 7.4.

Table 7.3 Definition of patient groups

Group	*No. of patients*	*% of total*
I: pain for < 1 year	7	9
II: pain persisting for < 1 year and lumbar surgery	15	19
III: pain for > 1 year	36	46
IV: pain persisting longer than 1 year and lumbar surgery	20	26
Total	78	100

The percentage of patients in each group who showed improvement in four of the parameters assessed at the beginning and end of the 3-week programme is shown in Figure 7.3. The best results were seen in groups I and II, with both objective and subjective measurements, all improving in over 80% of these patients who had had symptoms for less than 1 year. No differences in any of the measured parameters were observed between these two groups of non-surgical and surgical patients although it must be remembered that the numbers of patients (7 and 15, respectively) were small. As might be expected groups III and IV, with symptoms for longer than 1 year, fared less well. Pain improved in only 50% of the non-surgical and 30% of the surgical group. Surprisingly, function improved in just over 60% of patients in both groups despite the relatively poor relief of pain in the chronic post-surgical group.

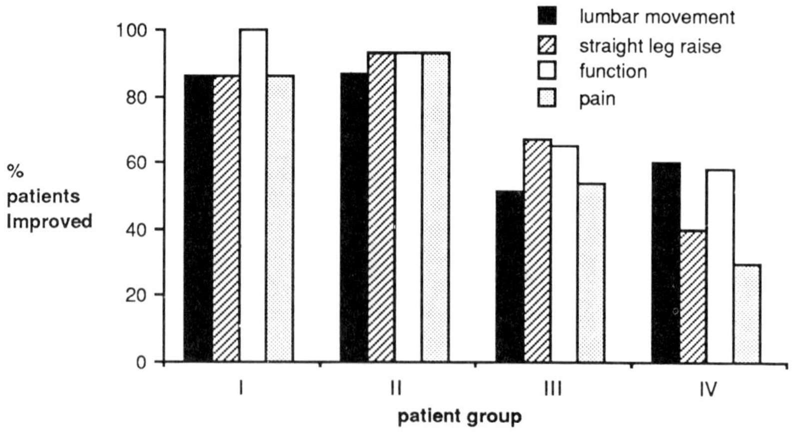

Fig 7.3 Assessment at end of 3-week programme

Table 7.4 Profile of patients in each group

Group	*M*	*F*	*Mean age*	*Age range*	*No. with neurological signs (%)*
I	5	2	39	20–57	3(48)
II	12	3	35	19–67	12(80)
III	17	19	37	22–55	10(28)
IV	7	13	40	24–55	10(50)
Total	41	37	38	19–67	35(45)

Patients were followed up after the programme for a variable period ranging from 6 weeks to over 1 year. No detailed assessment was made at these visits but subjective improvement in pain and ability to return to work or household duties was recorded. The percentage of patients showing improvement and their work status at the final out-patient visit is shown (Figure 7.4). Both groups I and II showed that improvement in pain had been maintained in over 80% of patients. A large proportion of patients had been working prior to their admission but again this was improved in both groups.

In both groups III and IV, the percentage of patients reporting improvement in pain at final follow-up had increased slightly and in both groups the percentage of patients working at follow-up compared with their pre-admission status had also improved. This was most marked in the post-

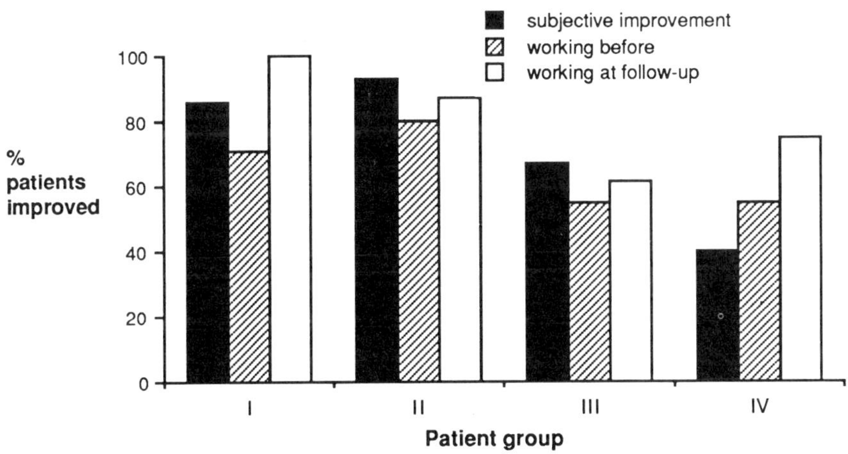

Fig 7.4 Benefit to the patient – subjective improvement, employment status before in-patient treatment and at follow-up

surgical group, where 20% of patients previously unemployed returned to work. Unfortunately this study does not enable any estimate of late improvement or relapse although the re-referral rate was low suggesting that the long-term success was high.

7.7 **Discussion**

Patients with chronic back pain form a heterogeneous group in terms of underlying pathology and the psychological interaction with their pain, which are both often poorly understood. Therefore, when assessing the response to a treatment in a cohort of patients, it may be more appropriate to try to group them rather than considering them as a whole. In this study patients have been grouped in terms of their chronicity (less than or more than 1 year) and previous lumbar surgery.

Perhaps not surprisingly, it was those patients with a shorter history, with or without surgery, who made the most dramatic response to the treatment. It is the presence of these two groups of relatively acute patients entered into the treatment programme that partly distinguishes this study from those previously described. A high rate of spontaneous improvement can be expected in such patients but the patients admitted to the programme were complaining of persistent problems despite their previous treatment. The vast majority were improved within 3 weeks and, even if the long-term spontaneous outcome was favourable, it would appear likely that recovery has been speeded up in a group of patients who were potentially heading for more chronic problems. The two groups (III and IV) of more chronic patients fared less well.

A sizeable group in this study consisted of patients who had not undergone surgery (55%). The proportion of patients in this category was larger than previously described American studies and the only recent British study by Wynn Parry & Girgis (1988). This is likely to reflect the fact that patients with back pain are six times more likely to have surgery in the United States (Mayer, 1983) and also the specialist nature of the Royal National Orthopaedic Hospital patients.

It is interesting that this patient group overall fared no better than those who had had previous surgery and indeed the ultimate outcome in terms of return to work was less good. From the accessible information it is not possible to comment on whether this relates to different underlying pathology or to the psychological factors.

The small number of patients suffering from ankylosing spondylitis included in group III tended to do well and if they were excluded the results for this group as a whole would probably have appeared even worse.

The failed post-surgical group were perhaps less severe than described in other studies (Wynn Parry & Girgis, 1988; Gottlieb *et al.*, 1982) in that just under 50% were working prior to entry into the programme. However Cambridge is an area of high employment and this may not only have influenced the pre-entry employment figure but also the fact that 20% of those previously unemployed achieved employment. This figure however remains encouraging when faced with those who appear to have failed to improve on all conventional forms of treatment.

The majority of patients in all groups appeared to benefit from treatment subjectively, objectively, and with respect to ultimate outcome (employment). Even the group with prolonged problems in spite of previous surgery benefited. The level of response is not greatly different from that achieved by Gottlieb *et al.* (1982). Indeed the response might have been even better if, as suggested by these authors, the course of treatment had been at least 4-weeks long.

The approach to treatment used also differs from most others in that it contains no clinical psychologist input and in many ways more closely resembles the Dallas programme of improved function and fitness through physical methods of exercise. This has been shown to be of benefit by Mayer *et al.* (1986) and a prolonged effect has been confirmed on long-term follow-up, as discussed recently by Mooney (1988). However, it differs from the Dallas approach as more direct pain-relief measures are included in the programme. Despite these differences, improvement in function and return to work was often achieved with no frank reduction in pain, particularly in groups III and IV. This disparity of response agrees with the findings of McArthur *et al.* (1987) and Mooney (1988). Improvement in other clinical measurements such as lumbar movement also did not seem to influence outcome. As suggested by Hall and Iceton (1983), it does not appear that previous lumbar surgery greatly influences the outcome of back rehabilitation programmes. However, there seems little doubt that the more chronic the back problem becomes, the less well the patient responds to such programmes. Although, in a group of patients who appear to have no hope of improving, a small but significant proportion can often be returned to a fulfilling lifestyle.

It is more than 150 years since Delpech started in-patient rehabilitation for chronic back pain and yet we are still far from understanding the underlying mechanisms and how best to manage such patients. In future better assessment of disability using standardised measures such as the Oswestry Disability questionnaire (see Chapters 12 and 13) and a clearer assessment of pain (see Chapter 9) may allow more conclusive results. It is most important that future studies should be both prospective and controlled if claims of efficacy are to be believed. Patients must also be fully assessed when reviewed, not just by questionnaire, and long-term follow-up must also documented. Only with this information can these programmes be satisfactorily assessed.

References

Aberg, J. (1984). Evaluation of an advanced back pain rehabilitation program, *Spine*, **9**, 317–8.

Cairns, D., Mooney, V. & Crane, P. (1984). Spinal pain rehabilitation: inpatient and outpatient treatment results and development of predictors for outcome, *Spine*, **9**, 91–95.

Delpech, J. M. (1828). *De L'orthomorphie*. Atlas, Gabon, Paris.

Gottlieb, H. J., Koller, R. & Alperson, B. L. (1982). Low back pain comprehensive rehabilitation program: a follow-up study, *Archives of Physical Medicine and Rehabilitation*, **63**, 458–61.

Hall, H. & Iceton, J. (1983). Backschools, *Clinical Orthopaedics and Related Research*, **179**, 10–17.

Jayson, M. (1987). Chronic inflammation and fibrosis in back pain syndromes. In: *The Lumbar Spine and Back Pain*, ed. M. Jayson, pp. 411–48. Churchill Livingstone, Edinburgh.

Mattingly, S. (1971). Rehabilitation of registered dock workers at Garston Manor, *Proceedings of the Royal Society. Medical*, **64**, 757–60.

McArthur, D. L., Cohen, M. J., Gottlieb, H. J., Naliboff, B. D. & Schandler, S. L. (1987). Treating chronic low back pain. I. Admissions to initial follow-up and II. Long-term follow-up, *Pain*, **29**, 1–39.

Mayer, T. G. (1983). Rehabilitation of the patient with spinal pain, *Orthopedic Clinics of North America*, **14**, 623–37.

Mayer, T. G., Gatchel, R. J., Kishino, N., Keeley, J., Mayer, H., Capra, P. & Mooney, V. (1986). A prospective short-term study of chronic low back pain patients utilizing novel objective functional measurement, *Pain*, **25**, 53–68.

Mooney, V. (1988). The failed back – an orthopaedic view, *International Disability Studies*, **10**, 32–36.

Peltier, L. F. (1983). The 'Back School' of Delpech in Montpellier, *Clinical Orthopaedics and Related Research*, **179**, 4–9.

Sandstrom, J. (1986). Clinical and social factors in rehabilitation of patients with chronic low back pain, *Scandinavian Journal of Rehabilitation Medicine*, **18**, 35–43.

Trief, P. M. (1983). Chronic back pain: A tripartite model of outcome, *Archives of Physical Medicine and Rehabilitation*, **64**, 53–56.

Wynn Parry, C. B. & Girgis, F. (1988). The assessment and management of the failed back, part II, *International Disability Studies*, **10**, 25–28.

Discussion

Frank (Northwick Park): If you are going to plan a prospective trial with a control group should you have people in hospital for 3 weeks doing something which is non-therapeutic?

Chard: Well that is the question. Do we compare to that or do we compare to a group of out-patients and follow them up and see who improves?

Glover (Swindon): I would suggest a control group using short-wave diathermy as a placebo.

Chard: We thought of comparing our in-patient rehabilitation programme with another treatment group, but it is a question of what we compare it against. For example, an out-patient backschool would be one possibility.

Morrison (Swindon): I really think if you are going to have an in-patient group you cannot compare it with an out-patient one because the two are so totally different. As far as I can see you could perhaps have a different programme within your rehabilitation programme, some having hydrotherapy, some not, some having a planned programme through the day and some doing some standard physiotherapy that would otherwise be done as an out-patient. I think you have got to compare in-patient with in-patient. You have already suggested that the treatment does them good and I think it is unethical to have a treatment group to which you do not give any treatment.

Roland (Cambridge): Mr Morrison is suggesting it is unethical to do a true controlled trial. I think it could be argued that it would be unethical not to do a true controlled trial as there is no method of proving that the treatment works without a controlled trial.

Swannell (Nottingham): I just want some information about the people didn't recover very well after surgery. Did you notice any difference in those patients compared with the others?

Chard: Yes. The group of post-surgical patients who were fairly acute, i.e. referred within a year of their surgery and were not mobilising well, did as well as patients with back pain of less than a year's standing who had not had surgery.

The chronic post-surgery group, i.e. those referred more than one year after surgery because of persisting symptoms, had as good a return to work as the chronic back pain group without surgery. The important point is that even in these groups of chronic 'no hopers' a small but important group can be rehabilitated by our programme and go back to work.

Moffett (Oxford): I agree that you certainly should do a controlled study and since admitting patients is a very expensive form of treatment it is important to look at this aspect of the treatment. Couldn't you have as your control group a similar treatment programme, bringing them in on a daily basis so they have the same programme, but as out-patients rather than in-patients. In that way it would be an awful lot cheaper and I would have thought more logical than admitting two groups of patients.

Chard: But it wouldn't tell us whether or not the intensity of the programme is useful. If both groups did well we would still be uncertain as to whether or not the treatment was as effective as nothing at all.

8 *C. C. Spanswick and C. J. Main*

The role of the anaesthetist in the management of chronic low back pain

8.1 Introduction

The origins of the anaesthetist's involvement in the treatment and management of chronic pain go back only to the late 1950s in the UK but as far back as the late 1940s in the USA (Bonica, 1973). Formal Pain Relief Clinics with their own clinic space and designated sessions are much more recent.

In the USA in Seattle, Bonica developed an interest in the treatment of chronic pain patients due to his experience of such patients in military hospitals in the post-war period. That interest has led, over the years, to the development of a large multidisciplinary clinic, involving a large number of specialists, ranging from neurosurgeons to psychologists. It was he who, with others, founded the International Association for the Study of Pain in 1973 following an International Symposium on Pain in Seattle.

In the UK Swerdlow led the way in 1958 (Swerdlow, 1967) with a clinic conducted very much on an informal basis, seeing and treating patients at the end of surgical lists, but eventually moving on to better things with the use of a room adjacent to theatres. Most of the patients seen had pain due to malignancies although a number of non-cancer patients were also treated. It was not until 1978 that a formal clinic with its own designated out-patient area was set up, allbeit in a Portacabin. The treatment options were largely confined to nerve-blocking techniques, using neurolytic agents in order to produce a more prolonged effect than that achieved with local anaesthetics. Neurolytic techniques proved to be very effective in the management of cancer pain but they were not without their complications. It was evident that there were a number of patients (presumably with non-cancer pain) who were not helped at all. Indeed the patient's general practitioner would often say that 'Nothing helps this patient'. Swerdlow went on to say that in such cases the use of neurolytic agents was best avoided (Swerdlow, 1967).

Today there are very few multidisciplinary clinics in the UK actively involving clinicians of different specialities on the same premises. Most are run single-handed by anaesthetists without the benefit of junior support. The referral pattern varies from clinic to clinic, although nowadays a smaller proportion of the patients are cancer patients and a larger proportion are people with chronic low back pain. In the Pain Relief Centre at Hope Hospital, Salford, chronic low back pain patients account for 45% of new referrals. Most of these have seen at least two different specialist teams, and half of them give a history of pain for more than 10 years. Like patients seen in other clinics, they have been confused by differing opinions from different doctors and consequently have become distressed and sometimes angry. Not infrequently they are labelled 'neurotic' or 'difficult', having failed to respond well to any of their previous treatment. At best, their past treatment has provided only short-term help, at worst it has compounded the clinical picture physically and certainly psychologically. They often show evidence of 'magnified illness behaviour' (Waddell *et al.*, 1984) and are more disabled than one might anticipate from objective physical assessment (Waddell & Main, 1984). This makes it very much more difficult for the doctor to see exactly what clinical problem lies behind the patient's apparent odd presentation and may then lead to either inappropriate physical treatment or an unnecessary psychiatric referral.

It is all too easy to blame the patients, in such circumstances, for insisting that 'something be done'. Doctors, however, must at least share the blame in this situation. They know from their own experience with similar patients that the likelihood of achieving a significant beneficial effect in such patients is very small. It has been shown (Chapman & Brena, 1982) that chronic back pain patients who are fixed in their focus on their pain, and have high levels of pain-related behaviours, respond poorly to physical therapy (in the form of injections), and that physical therapies should include other measures to reduce their helplessness. Continued physical therapy alone will tend to reinforce the patient's chronic consulting behaviour. It will also tend to reinforce the patient's belief that there is a purely physical solution to their problem. Such therapy, however, may not only make little change to their pain but may, in fact, make the patient worse, both physically and psychologically.

What treatment options does the anaesthetist have available? These can be divided into:

Pharmacological intervention
Non-invasive physical methods

Invasive physical procedures
Pain management.

8.2 **Pharmacological intervention**

The drugs that are commonly used in chronic pain relief clinics may be divided into a number of different groups based on their action. These obviously include analgesic preparations, but also include a number of drugs which would not normally be considered analgesics but do appear to have some effect on pain. For ease of discussion they have been divided into standard pharmacological categories.

8.2.1 *Non-narcotics*

Paracetamol is by far the commonest non-narcotic prescribed. It appears not to be addictive although it is well known to cause liver problems (which can be fatal) if taken in overdose. The major problem with paracetamol is its inclusion with weak narcotic drugs in combination preparations. Inadvertent overdose is quite possible if the patient is not made aware that such preparations contain paracetamol. Stronger non-narcotic analgesics such as nefopam are sometimes used. Although nefopam does not appear to be addictive, it is potent and side effects do cause problems in a significant proportion of patients. Its exact mode of action is unknown, but is probably central.

8.2.2 *Narcotics*

Of patients attending the Pain Relief Centre at Salford 60% are taking preparations containing narcotics. Occasionally they are not aware of it. Many patients are certainly not aware of the potential of developing tolerance and addiction. It is interesting to note that a number of doctors are unwilling to prescribe strong narcotic drugs such as morphine for cancer patients (who obviously have a limited life expectancy) but seem to be prepared to prescribe other narcotics for patients with a normal life expectancy for prolonged periods, even when the evidence suggest that they are not producing any therapeutic benefit. There is no evidence to show that prolonged use of narcotic drugs is beneficial in the management of chronic benign pain.

8.2.3 *Non-steroidal anti-inflammatory drugs*

Non-steroidal anti-inflammatory drugs (NSAIDs) are commonly used in painful acute inflammatory conditions. There is evidence to show that they can be of use in the treatment of acute episodes of low back pain (Orava, 1986; Amlie, 1987). Although such drugs do seem to have an analgesic effect, which may be separate from their anti-inflammatory action, their efficacy in the treatment of *chronic* low back pain is equivocal (Hickey, 1982; Videman & Osterman, 1984). Some studies purporting to show benefit from NSAIDs include only short-term follow-up (for 4 to 6 weeks) while other studies show them to be of no greater value than placebo (Berry *et al.*, 1982). The choice of which NSAID to use becomes difficult when evidence of efficacy is either not forthcoming or contradictory (Hurme & Himanen, 1986). The lack of side effects may well be the deciding factor as to which drug to use. Most of these drugs have significant side effects (particularly in the elderly). In addition to the expected gastric irritation, side effects include significant central effects, giving a sense of generally feeling unwell, possible exacerbation of lower bowel disease and significant drug interactions with some antihypertensives (Schwartz, 1981; Wong *et al.*, 1986).

8.2.4 *Antidepressants*

These are used frequently in pain relief clinics, not only for their mood elevating effect but also for their apparent analgesic activity in some patients. Their pain-relieving activity may well be independent of their antidepressant activity, although it is well known that pain tolerance is increased in depressed patients if their mood is elevated (Bond, 1984). There are considerable variations in the diagnostic groupings in different studies thus making interpretation of findings difficult. Pilowsky *et al.* (1982) showed there to be no difference between placebo and amitriptyline, but the group of patients were highly selected, being patients who had pain for which 'no substantial organic cause could be demonstrated'. Ward (1986), however, demonstrated the effectiveness of desipramine and doxepin in patients with chronic low back pain. This effect seems to be most likely to be serotonergic and not related to mood elevation.

It is common practice to use low dose tricyclic antidepressants to enhance the effect of transcutaneous nerve stimulation. In clinical practice this seems to work, and it is currently under investigation in this clinic in a double-blind cross-over study.

8.2.5 *Anti-epileptic agents*

These drugs have been in use for some time for the treatment of shooting and so-called 'lancinating' pain (Swerdlow, 1980, 1981). They appear to be of considerable benefit in neurogenic pain of this type. Carbamazepine has been used for many years in the treatment of trigeminal and glossopharyngeal neuralgia. It does have the disadvantage of producing significant side effects in some patients, particularly the elderly. Sodium valproate is the commonest anti-epileptic used for other pain syndromes in pain relief clinics. It is sometimes used in combination with tricyclic antidepressants, especially in the management of post-herpetic neuralgia (Raftery, 1979).

These drugs are also of use in the managment of root distribution pain (post-laminectomy), particularly where further surgery is inadvisable.

8.3 **Non-invasive physical methods**

The two major non-invasive measures used in pain clinics in the UK are transcutaneous electrical nerve stimulation (TNS or TENS) and acupuncture. Both of these have significant advantages over other methods of pain relief in that they are non-invasive, have little in the way of side effects and, in the long term, are relatively cheap.

8.3.1 *TENS*

Melzack and Wall first described their 'gate theory' of pain control in 1965 (Melzack & Wall, 1965). They suggested that it would be possible to modulate incoming pain signals, transmitted via unmyelinated and small myelinated fibres at relatively slow speeds (C and A delta fibres), by stimulating thicker fibres (A beta fibres) whose transmission speed is much faster. Machines capable of producing transcutaneous stimulation first became clinically available in the early 1970s (Long & Hagfors, 1975). Originally such machines were used to assess patients for suitability for implantation of dorsal column stimulating electrodes. It was discovered that a number of patients benefited significantly from cutaneous stimulation alone, without the necessity to go on to implant electrodes. The settings on the machines (frequency of stimulus and voltage) were entirely empirical. Some of their original data is quite interesting (see Table 8.1).

This confirms the findings of others (Richardson *et al.*, 1981) that TENS works well in organic pain patients but that the long-term response is poor in people who display a considerable amount of abnormal illness behaviour (these may well be classified as 'functional' by other authors). The initial response rate is variable but may be as high as 70% in unselected patients and will reduce to about 40% after 2 months or so, when the placebo effect has worn off in some patients. The fact that TENS works in other pain

Table 8.1 Pain relief with transcutaneous nerve stimulation (chronic low back pain patients)

Patient group	*n*	*Excellent*	*None*
Chronic low back pain	221	32%	17%
Chronic low back pain (without multiple operations)	50	42%	32%
Psychogenic pain	30	3%	97%

Adapted from Long & Hagfors (1975), Table 1.

syndromes is not in doubt (Nathan & Wall, 1974; Gessler & Struppler, 1983) but it also appears that it has a place in the management of some patients with chronic low back pain (Fox & Melzack, 1976; Melzack *et al.*, 1983).

8.3.2 *Acupuncture*

The practice of acupuncture goes back several millennia. The first written descriptions of acupuncture and the philosophy surrounding it are to be found in *The Yellow Emperor's Classic of Internal Medicine*, which was written between the 8th and 5th centuries BC. The first use of acupuncture in Europe was in the 17th century, very much earlier than might have been anticipated.

In his article describing his visit to the People's Republic of China, Bonica recounts that even in China little or nothing had been done in the way of controlled trials of acupuncture (Bonica, 1974). In the West things are little better. Several clinical trials have been done but there are considerable methodological problems. The trials differ in their choice of placebo, some of which may produce quite a potent placebo effect. This makes it more difficult to demonstrate effect greater than placebo. This has been well reviewed by Vincent and Richardson (1986).

It has been shown that acupuncture has a significant effect in the treatment of a variety of clinical syndromes including low back pain (Dowson *et al.*, 1985; MacDonald *et al.*, 1983). Many of the studies, however, only follow up patients for a relatively short period of time and there has yet to be shown a significant long-term beneficial effect. Some studies have shown there to be little or no difference between acupuncture and placebo, especially when interaction between the therapist and the patient is kept to a minimum (Mendleson *et al.*, 1978; Murphy, 1979). On balance it seems there is a significant improvement of pain with acupuncture although this may well be short lived. Acupuncture used for the relief of chronic pain still requires further controlled studies (Richardson & Vincent, 1986).

8.4 **Invasive physical procedures**

Many anaesthetists, perhaps unsurprisingly, have a preference for invasive techniques for the treatment of chronic pain patients. This is largely as a result of their training in the use of regional blocks, spinal and epidural injections for providing good analgesia in the short term for some patients undergoing surgery. This was put to good use in the earlier clinics where the treatment of cancer pain was the major part of their work, and neurolytic agents such as phenol and chlorocresol were used instead of local anaesthetics. The use of such techniques in the management of chronic benign pain, especially chronic low back pain, may well be contraindicated on the basis of already published scientific data (Quebec Task Force,

1987). It has been shown that peripheral nerve damage, of whatever cause, leads to significant changes in the nervous system more centrally, resulting in a loss of inhibitory control of sensory input, thus leading to potentially more pain problems rather than less in the long term (Wall & Devor, 1981). There is, therefore, no logical basis for denervation techniques in the management of chronic pain in patients with a normal life expectancy. Indeed even those who advocate such techniques advise caution. Shealey (1975) in one of his original papers on facet denervation says: 'Furthermore, when the patient is indeed an invalid, the facet denervation procedure alone is quite inadequate to get most patients rehabilitated and a more aggressive approach of physical exercise and psychophysiological rehabilitation is necessary.' It would seem that not only is denervation of limited value in the management of chronic low back pain but that it is contraindicated.

8.4.1 *Facet joint injection*

Mooney and Robertson (1976) have shown facet joint injections to be of considerable benefit, but since the injected volume was up to 5 ml this will have affected other structures as well as the facet joint. Volumes as large as this were either not injected into the joint capsule or the capsule will have been ruptured, thus invalidating the diagnostic accuracy of the technique. In addition they relied on the self-report of pain as the outcome measure, and it has been recently shown (Waddell *et al.*, 1986) that reliance on self-report of pain as an outcome measure is of limited value.

Other work by Raymond and Dumas (1984) has shown that if the volume injected into the facet joint is limited to less than 2 ml the response rate fell to 16%, compared to 62% initial response in the Mooney & Robertson study. When injecting volumes larger than 2 ml into facet joints there will be a significant spillover into the epidural space. In addition the placebo effect has been shown to be potentially very powerful, as high as 85% (Cobb *et al.*, 1959). This is not patient-dependent but more related to the sophistication of the procedure and the enthusiasm of the therapist (Richardson, 1988).

8.4.2 *Epidural injections*

Epidural injection has been an established anaesthetist skill for some considerable time. Although well-established as a practice in the management of labour pain using an indwelling epidural catheter, the use of epidural injections in the management of chronic low back pain is by no means new. The use of local anaesthetics given epidurally for back pain goes back at least five decades (Evans, 1930). The use of epidural steroids is more recent. There have been reports, also recent, of using combinations of epidural narcotics and steroids together (Dallas *et al.*, 1987), however their long-term effects have yet to be established.

The use of epidural injections is a common practice in pain relief clinics for a number of clinical conditions including low back pain and sciatica. There have been a number of clinical trials with variable results. Some authors have found them to be 'useless' and indeed have warned strongly of the potential complications due to the vehicle in which the steroids are dissolved, which may cause arachnoiditis (Andersen & Mosdal, 1987). Others, having reviewed the literature, condemn the use of epidural injections outright as being potentially dangerous and without any established long-term beneficial effect (Kepes & Duncalf, 1985). There is evidence, however, to show that epidural injections of local anaesthetic and steroids are of some value in the management of leg and root distribution pain, although they are less effective in the very chronic patient (Brevik, 1976; Bermen *et al.* 1984).

Epidural injections of local anaesthetic and steroids are used in the Pain Relief Centre for patients with root distribution pain. In agreement with Shealey, the injections are combined with an active rehabilitative programme since the injections by themselves are only part of the management of the patient.

8.5 **Pain management**

The fundamental difference between pain management and any other form of therapy is that it requires the active participation of the patient. Most if not all other treatment modalities merely require the patient to be in receipt of therapy given by somebody else. Pain management is not aimed at treating 'the pain' but more at 'the patient' – helping them to accept their pain (i.e. to live with it rather than just tolerate it) and to begin to restore their levels of functioning as much as possible within the bounds of their medical problem. The management is aimed at several aspects of their life which may have been affected by their pain: physical, emotional, social, marital and many others. They should be at the end of 'sensible' medical and surgical treatment, but just being at the end of treatment is not a reason in itself for such referral. It is not just something else to do when all else fails, since the management is aimed at reducing unnecessary disability and high levels of distress. This aspect of the management of patients with chronic pain is discussed further in Chapter 9.

8.6 **Patterns of drug usage in chronic low-back pain patients; a prospective study**

8.6.1 *Introduction*

A significant proportion of patients referred to pain relief clinics appear to be consuming a considerable amount of medication. These include psychotropic agents as well as analgesics of different classes. It is apparent that a number of patients, quite unaware of the addictive potential of some drugs, have been exceeding the maximum recommended doses. This problem is not always the fault of the patient; some doctors have been prescribing regimes of such medication for very long periods, occasionally more than 10 years.

Even in such circumstances there may have been no attempt to counsel the patient or to advise the patient to withdraw the medication despite the fact that it may well not be providing any significant help.

Patients who consume large quantities of medication appear to be more disabled and distressed than the average chronic pain patient, yet do not seem to differ on objective physical assessment. A pilot study (Spanswick & Main, 1987) demonstrated a close relationship between measures of drug usage and levels of distress, with no demonstrable correlation with objective physical measures. A prospective study of the use of medication by chronic low back pain patients was therefore designed to test the hypothesis that patients' increasing use of medication is a symptom of distress rather than increasing levels of physical damage.

8.6.2 *Aims*

The aims of the study were:

(1) to determine the degree and pattern of usage of drugs by patients with chronic low back pain referred to the Pain Relief Centre, Hope Hospital, Salford, or the The Salford Pain Management Programme;

(2) to examine the relationship of drug use to a number of parameters including clinical history, objective physical impairment, distress, disability, magnified illness behaviour, cognition, work loss, litigation, and current level of benefits.

8.6.3 *Method of assessment*

It has been shown (Waddell *et al.*, 1984) that assessment only in terms of physical examination and self-report of pain is insufficient, especially for the chronic patient (Waddell *et al.*, 1984). There are many factors which influence self-report of pain and responses to physical examination other than organic disease. Indeed Waddell (1987) implies that we should regard chronic low back pain as an illness, rather than a disease for which there must be a single cause, and that, unlike traditional medical practice, treatment should be directed at the illness rather than a postulated underlying disease. It was decided, therefore, to assess patients using the broadly based assessment which has been developed systematically and progressively over the last decade. The methods of assessment can be broadly divided into five categories.

Social, demographic and occupational information: This includes details of age, gender, work status, total work loss, work lost in the previous year, current levels of benefits received, and any outstanding litigation or compensation claims.

Clinical history and presenting symptomatology: This includes a number of factors elicited from the history and is based on previously published work (Waddell & Main, 1984): time from first onset of symptoms; the length of present episode (if different); the time pattern of the pain (acute, chronic or recurrent); the pain pattern (back pain only, back and leg pain or root pain); the number and type of back operations; the number of different specialists consulted; the reported level of disability on a 9-point scale (Waddell & Main, 1984) and inappropriate symptoms (Waddell *et al.*, 1984).

Physical examination: Following the interview the patients were examined in a standardised manner looking for inappropriate responses to physical examination (Waddell *et al.*, 1980) in addition to lumbar flexion – by skin marking technique (Waddell, 1982) – straight leg raising and signs of root irritation or compression.

Psychological tests: These were used to measure levels of distress and the patients beliefs about pain and included the pain drawing, the Modified Zung (Main & Waddell, 1984), the Modified Somatic Perception Questionnaire (Main, 1983), and the Pain Locus of Control (Main, in preparation). The rational for their use is discussed in depth in Chapter 9.

Current drug status: In order to make sense of assessing current medication consumption, only some groups of drugs have been considered. They have been divided up into their pharmacological families depending on their mode of action and reasons for prescribing.

The analgesics were, therefore, divided into non-steroidal anti-inflammatory agents, narcotic analgesics and non-narcotic analgesics. Narcotic-analgesics were those which included morphine buprenorphine, pentazocine, dihydrocodeine, dextropropoxyphene or codeine. The modes of action of these different groups are well known and sufficiently different to be worth considering separately. The narcotics in particular have significant central effects and all narcotics have the potential for developing tolerance and addiction.

Psychotropic drugs were divided into tranquillisers, antidepressants and hypnotics. Although, structurally, hypnotics and tranquillisers are similar, their use is very different and they are prescribed for different reasons. Again, tolerance and dependence is a significant problem with these drugs when used for prolonged periods. Antidepressants cover a number of different groups of drugs including tricyclic and tetracyclic antidepressants as well as mono-amine oxidase inhibitors.

The factors relating to drug consumption included: the frequency of consumption, the clinical effect, the occurrence of side effects and the contingency of consumption.

(1) Frequency. Each group of drugs was scored from 0 to 4 as:
0 = not taking
1 = taking on an irregular basis (i.e. some days without)
2 = taking on a regular basis (i.e. never misses a day)
3 = occasionally takes more than the maximum recommended dose
4 = regularly takes more than the maximum recommended dose.

(2) Effect. The effect was scored in the following manner:
1 = made the symptoms worse
2 = no effect, or useless
3 = slight effect, or 'just takes the edge off the pain'.
4 = considerable help.
Although a crude scale, this represents the best information realistically obtainable from most patients about drug efficacy.

(3) Side effects. These were scored as:
0 = none
1 = some, but not troublesome
2 = significant.

(4) Contingency. This was scored on the basis of how the patient used the medication. Many patients only take medication when they get pain. This may work well for acute pain episodes but often is not helpful in chronic pain states. This was scored as:
0 = not pain contingent (i.e. taken regularly by the clock)
1 = pain contingent (i.e. taken when the pain gets bad).

The consumption of other drugs was recorded but not computed. The information was gathered from the patients by interview. The technique of interview is important as the details need to be gathered in a non-threatening way. The patient must be allowed to admit that they may have taken more than the recommended dose. A useful way of doing this is to ask how many tablets the pain makes them take (i.e. the pain is to blame rather than themselves).

8.6.4 *Selection of subjects*

Consecutive referrals of patients with chronic low back pain (pain for more than 6 months) to the Pain Relief Centre or the Pain Management

Programme were assessed by the authors. The inclusion/exclusion criteria were:

(1) English as first language;

(2) aged between 18 and 65 years;

(3) able to read and write;

(4) exclusion of major spinal pathology (e.g. tumour and spinal fractures);

(5) not undergoing investigation or treatment for other medical problems;

(6) excluding major psychiatric illness.

Each patient was sent a letter with their first appointment explaining the nature of the assessment that would take place at their first interview. This was to enable them to make appropriate domestic arrangements to allow them to be in the clinic for approximately 2 hours. They were asked to bring with them all medication that they were currently taking and their spectacles (if they used them) to enable them to answer some questionnaires. By the use of such a letter, the patient compliance was 100%.

On arrival at the Pain Relief Centre the patients were greeted by the clinic sister and shown into a separate room and asked to complete the questionnaires unassisted. Following completion of the questionnaires the patients were then interviewed and examined by one of the authors (CCS).

8.6.5 *Results*

A general description of the patients is presented in Table 8.2. The mean age, length of history and gender distribution are broadly similar to other groups that we have studied (Main *et al.*, 1986; Spanswick & Main, 1987). These patients have had their symptoms for some considerable time and have seen a number of different specialists before reaching the Pain Relief Clinic or the Pain Management Programme.

Table 8.2 Salford drug study: general description of patients ($n = 172$)

Gender: male	44.2%
female	55.8%
Age (years)	45.0 (9.3)
Time since first onset (years)	10.6 (8.4)
Present episode (months)	62.5 (66.6)

Apart from gender, values are means (SD).

Table 8.3 Salford drug study: patients' drug consumption (n = 172)

Number of drugs	*Percentage of patients*
None	13.1
1	38.3
2	28.8
>2	18.4

The use of drugs is presented in Table 8.3. As can be seen most patients were taking either one or two different drugs in the above classification. A proportion of patients (13.1%) were taking no drugs at all. The most common reason given was that 'nothing works'. It is interesting that there were a number of patients who were still taking medication despite gaining little or no relief of pain. This applied to those taking drugs in excess of the maximum recommended doses as well as those on 'normal' doses. Quite a large proportion, nearly one in five patients were taking two or more drugs.

The pattern of consumption is shown in Table 8.4 and a number of facts become evident when it is examined. Perhaps unsurprisingly to the experienced clinician, nearly 60% of patients were taking narcotic-containing analgesics. Quite a high proportion (13.8%) admitted to taking them in doses greater than the recommended maximum. Despite this increased consumption, these patients seemed to gain no greater effect from their narcotics than those who used them at lower doses. There seemed to be much less misuse of the other groups of drugs, although there were anecdotal cases which were quite surprising (e.g. one patient consuming 25 mg of Nitrazepam during the daytime to try to help his pain). Relatively few patients (29.3%) were using NSAIDS for analgesia, either because they were not so effective or because of side effects. A small number of patients were using tranquillisers and antidepressants. Unfortunately this is too small a number to be able to come to any conclusions.

Table 8.4 Salford drug study: pattern of drug consumption in percentages of patients (n = 172)

	Narcotics	*Non-steroidal anti-inflammatory drugs*	*Tranquillisers*	*Anti-depressants*	*Night sedation*
Not taking	39.6	70.7	89.9	84.8	81.6
Irregularly	21.4	8.9	1.3	2.5	3.8
Regularly	25.2	18.5	7.0	12.7	12.7
>Max	13.8	1.9	1.9	0.	1.9

Table 8.5 Salford drug study: drug consumption I. Relationship with demographic and occupational data ($n = 172$)

	Narcotics	*Non-steroidal anti-inflammatory drugs*	*Tranquillisers*	*Anti-depressants*	*Night sedation*
Age					23
Gender					
Work lost (tot.)	20			22	21
Work lost (in last year)			23		
Litigation					
Current benefits	30*			24	

Values are Pearson Correlation Coefficients (×100). Only significant correlations are shown ($p > 0.05$); * $p > 0.001$.

The relationship of demographic and occupational information to drug history is shown in Table 8.5. As one might expect, the use of night sedation relates to age. This group of patients are not only sleeping poorly but are in pain at the same time and their insomnia, therefore, presents more of a problem. It is well know that habituation to benzodiazepines develops quickly and these patients gain little in terms of long lasting benefit with continued use of hypnotics.

Work lost (either total or that in the last year) correlates well with the use of most of the groups of drugs. The loss of work and potential loss of job is very anxiety producing. It is not surprising that psychotropic drugs are prescribed to try and help patients through these sorts of problems. The longer people are out of work, the less likely they are to return to work (Waddell, 1987). These patients necessarily become more and more distressed. This will contribute to the overall clinical presentation and lead to further consultations with a greater likelihood of more prescriptions for analgesics and psychotropic drugs.

Current levels of benefits correlate well with antidepressant usage and very highly with narcotic usage. Patients who have been 'in the system' for long enough become more and more distressed and hopeless. Perhaps unsurprisingly their mood tends to go down. As mood drops, pain tolerance reduces and so a cycle is set up of pain and lowering of mood. It is difficult to exclude the fact that chronic narcotic consumption may lead to a fall in mood. With increasing level of benefits goes continual medical examinations to 'prove' that they need such benefits, these patients thus become more and more entrenched in their illness behaviour and tend to rely more and more on others (or drugs) to help solve their problems.

Table 8.6 Salford drug study: drug consumption II. Relationship with clinical history and physical examination ($n = 172$)

	Narcotics	*Non-steroidal anti-inflammatory drugs*	*Tranquillisers*	*Anti-depressants*	*Night sedation*
Time since first onset (years)					
Present episode (months)					
No. of specialists					
Previous lumbar surgery					
Objective physical impairment					
Lumbar flexion	21				
Disability	30*				

Values are Pearson Correlation Coefficients (×100). Only significant correlations are shown ($p > 0.05$); * $p > 0.001$.

The relation of features of the clinical history and physical examination to drug usage is shown in Table 8.6. The usage of drugs in general, and narcotics in particular, does not correlate with overall levels of objective physical impairment. The only factors that correlate with drug, and in particular narcotic, usage are lumbar flexion and disability. This group of patients are more disabled than might be anticipated, and it has been shown that physical measures alone do not explain these patients' disability (Waddell, 1987). Disability correlates better with measures of distress than objective physical measures, suggesting alternative explanations for the patients' use of drugs.

The relationship of distress, magnified illness behaviour, and beliefs about pain are shown in Table 8.7. Narcotic usage in particular correlates well with a number of measures of distress. Patients who feel that they bear little responsibility for how pain affects them also tend to have a higher consumption of narcotics. These patients do not feel they can gain any control over their pain and in particular rely on others to help their pain. The others include drugs and they tend to adopt the pain/pill philosophy.

8.7 **Discussion**

The straightforward medical model approach to the management of patients with acute medical problems works extremely well. It is quite apparent that in chronic illness, in particular chronic low back pain,

Table 8.7 Salford drug study: drug consumption III. Relationship with distress, magnified illness behaviour and cognitions ($n = 172$)

	Narcotics	*Non-steroidal anti-inflammatory drugs*	*Tranquillisers*	*Anti-depressants*	*Night sedation*
Inappropriate symptoms	22				
Inappropriate signs	31*				22
Somatic anxiety					
Depressive symptoms	24				
Cognitive control					
Pain responsibility	20				

Values are Pearson Correlation Coefficients (×100). Only significant correlations are shown ($p > 0.05$); * $p > 0.001$.

there are a number of factors other than nociception that influence the patients' self-report of pain and their level of disability. Waddell (1987) has proposed a biopsychosocial model for low back pain. Indeed it is because the medical model approach has failed that patients ultimately appear at pain relief clinics.

As has already been mentioned, our previous work (Main *et al.*, 1985; Spanswick & Main, 1987) has demonstrated increasing levels of distress and drug usage, the longer that patients are in the health care system. It seems that the health care system may not only not be helping them, but actually adding to their levels of distress. By continuing to treat patients purely with physical measures, their passive behaviour is being reinforced. They are being taught that they need do nothing, but that if they continue to consult, someone eventually will be able to provide a cure. This is patently not true. The more specialists they consult, the larger the number of differing opinions they receive and the more confused and distressed they become. Their presentation often becomes more and more bizarre and this clouds the clinical issues even more, making the differentiation of signs of organic disease from signs of distress very difficult. The likelihood of then receiving appropriate physical therapy, as well as psychological help, diminishes considerably.

It is at this stage that they will often be labelled 'neurotic' or 'functional' and will receive either inappropriate physical therapy, in an effort to appease them, or inappropriate psychiatric referral.

There is little scientific evidence supporting the efficacy of many of the commonly prescribed therapies for chronic low back pain (Quebec Task Force, 1987). Indeed the scientific evidence actually contraindicates some therapies (e.g. denervation). Chronic low back pain patients learn to depend on doctors and others largely because continuous treatment is offered, if not by the same clinician then certainly by another. Waddell has shown that low back pain is universal in most societies, but only in societies where Western medicine is practised do patients become disabled and stop working (Waddell, 1987). Much of low back pain patients behaviours suggests a 'learned helplessness'. They have been taught that they need not bear any responsibility for how their pain effects them.

Chapman and Brena (1982) have shown that patients develop learned helplessness as a response to injection therapy for back pain. This helplessness correlates well with measures of drug dependence, low activity levels and elevated MMPI scores on the hypochondriasis, depression and hysteria scales. McCreary and Colman (1984) have shown that multiple drug users (including narcotics and others) tend to report more pain and scored highly on the hypochondriasis and hysteria scales of the MMPI. They showed that there is a close relationship between medication usage, emotional disturbance and pain behaviour. Our study confirms this. The level of narcotic consumption, in particular, relates to levels of distress and not to measures of objective physical impairment, and again can be thought of as a degree of learned helplessness reinforced by prescribing habits. It is interesting to note that many doctors are reluctant to prescribe strong narcotics for patients with cancer for fear of producing addiction, but will happily continuously prescribe other opioids of equal addictive potential for patient with pain of non-malignant origin.

Although some authors (Portenoy & Foley, 1986) have advocated the use of opioids in non-malignant pain when there is no other alternative therapy, there is no evidence even in their study to show that the use of such drug regimes are efficacious, improve disability, or allow the patient to return to work. Their methodology does not stand up to critical appraisal (Sternbach, 1987).

In the present study increasing use of narcotics was not paralleled by an increase in pain relief or any change in disability. There are no pharmacological reasons for the continuous use of opioids in non-malignant pain. Tolerance develops, total relief of pain does not occur, and in fact the chronic use of such drugs may well perpetuate chronic benign pain (Gildenberg, 1987). Most available narcotic-containing drugs have a short duration of action and even if taken on a regular basis will lead to considerable variations in plasma levels. This causes periods of withdrawal each day producing more pain, accentuating pain rather than helping it. Such drugs are actually contraindicated as far as effects on pain are concerned and of course patients generally report feeling better when not taking such toxic drugs. Although patients may get some short-term increase in their pain while withdrawing (in addition to the other withdrawal symptoms), like all withdrawal effects this eventually subsides and when they are drug free their pain levels are usually considerably lower than when they were taking opioid drugs.

8.8 **Conclusion**

The increasing use of narcotic analgesics may be interpreted as a distress sign and is not related to objective measures of physical damage.

The inappropriate use of narcotic analgesics is a learned helplessness which is compounded by prescribing habits. The continuous use or prescribing of narcotic analgesics is contraindicated for chronic non-malignant pain as it may actually perpetuate pain and will produce significant unnecessary dependence.

The role of the anaesthetist should be seen not so much as a provider of injections but as a specialist who, by developing communication skills, can separate distress from treatable pathology and thus provide appropriate intervention whether in the form of counselling, drug management or, indeed, injection therapy.

Acknowledgement

We would like to thank Sister M. Hunter (Sister in charge of the Pain Relief Centre, Hope Hospital, Salford) for her considerable help in this research.

References

Amlie, E., Weber, H. & Holme, I. (1987). Treatment of acute low-back pain with Piroxicam: Results of a double-blind placebo-controlled trial, *Spine*, **12**, 473–6.

Andersen, K. H. & Mosdal C. (1987). Epidural application of cortico-steroids in low-back pain and sciatica, *Acta Neurochirurgica (Wien)*, **87**, 52–53.

Benzon, H. T. (1986). Epidural steroid injections for low back pain and lumbosacral radiculopathy, *Pain*, **24**, 277–95.

Berman A. T., Garbarino, J. L., Fisher, S. M. & Bosacco, S. J. (1984). The effects of epidural injection of local anaesthetics and corticosteroids on patients with lumbosciatic pain, *Clinical Orthopaedics and Related Research*, **188**, 144–51.

Berry, H. Bloom, B., Hamilton, E. B. D. & Swinson, D. R. (1982). Naproxen sodium, Diflunisal, and placebo in the treatment of chronic back pain, *Annals of the Rheumatic Diseases*, **41**, 129–32.

Bonica, J. J. (1974). Acupuncture anaesthesia in the People's Republic of China. Implications for American medicine, *The Journal of the American Medical Association*, **229**, 1317–25.

Bonica, J. J. (1974). Therapeutic acupuncture in the People's Republic of China. Implications for American medicine, *The Journal of the American Medical Association*, **228**, 1544–51.

Bonica, J. J. (1983). IASP Presidential Address, Pain research and therapy: Achievements of the past and challenges of the future. In: *Advances in Pain Research and Therapy*, eds. J. J. Bonica *et al.*, Vol. 5, pp. 1–36. Raven Press, New York.

Breivik, H. (1976). Treatment of low back pain and sciatica: Comparison of caudal epidural injections of bupivacaine and methylprednisolone with bupivacaine alone followed by saline. In: *Advances in Pain Research and Therapy*, Vol. 1, pp. 927–32. Raven Press, New York.

Cobb, L. A., Thomas, G. I., Dillard, D. H., Merendino, K. A. & Bruce, R. A. (1959). An evaluation of internal mammary ligation by a double blind technique, *New England Journal of Medicine*, **260**, 1115–18.

Chapman, S. L. & Brena, S. B. (1982). Learned helplessness and responses to nerve blocks in chronic low back pain patients, *Pain*, **14**, 355–64.

Dallas, T. L. (1987). Epidural morphine and methylprednisolone for low-back pain, *Anaesthesiology*, **67**, 408–11.

Dowson, D. I., Lewith, G. & Machin, D. (1985). The effects of acupuncture versus placebo in the treatment of headache, *Pain*, **21**, 35–42.

Evans, W. (1930). Intrasacral epidural injection in the treatment of sciatica, *Lancet*, **2**, 1225–29.

Fox, E. & Melzack, R. (1976). Comparison of transcutaneous electrical stimulation and acupuncture in the treatment of chronic pain. In: *Advances in Pain Research and Therapy*, Vol. 1, pp. 797–801. Raven Press, New York.

Gessler, M. & Struppler, A. (1983). Relief of phantom pain following modification of phantom sensation by TNS. In: *Advances in Pain Research and Therapy*, Vol. 5, pp. 591–4. Raven Press, New York.

Gildenberg, P. L. (1987). *Pain and Headache*, Vol. 7. ed. R. A. De Vaul, *The Chronic Pain Patient*. Karger, Basel.

Hickey, R. F. J. (1982). Chronic low back pain: A comparison of difunisal with paracetamol, *New Zealand Medical Journal*, **95**, 312–14.

Hurme, M. & Himanen, P. (1986). Diflunisal in the treatment of low back pain in a multicentre trial, *The International Journal on Clinical Pharmacology and Research*, **6**, 53–58.

Kepes, E. R. & Duncalf, D. (1985). Treatment of backache with spinal injections of local anaesthetic, spinal and systemic steroids. A review, *Pain*, **22**, 33–47.

Lewith, G. T., Field, J. & Machin, D. (1983). Acupuncture compared with placebo in post-herpetic pain, *Pain*, **17**, 361–8.

Lewith, G. T. & Machin, D. (1983). On the evaluation of the clinical effects of acupuncture, *Pain*, **16**, 111–27.

Long, D. M. & Hagfors, N. (1975). Electrical stimulation in the nervous system. The current status of electrical stimulation of the nervous system for the relief of pain, *Pain*, **1**, 109–23.

McCreary, C. & Colman, A. (1984). Medication usage, emotional disturbance, and pain behaviour in chronic low back pain patients, *Journal of Clinical Psychology*, **40**, 15–19.

MacDonald, A. J. (1983). Superficial acupuncture in the relief of chronic low back pain, *Annals of the Royal College of Surgeons of England*, **65**, 44–46.

Main, C. J. (1983). The modified somatic perception questionnaire, *Journal of Psychosomatic Research*, **27**, 503–14.

Main, C. J. & Waddell, G. (1984). The detection of psychological abnormality in chronic low back pain using four simple scales, *Current Concepts in Pain*, **2**, 10–15.

Main, C. J., Spanswick, C. C., Berger, S. M. & Wood, P. L. (1986). Low back pain, psychological disturbance and the health care system. Paper presented at *1st World Congress on Low Back Pain*, Vienna.

Main, C. J. & Waddell, G. (1987). Personality assessment in the management of low back pain, *Clinical Rehabilitation*, **1**, 139–42.

Melzack, R., Vetere, P. & Finch, L. (1983). Transcutaneous nerve stimulation for low back pain. A comparison of TENS and massage for pain and range of movement, *Physical Therapy*, **63**, 489–93.

Melzack, R. & Wall, P. D. (1965). Pain mechanisms, a new theory, *Science*, **150**, 971–9.

Mendelson G., Kidson, M. A., Loh, S. T., Scott, D. F., Selwood, P. S. & Kranz, H. (1978). Acupuncture analgesia for chronic low back pain, *Clinical and Experimental Neurology*, **15**, 182–5.

Mooney, V. & Robertson, J. (1976). The facet syndrome, *Clinical Orthopaedics and Related Research*, **115**, 149–56.

Murphy, T. M. (1976). Subjective and objective follow-up assessment of acupuncture therapy without suggestion with 100 chronic pain patients. In: *Advances in Pain Research and Therapy*, Vol. 1, pp. 811–815. Raven Press, New York.

Nathan, P. W. & Wall, P. D. (1974). Treatment of post-herpetic neuralgia by prolonged electrical stimulation, *British Medical Journal*, **3**, 645–7.

Orava, S. (1986). Medical treatment of low back pain. Diflunisal compared with indomethacin in acute lumbago, *International Journal on Clinical Pharmacology and Research*, **6**, 45–51.

Pilowsky, I., Hallett, E. C., Bassett, D. L., Thomas, P. G. & Penhall, R. K. (1982). A controlled study of amitriptyline in the treatment of chronic pain, *Pain*, **14**, 169–79.

Portenoy, R. K. & Foley, K. M. (1986). Chronic use of opioid analgesics in non-malignant pain: Report of 38 cases, *Pain*, **25**, 171–86.

Quebec Task Force (1987). Scientific approach to the assessment and management of activity-related spinal disorders. A monograph for clinicians. Report of the Quebec Task Force on Spinal Disorders, *Spine*, Supplement **12**, S1-S59.

Raftery, H. (1979). The management of post-herpetic pain using sodium valproate and amitriptyline, *Irish Medical Journal*, **72**, 399–401.

Raymond, J. & Dumas, J-M. (1984). Intraarticular facet block: Diagnostic test or therapeutic procedure, *Radiology*, **151**, 333–6.

Richardson, P. H. (1988). Placebos: Their effectiveness and modes of action. In: *Health Psychology* ed. A. K. Broome, Croom-Helm, London.

Richardson, P. H. & Vincent, C. A. (1986). Acupuncture for the treatment of pain: a review of evaluative research, *Pain*, **24**, 14–40.

Richardson, R. R., Arbit, J., Sequeira, E. B. & Zagor, R., (1981). Transcutaneous electrical neurostimulation in functional pain, *Spine*, **6**, 185–8.

Saunders, C. M. (1967). *The Management of Terminal Illness*. Edward Arnold, London.

Schwartz, H. A. (1981). Lower gastrointestinal side effects of nonsteroidal anti-inflammatory drugs, *Journal of Rheumatology*, **8**, 952–4.

Shealey, N. C. (1976). Facet denervation in the management of back and sciatic pain, *Clinical Orthopaedics and Related Research*, **115**, 157–64.

Spanswick, C. C. & Main, C. J. (1987). Referral to the pain management programme for low back pain in Salford. Poster presented at the *5th World Congress of the International Association for the Study of Pain*, Hamburg.

Sternbach, R. A. (1987) Letter, *Pain*, **29**, 257–8.

Swerdlow, M. (1967). 4 years pain clinic experience, *Anaesthesia*, **22**, 568–74.

Swerdlow, M. (1980). The treatment of 'shooting' pain, *Post Graduate Medical Journal*, **56**, 159–61.

Swerdlow, M. & Cundill, J. G. (1981). Anticonvulsant drugs used in the treatment of lancinating pain. A comparison, *Anaesthesia*, **36**, 1129–32.

Toomey, T. C., Taylor, A. G., Skelton, J. A. & Carron, H. (1982). Stability of self-report measures of improvement in chronic pain: A five year follow-up, *Pain*, **12**, 273–83.

Twycross, R. G. (1974). Clinical experience with diamorphine in advanced malignant disease, *International Journal of Clinical Pharmacology*, **9**, 184–98.

Videman T. & Osterman K. (1984). Double-blind parallel study of piroxicam *versus* indomethacin in the treatment of low back pain, *Annals of Clinical Research*, **16**, 156–60.

Vincent, C. A. & Richardson, P. H. (1986). The evaluation of therapeutic acupuncture: Concepts and methods, *Pain*, **24**, 1–13.

Waddell, G. (1982). A approach to backache, *British Journal of Hospital Medicine*, **28**, 187–219.

Waddell, G. (1987). A new clinical model for the treatment of low-back pain, *Spine*, **12**, 632–44.

Waddell, G., McCulloch, J. A., Kummel, E. & Venner, R. M. (1980). Nonorganic physical signs in low back pain, *Spine*, **5**, 117–25.

Waddell, G. & Main, C. J. (1984). Assessment of severity in low back disorders, *Spine*, **9**, 204–8.

Waddell, G., Main, C. J. Morris, E. W., Di Paola, M. & Gray, I. C. M. (1984). Chronic low back pain, pyschological distress and illness behaviour, *Spine*, 9, 209–13.

Wall, P. D. & Devor, M. (1981). The effects of peripheral nerve injury on dorsal root potentials and on transmission of afferent signals into the spinal cord, *Brain Research*, **209**, 95–111.

Ward, N. G. (1986). 1986 Volvo Award in Clinical Sciences. Tricyclic antidepressants for chronic low-back pain. Mechanisms of action and predictors of response, *Spine*, **11**, 661–5.

Wong, D. G. Spence, J. D., Lamki, L., Freeman, D. & McDonald, J. W. D. (1986). The effect of nonsteroidal anti-inflammatory drugs on control of hypertension by beta blockers and diuretics, *Lancet*, **1**, 997–1001.

9 *C. J. Main and H. Parker*

The evaluation and outcome of pain management programmes for chronic low back pain

9.1 Introduction

Recent statistics in the United Kingdom (OHE, 1985) demonstrate that musculoskeletal disorders, dorsopathies and back strains together account for approximately 25% of annual work loss (360 million days). Of the estimated 23 million episodes of back pain annually in the general population, about one tenth will lead to consultations with general practitioners and of those about one seventh will be referred to hospital specialists. About one fifth of the latter will in turn be admitted to hospital for specialist investigation. Although the number of spinal operations may be decreasing, in 1982 there were approximately 10 000 such operations. The total annual cost of such wide-ranging investigation and treatment was estimated at £156 million, which at that time was equivalent to opening 18 new District General Hospitals.

The costs of low back pain are economically staggering, not only indirectly in terms of work loss, invalidity allowances, disability awards and mobility payments, but also more directly in the cost of treatment and investigation.

There is of course a further cost, *viz.* the pain, suffering and associated disability to the individual patient and his or her family. Chronic pain and limitation in activities of daily living, as with any other life stress, will eventually have a psychological impact. Once the pain has progressed beyond the acute phase, the chronic pain patient becomes progressively more demoralised and angry (Sternbach, 1974). Unfortunately, the effects of repeated investigations and failed treatment magnify the distress still further and may lead to magnified illness presentation in the form of inappropriate responses to physical examination (Waddell *et al.*, 1980) or inappropriate symptomatology (Main & Waddell, 1982; Waddell *et al.*,

1984a). In addition to distress, anger and inappropriate illness behaviour, confusion and misunderstanding may arise. Patients find it profoundly difficult to accept that scientific technology has advanced far enough to enable a lunar landing, yet modern technological medicine offers successful treatment for only a minority of back pain sufferers. Even in patients admitted to hospital for specialist investigation of low back pain, at the time of discharge or death no definite diagnosis has been made in almost 60% of cases (OHE, 1985). Patients do not realise that much treatment is purely empirical and do not understand why patients with apparently similar symptoms may be offered quite different investigations or treatment.

It is against such a complex background that a patient's likelihood of benefiting from a pain management programme (PMP) has to be appraised. The decision to offer a course of treatment (of whatever nature) must be based on an adequate assessment of the patient. Before discussing PMPs therefore it will be necessary to consider the nature of psychological factors in low back pain and various approaches to psychological assessment.

9.2 The nature of psychological factors

Had the treatment of low back pain been more successful, then interest in psychosocial factors might well not have gathered its current momentum. For the last two decades, however, the rising costs of chronic disability has led to attempts to explain differences in levels of functional disability (in patients with seemingly comparable levels of physical impairment) on psychological grounds.

There are a number of ways of investigating psychological features in low back pain, but these can be classified into three general approaches:

(1) assessment of pain;

(2) psychological tests (primarily self-report questionnaires);

(3) pain behaviour (which can be assessed in a number of ways).

Each of these general approaches will be considered briefly and then a comparison of their relative importance in understanding chronic low back pain disability will be made from recent UK studies.

9.2.1 *The assessment of pain*

Pain can be assessed either experimentally or clinically. Typically, experimental methods involve the controlled administration of a painful stimulus in a laboratory setting. There are a variety of laboratory pain induction methods, but perhaps best known is the tourniquet test (Smith *et al.*, 1966) which produces ischaemic pain when a tourniquet is fixed to the upper arm and the arm is drained of blood. The principal advantage of such methods lies in the accurate control of the painful stimulus, thus permitting comparison of subjects on parameters such as pain threshold and pain tolerance, often analysing the results using signal detection theory (Grossberg & Grant, 1978). Unfortunately, patients tend to respond differently to different experimental methods (Lynn & Perl, 1977), and anxiety can have a marked effect on test results (Von Graffenfried *et al.*, 1978). Furthermore, it has been shown recently (Coppola & Gracely, 1983) that patients' discrimination of painful stimuli is influenced by both sensory and non-sensory factors so that, for example, in drug trials, it is impossible to distinguish true analgesic effects from inconsistency in patients' ability to make judgments. The incorporation of such methods into general clinical practice therefore is problematic and, however apparently attractive, differences in experimentally derived measures of pain threshold and pain tolerance cannot be given a clear clinical interpretation.

Of wider applicability are self-report measures such as the pain thermometer or visual analogue scale (VAS), a number of different versions of which have been compared (Jensen *et al.*, 1976). Unfortunately, perceived pain is multidimensional rather than unidimensional (Reading, 1980); ratings are affected by mood (Shacham *et al.*, 1984); and by degree of perceived control over pain (Weisenberg *et al.*, 1985). Although such limitations make comparison of patients difficult, the VAS may be of more use in the individual case (e.g. in assessing change), since, presumably, non-sensory influences on the report of pain will remain relatively constant. VAS are frequently incorporated into pain diaries (Fordyce *et al.*, 1984).

The pain drawing (Ransford *et al.*, 1976) has also been used in low-back pain as a measure of psychological overlay or distress. The original scoring system has been criticised both in terms of poor reliability (Main, 1984) and clinical validity (Von Baeyer *et al.*, 1983). A different scoring system has recently been proposed (Margolis *et al.*, 1986). In summary, the identification of distress from patients' drawings of their pain would seem to have some intuitive validity and a degree of scientific support, but a satisfactory method of differentiating 'appropriate' representations of pain from those suggestive of distress has still to be devised.

The most widely used pain measure to identify psychological overlay is the McGill Pain Questionnaire (MPQ) (Melzack, 1975). Patients are asked which of 78 words describe their pain and the answers yield scores (principally) on Sensory, Affective and Evaluative dimensions. (There are a variety of scores in current use.) Different studies have produced differing factor structures (or underlying dimensions) from the basic list of words. There would seem to be some general support at least for the distinction between Sensory and Affective dimensions but the precise distinction is unclear and variable in studies reporting use of the MPQ.

Nonetheless, the MPQ has been used with a wide variety of diagnostic groups and in a large number of settings. It has also been translated into several languages. But the MPQ has been criticised for the scaling of the individual items (Reading *et al.*, 1982) and for its dependence on verbal skills (Walsh, 1984). More seriously, it has been shown that chronic pain patients do not use pain descriptors in a precise or systematic manner (Atkinson *et al.*, 1982).

An explanation for some of the inconsistencies in research on the MPQ has been offered. Pain vocabulary may be useful to varying degrees, depending on whether it is being used to classify pain, evaluate treatment or predict outcome (Carlsson, 1984). A recent version of the questionnaire containing only 15 words (primarily Affective) and allowing each word to be rated on a 4-point scale has been published (Melzack, 1987). This may be an improvement on the original questionnaire, but seems to have limitations in that the emotionally laden content of the words is clearly apparent (and may lead to bias in response).

9.2.2 *The use of psychological tests*

Many early investigators into the role of psychological factors in physical illness were heavily influenced by psychosomatic formulations derived essentially from psychoanalytic theory. Although the derivation of projective tests such as the Rorschach ink-blot tests purported to be more objective than psychoanalytic speculation, it was not until statistical methodology derived essentially in the field of educational psychology was incorporated into the assessment of personality that the modern personality test was derived.

The most widely used personality test is the Minnesota Multiphasic Personality Inventory or MMPI (Dahlstrom & Welsh, 1960). The original inventory comprised 566 items, yielding scores on ten clinical scales and three validity scales. Although a number of shorter versions have been produced, these are not entirely satisfactory clinically (Hoffman & Butcher, 1975). The MMPI has been used in a number of ways ('diagnostically', descriptively and predictively). Many studies have tried to classify low back patients into 'functional' or 'organic' on the basis of the questionnaire, but the insensitivity of the test and the high misclassification rate would seem to preclude its use in the individual case for such a purpose (Cummings *et al.*, 1979). Attempts to rediscover the low back pain personality profile described by Hanvik (1951) have not been successful. The questionnaire is clearly capable of picking up some sort of distress in a proportion of patients, but it may be identifying no more than the emotional disturbance associated with chronic limitation and disruption of activity (Naliboff *et al.*, 1982). It thus lacks both diagnostic and descriptive accuracy.

Methodological problems bedevil many of the studies using the MMPI as a predictive tool. In one of the better designed studies (Strassberg *et al.*,

1981), three of the MMPI scales added significantly to the prediction of subjective outcome, but only for patients clearly identified as needing, and subsequently receiving, psychiatric treatment. Since the test was originally designed to identify 'psychiatric cases', the finding is not surprising. More importantly, for the general hospital patients, the test was of no predictive value. A new MMPI four-cluster typology has recently been proposed (Costello *et al.*, 1987), and this classification may simplify the use of the test predictively, but even the most elegant statistical superstructure is rendered vulnerable by weak theoretical foundations.

The Eysenck Personality Questionnaire or EPQ (Eysenck & Eysenck, 1975) is the latest in a series of British personality tests. It has been used in the UK in studies of cancer pain (Bond, 1971, 1973), and, although it has not been used specifically with low back pain patients, it at least has normative British data. It yields scores on Extraversion, Neuroticism, 'Psychoticism' and incorporates a Lie scale.

A number of other general personality tests such as the SCL-90 (Derogatis, 1977) are available but have not as yet been used widely in research.

A more specific questionnaire is the Illness Behaviour Questionnaire or IBQ (Pilowsky & Spence, 1975). The latest version consists of 62 items giving scores on seven different scales of which the best known are perhaps General Hypochondriasis and Disease Conviction. The scales have been used widely in studies of pain patients and in general discriminate pain patients from normals. A recent study in the UK (Main & Waddell, 1987) has highlighted major statistical problems in the construction of the scale and the IBQ would certainly seem to be of only limited use with British low back pain patients.

Unfortunately many psychological tests are used for purposes for which they were never originally designed, or have not been subjected to the sort of statistical appraisal which is necessary to remove measurement inaccuracy. This may explain in part the conceptual confusion evident in the literature about the nature and significance of psychological features in low back pain patients. In the UK, two much simpler tests have been designed to evaluate aspects of patients' distress. The Modified Somatic Perception Questionnaire or MSPQ (Main, 1983) was designed specifically to identify somatic anxiety in chronic low back patients. The Modified Zung Questionnaire (Main & Waddell, 1984), a slightly modified version of the original Zung questionnaire (Zung, 1965), gives an evaluation of depressive symptomatology and recently has been compared favourably with other self-report screening measures for depression in chronic pain syndromes (Turner & Romano, 1984). UK normative data is also available on this instrument. Although these tests in no sense provide a comprehensive psychological evaluation, they represent a move to a simpler level of conceptualisation and may serve as a foundation for more complex model-building.

There are many other psychological tests and screening instruments currently in use, but space precludes their discussion.

9.2.3 *Pain behaviour*

Psychological investigations have also included investigations of various aspects of pain behaviour. Such methods have their origin in experimental animal work, such as classical conditioning experiments (Pavlov, 1927) which showed that certain aspects of behaviour were under the control of their antecedents. The theoretical basis of such relationships was systematised in Learning Theory. Later experimental work demonstrated that behaviour patterns could also be established and maintained by manipulation of the consequences of the particular behaviour (Thorndike, 1931; Skinner, 1938). Perhaps surprisingly, the general principles of Learning Theory were found to be applicable to human behaviour and the experimental analysis of behaviour has assumed particular importance in the design of psychological treatments for many different psychiatric disorders such as the treatment of phobias, obsessions or more generalised anxiety (Wolpe, 1958) or in the reinstatement of normal behaviour as with chronic schizophrenic patients (Baker *et al.*, 1974). Behavioural analysis of problems of chronic pain and invalidism has led to treatment programmes designed to replace inappropriate behaviour patterns with more adaptive (and appropriate) responses to chronic pain and disease. The general approach is well described elsewhere (Fordyce, 1976).

There are both experimental and clinical approaches to the assessment of illness behaviour in low back pain. Keefe and his colleagues (Keefe & Block, 1982) have developed an observational method incorporating a 10-minute standardised sequence of movements which are videotaped and rated according to a set of pain behaviour categories (such as grimacing and guarding) by trained observers. This method is now being used in studies of low back pain and of rheumatoid arthritis (Anderson *et al.*, 1987). There are a number of behavioural checklists currently available, but these tend to be much too heterogeneous for routine clinical application.

In low back pain a set of inappropriate responses to physical examination have been identified (Waddell *et al.*, 1980) and integrated into a systematic assessment of the patient. The inappropriate signs test, in conjunction with an assessment of inappropriate symptomatology (Waddell *et al.*, 1984a), provides an overall assessment of magnified illness presentation or inappropriate illness behaviour which can be carried out during a routine examination of the low back pain patient. In general these signs and symptoms are vague, ill-localised and lack the expected relationships with time, physical activity and anatomy. They are best interpreted as signs of distress.

9.2.4 *A comparison of different types of psychological information*
Following the construction of scales measuring objective physical impairment (OPC) and functional disability (Waddell & Main, 1984), the relative importance of different sorts of psychological information has been examined in a study of 200 British patients with chronic low back pain.

In this study the dependent variable was subjectively reported disability using the 9-item disability index. Various sorts of psychological information were compared, both directly in the prediction of disability scores and also after allowance had been made statistically for differences in the level of physical impairment and for gender differences. The results are shown in Figure 9.1.

In column A, general personality variables (such as Neuroticism and Extraversion from the EPQ) and Hypochondriacal scales (from the IBQ) in combination initially explain 13–14% of the variance in disability, but

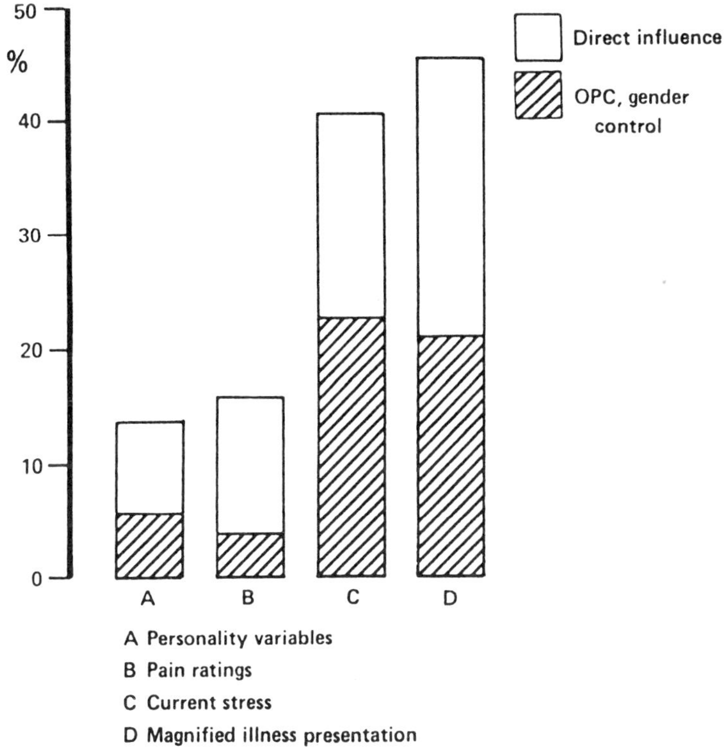

Fig 9.1 Comparison of usefulness of different sorts of psychological information in predicting disability scores: (A) personality variables; (B) pain ratings; (C) current stress; (D) magnified illness presentation. *Ordinate*: % of variance in disability scores accounted for by psychological variables

controlling for gender and objective physical impairment (OPC), this falls to 7–8%.

In column B, pain ratings (VAS Pain Drawing) initially predict 15–16% of the disability score, but this falls to 4–5% when controlled for OPC and gender differences (i.e. these variables add only very little to the information obtained from the physical examination).

It can be seen in columns C and D, however, that psychological distress (in the form of somatic anxiety and depressive symptoms) and magnified illness presentation (as represented by inappropriate signs and symptoms) are of much more significance, both initially and after controlling for physical impairment and gender differences. The key elements of this Glasgow Illness Model (Waddell *et al.*, 1984b) have been replicated in further studies, both in Glasgow (Waddell, 1987), in other parts of the UK (Wood & Main, in preparation), and in Canada (Reesor & Craig, 1987). Distress and illness behaviour have also been identified in the outcome of surgery for low back pain (Waddell *et al.*, 1986) and in patients' use of narcotics (Spanswick & Main, Chapter 8).

Finally, it has been shown that the effect of distress and inappropriate illness behaviour increases with duration of symptomatology (Wood & Main, 1985), and with the number of specialists seen (Main *et al.*, 1985), and that levels of inappropriate symptomatology are a function of the amount of previous unsuccessful conservative treatment (Waddell *et al.*, 1984b).

In conclusion, psychological factors are certainly of importance in explaining patients' levels of disability and in predicting the outcome of treatment. The key elements are not long-standing personality traits or clearly hypochondriacal beliefs, but depressive symptoms and somatic anxiety (both measures of the impact of the back pain and its associated disability on the patient). Hysterical or hypochondriacal features identified in other studies have been found mainly in psychiatric patients presenting with pain problems rather than low back pain patients with distress. Magnified illness presentation may be in part a response to the patient's desire to convince the doctor that some effective treatment is required, but may be understood also as learned patterns of behaviour, shaped by successive consultations and ineffective treatment.

9.3 **Pain management programmes**

9.3.1 *Approaches to rehabilitation*

The modern pain management programme (PMP) consists of a variety of approaches and procedures which have their origins partly in preventative programmes in industrial settings and partly in rehabilitation programmes in health care settings. The goal of most PMPs is rehabilitation rather than cure (Follick, 1986) and patients are not usually offered cures for their pain, although they may have been made many such offers by specialists prior to their consideration for a PMP. The general emphasis is on improving functional capacity while at the same time trying to reduce specific illness related behaviours.

There are similarities between PMPs and backschools, but also important differences. Backschools have been described in Chapter 2 and have been reviewed by Andersson (1987).

The Canadian approach seems best suited to patients with chronic low back pain and is similar to a PMP in its breadth of content. The general educational component is found in almost any sort of rehabilitation programme, but in occupational rehabilitation programmes, such as those funded by the Workmens' Compensation Board in Canada or the Rehabilitation Institute in Helsinki, much more emphasis is placed on the restoration of physical condition. Such emphasis is understandable given the explicit purpose of such programmes, and a 'robust' approach undoubtedly is effective at certain stages in illness.

9.3.2 *Development of pain management programmes*

Multidisciplinary PMPs vary widely in terms of administration, type of patient, funding, philosophy and clinical content (Ng, 1981). Most PMPs, however, contain a variety of psychological techniques designed to reduce patients' levels of distress, build their confidence, and offer specific training in problem-solving techniques. Stress reduction techniques include psychophysiological approaches in which patients are shown how to reduce muscle tension and normalise their breathing patterns, sometimes with the aid of physiological equipment which feeds back information to the patient about his physiological functioning thus enabling an increased degree of control over it.

The first true PMP was pioneered in the Department of Rehabilitation Medicine at the University of Washington in Seattle (Bonica & Fordyce, 1974). The general emphasis was clearly behavioural. The programme begins with a behavioural analysis of the patient's pain problem on the basis of which specific targets for change are agreed and set as objectives. Behavioural techniques are then employed specifically to eliminate or minimise undesirable pain behaviours and re-establish or introduce more acceptable behaviours relevant to various aspects of the patient's life. The behaviour modification programme is offered as a 3- or 4-week in-patient programme. Many such PMPs have been established, particularly in North America, during the last two decades. Almost all include mobility and fitness training as well as some sort of behaviour modification. Some PMPs operate almost entirely as 3- or 4-week in-patient programmes, while others are offered as out-patient programmes.

In the last decade, a more psychological focus has become apparent in many PMPs. This derives essentially from cognitive therapy (Beck, 1976), a form of psychotherapy devised originally for the treatment of depression and based on the 'learned helplessness' model (Seligman, 1975). The newer cognitive-behavioural therapy contains ingredients of both behaviour therapy and cognitive psychotherapy and allows a fairly broad approach to the patient (Turk *et al.*, 1983).

9.3.3 *A comparison of pain management programmes, backschools and the general medical approach*

The modern PMP is compared with backschools and the general medical approach in Table 9.1.

Most general medical approaches are designed primarily (and appropriately) to treat low back pain. A lot of backschools, particularly in

Table 9.1 Comparison of general medical approach (GMA), backschools (BS), and pain management programmes (PMP)

	GMA	*BS*	*PMP*
I General Objective			
General aim	Treatment	Primary prevention or prevention of relapse	Rehabilitation
Stage in illness	Acute-chronic	Pre-acute and semi-chronic	Chronic
Professional input	Individual or Multi-disciplinary	Multidisciplinary	Inter-disciplinary
Method of delivery	Individual	Group	Group
II Therapeutic Objectives			
Pain reduction	Major	Minor	Minor
Disability and mobility	Minor	Major	Major
Reduction of distress	None	Minor	Major
Reduction of invalidism	None	Minor	Major
Giving coping skills	None	Minor	Major
III Philosophy of Care			
Education	None	Major	Major
Patient involvement in treatment	Passive	Mixed	Active
Patient involvement in decision making	None	Minor	Major

industrial settings, are concerned with primary prevention or in the prevention of relapse. Research on backschools suggests that while they may be appropriate for acute or semi-acute back problems, they have little impact on chronic back pain (Nordin, 1985). PMPs deal almost exclusively with the chronic back patient. Professional input in general medical approaches tend to be either by a single professional or involve multidisciplinary input by a sequence of different professionals; in the general medical approach patients are seen by one specialist at a time. Interdisciplinary input, however, requires close communication among the professionals, frequently on the basis of shared expertise, and is much less likely to lead to the delivery of inadequate or even conflicting advice being given to the patient. The other approaches normally involve a large proportion of group teaching, training and counselling; not simply for reasons of economy of effort, but because patients derive considerable benefit from being part of a group and being able to talk to each other.

The importance of various therapeutic objectives is also presented in Table 9.1. While pain reduction is the explicit purpose of most general medical approaches, reduction in disability and improvement in mobility are more important in backschools and PMPs. Many hospital specialists are not particularly expert either at recognising or in dealing with distress; indeed they would not claim to be so, believing that the management of distress is the responsibility either of the patient's general practitioner or of another hospital specialist. While some reduction of distress may be achieved with good and sensitive communication both in general medical approaches and backschools, it is of particular importance in PMPs, and is recognised as such. Reduction of invalidism may necessitate the involvement of spouses or even families in the treatment programme and, although sometimes difficult to achieve, such involvement is considered to be important in most PMPs. Finally, although many professionals would claim to be offering coping skills to patients, a wider range of skills with more specific training is usually offered in PMPs.

There are clear differences among the three approaches as far as philosophy of care is concerned. Although doctors are becoming aware of the importance (at least) of correcting major misunderstandings, education is taken much more seriously by backschools and PMPs. General medical approaches are characterised by an extremely active approach by the doctor, often prescribing a succession of fairly empirical treatment procedures of which the patient is a passive recipient. Backschools contain a mixture of active and passive approaches (as far as the patient is concerned), but it is usually only in the PMPs that the patient has to become actively involved in almost all aspects of treatment. This difference is also evident in the taking of decisions. In the general medical approach it is usually considered awkward or embarrassing if the patient asks the doctor too many questions, or tries to become too involved in decisions at early stages of treatment. The longer the back pain has continued, however, and the more failed treatment the patient has undergone, the more appropriate, and indeed necessary, it becomes to involve the patient explicitly in decision making.

9.4 The Salford Pain Management Programme: an evaluation

9.4.1 *Development and general description*

The Salford PMP, the first in the UK established specifically for patients with low back pain, was established in 1983 initially as an assessment and counselling service for out-patients seen on an individual basis. Then two small group treatment programmes were run on very similar lines to the Canadian back school described in Chapter 2, 2.5, placing emphasis primarily on the educational aspects of rehabilitation. Since then, the Salford PMP has been developed progressively. At present (1988) it consists of an assessment and counselling service for individual out-patients; the group PMP for 10–14 out-patients at a time; and a small in-patient programme (still very much at a 'pilot stage') for patients who are particularly disabled. The PMP is part of a wider range of treatment services at the pain clinic (Spanswick & Main, Chapter 8).

Patients are considered for the PMP if their primary presenting symptom is low back pain. Patients with serious pathology or major structural abnormalities are excluded. About 45% of patients are referred from Salford itself, but an increasing proportion of patients are referred from other parts of NW England and from other parts of the UK. At present patients below 18 years, above 65 years, in whom English is not their first language, of below normal intelligence or with major psychiatric illness are not considered for the PMP. All other patients are given a standardised medical and psychosocial assessment, including physical examination, a clinical and drug history, a number of psychological questionnaires and a structured interview. (The various elements of this assessment are the basis of a video-based training workshop for pain specialists.) The patient is assessed both by the pain specialist (anaesthetist) and by one of the clinical psychologists. The spouse usually will be interviewed, at least briefly, and the patient may be asked to keep a Pain Diary for 2 or 3 weeks. If the patients are actively involved in physical treatment at the time of initial assessment, the full assessment may not be carried out until a later date. Patients currently involved in medico-legal proceedings will be assessed, but are less likely to be offered a place on the PMP and a decision regarding their suitability is sometimes deferred until legal proceedings are concluded.

9.4.2 *Salford PMP: selection for treatment*

The patient may then be offered an individual programme (Including education, general counselling possibly including stress reduction, and simple ergonomic advice) by one of the psychologists; a joint appointment with the physiotherapist, which may lead to an individualised physiotherapy or an isometric programme; training in self-hypnosis; or marital therapy (if there appear to be serious interpersonal difficulties likely to hinder or prevent progress in rehabilitation). Extremely immobile patients may be offered a place on the in-patient programme, sometimes with a view to considering them for the group out-patient programme.

Patients may be considered unsuitable for treatment either because they are coping well and not felt to need a comprehensive programme, or because they are still seeking a 'miracle cure' and are not prepared to consider a self-help approach.

The treatment plan of choice is the group programme, but to be considered suitable for this, patients must show signs of distress (whether depressive symptoms, somatic anxiety or, sometimes, anger), a degree of unnecessary disability (i.e. potentially recoverable function) or excessive pain preoccupation, and be willing to make a clear open-minded commitment to rehabilitation once the nature of the PMP has been described to them. Much of the initial assessment has to be carried out sensitively to enable an honest and realistic discussion about the range of rehabilitation objectives which might be considered for that patient.

9.4.3 *Salford PMP: content of group programme*

Patients selected for the group programme attend the physiotherapy gymnasium once per week for about 3 hours on 7 consecutive weeks, although they may be asked to attend for a video-assessment of movement before and after the programme. They are assessed prior to the programme; at the end of the programme; at 6-week follow-up and (latterly) at 6-month follow-up. Each session consists of a mobility evaluation on three pieces of equipment (patients are required to increase their tolerance for exercise successively throughout the programme); individual physiotherapy (monitoring exercises which they have been set); practice in stress reduction (using a variety of techniques); formal teaching on set topics; and small group problem-solving on various aspects of low back pain and its effects. Discussion of more sensitive 'psychological' topics is deferred until later in the programme. There are 10–14 patients in the PMP. At times they will be seen individually, at times in pairs, at times in small groups of four or five patients and sometimes all in one group. In addition to the weekly sessions, patients are set homework targets which will include increasing fitness and mobility, practising stress reduction, appraising certain aspects

Table 9.2 Salford Pain Management Programme: educational and clinical content

Education:	1. Nature of low back pain 2. Correcting misunderstandings 3. Setting realistic goals
Reducing invalidism:	1. Increasing mobility and fitness 2. Eliminating inappropriate illness behaviour 3. Decreasing medication use 4. Decreasing consulting behaviour
Skills acquisition:	1. Stress reduction 2. Problem analysis and problem solving
Counselling:	1. Reducing anger and distress 2. Building confidence 3. Taking responsibility

of their disability and reading the relevant sections from the patient manual prior to teaching on a particular topic or to revising teaching already received. The general content of the programme is summarised in Table 9.2.

9.4.4 *Salford PMP outcome evaluation: research design*

As already indicated, the Salford PMP has been developed progressively over the last 5 years. During the course of the first four programmes, clinical content was gradually expanded and modified in the light of experience. The assessment system has also been gradually developed. This has had the unfortunate but inevitable consequence that more information has been obtained on some patients than on others and a more comprehensive assessment is available on the later PMPs. Relatively complete psychometric information is available on the last 49 patients, but changes in mobility (a critical outcome measure) have been obtained only on the last 34 patients. Similarly, follow-up clinics have been introduced, but at this juncture a relatively limited database on follow-up (6-week and 6-month) has been collected and so the data will not be presented as part of this study.

9.4.5 *Salford PMP outcome evaluation: assessment materials*

Patients entering the PMP are assessed medically and psychosocially prior to the programme and various aspects of the assessment are repeated at the end, at 6 weeks or at 6 months. Resources so far have not permitted a complete reassessment for each patient at each stage.

Self-reported pain was assessed using a 100 mm horizontal Visual Analogue Scale (VAS) with 'anchor' phrases at either end of the line. Mobility was assessed by means of performance on three pieces of gymnasium equipment. Treadmill tolerance was assessed by asking patients to continue walking on the treadmill 'as long as they could'. Bike time is the time taken to cycle 0.5 km on an exercise bicycle and is therefore a measure of speed. The number of step-ups per minute was assessed with left leg leading (for 30 s) then right leg leading (for 30 s) on a set of gymnasium steps. The total score is presented in the results. Distress was evaluated using the MSPQ and the Modified Zung (described earlier).

Beliefs about pain were assessed using the Pain Locus of Control Questionnaire (PLC), a 20-item 4-point questionnaire yielding two scores: the A27 scale (cognitive control) and the B18 scale (pain responsibility), the first of which (A27) examines patients' beliefs about being able to affect their pain levels, and the second the extent to which they believe that managing pain should be the doctor's responsibility or something for which they have to take a degree of responsibility (B18). The PLC has been devised specifically for pain patients and so far has been standardised in the UK primarily for use with low back patients, although it has wider applicability (Main *et al.*, submitted for publication).

Finally, patients' appraisal of various aspects of the programme was assessed using the Self Evaluation Questionnaire (SEQ), a new instrument containing 27 VAS concerning different aspects of the programme. Since this instrument is as yet at an early stage of development, it will be discussed only briefly.

9.4.6 *Salford PMP evaluation: initial description*

The initial description of patients is presented in Table 9.3. The age and gender distribution is similar to back pain clinics. The patients are slightly older on average than patients attending routine orthopaedic out-patient clinics. A high level of chronicity is indicated by the time since their first onset of back pain (leading to consultation) and by the mean length of the present episode. The average number of specialists seen during the present episode prior to attending the present clinic is interesting. More than one sixth of the patients had already seen more than three specialists. As might be expected with this level of chronicity, a lot of time has been lost from work.

The major physical features are shown in Table 9.4. Only 20.6% of the group have had previous lumbar surgery. This is a smaller proportion than reported in previous studies in the UK (Waddell *et al.*, 1979) and may be a reflection of the decrease in the number of spinal operations for 'simple' back pain over the last decade. The values for lumbar flexion, straight leg raising and root compression signs are comparable to other reports (Waddell & Main, 1984).

Drug usage is displayed in Table 9.5. 40% of the patients are taking two or more drugs when initially seen, with 80.6% taking at least one drug. The

Table 9.3 Initial description of patients in Salford Pain Management Programme: demographic and occupational data

		Ranges of scores	
	Mean	*Min*	*Max*
Age (years)	44.09	25	59
Duration (years)	9.12	2	20
Present episode (months)	54.12	6	240
Work loss this episode (months)	34.17	0	72
Work loss in last year (weeks)	42.73	0	52
No. of specialists	3.08	1	9

Number of patients = 34: 22 female; 12 male.

Table 9.4 Initial description of patients in Salford PMP: physical characteristics ($n = 34$)

Previous lumbar surgery	None: 79.4%	One: 20.6%
Pain pattern	Intermittent: 12.1%	Continuous: 87.9%
Root compression signs	None: 83.9%	Present: 16.1%
Lumbar flexion	[a] 3.77 (1.5) cm	
Straight leg raising:		
left	[a] 69.86 (13.57)°	
right	[a] 71.61 (12.48)°	

[a] Values are means (SD).

Table 9.5 Initial description of patients: drug usage (% taking; $n = 34$)

	Not-taking	*Taking irregularly*	*Taking regularly*	*Exceeding maximum*
Narcotics	34.4	25.0	28.1	6.3
NSAIDs	77.4	6.5	16.1	0
Antidepressants	77.4	3.2	19.4	0
Tranquillisers	93.5	0	6.5	0
Night sedation	90.3	0	9.7	0

Number of drugs taken: none, 19.4%; 1, 41.9%; 2, 22.6%; > 2, 16.1%.

Table 9.6 Initial description of patients: pain, disability and mobility (n = 34)

	Mean	*Standard deviation*
Pain (now)	53.88	18.73
Pain (last week)	60.53	18.26
Treadmill tolerance	0.89 min	0.40 min
Bike time	1.41 min	0.61 min
Step-ups/min	19.44	5.30
Disability index (score out of 9)	5.30	2.30

Table 9.7 Initial description of patients: distress and beliefs about pain (n = 34)

	Mean	*Standard deviation*
Depressive symptoms (Modified Zung)	33.13	8.49
Somatic anxiety (MSPQ)	10.29	5.26
Cognitive control (PLC A27)	5.13	4.70
Pain responsibility (PLC B18)	5.97	2.76
Magnified illness presentation:		
inappropriate signs (score out of 7)	3.00	2.31
inappropriate symptoms (score out of 7)	2.82	1.53

most commonly taken drugs are narcotics which include codeine, dihydrocodeine, pentazocine, dextropropoxyphene, buprenorphine and morphine. The relationship between drug use and other features at initial presentation are discussed elsewhere in Chapter 8.

Initial levels of pain and mobility are shown in Table 9.6. These data were collected primarily for comparative purposes (pre- and post-PMP). The values on the disability index indicate a slightly higher level of disability than even secondary back referrals seen in out-patient orthopaedic clinics (Waddell & Main, 1984).

Patients' initial levels of distress are shown in Table 9.7. Both the levels of depressive symptomatology and of somatic anxiety are higher than in routine orthopaedic clinics. Their optimism about being able to control pain and degree of perceived responsibility for it are comparable to patients presenting initially in other clinics.

As might be expected given the chronicity and amount of previous treatment (not presented here), the patient group showed higher levels of magnified illness presentation (inappropriate signs and symptoms) than normal.

The relationship between values at the start of the PMP and other descriptive information was examined. Initial pain levels are correlated positively with age, use of non-steroidal anti-inflammatory agents, inappropriate symptoms and (negatively) with length of present episode. Mobility levels are all correlated with initial scores on the disability index. The only other clear relationships are between total amount of work loss and three of the psychometric variables. The relationship between locus of control (cognitive control and pain responsibility) and work loss is unsurprising, but the negative relationship between depressive symptoms and work loss is difficult to explain unless people would rather not be working! The relationship requires further analysis on a larger data set.

9.4.7 *Salford PMP: outcome evaluation – missing data*

Of the 34 patients initially selected and assessed, three dropped out after the first session and two after the second session. It was soon clear that four of these five patients were entirely unsuitable for the PMP (and had not in fact been assessed by the psychologists who run the group programme). The fifth dropout was acknowledged as a 'calculated risk' and of course it is necessary to take risks, as some patients improve far more than expected. There is not yet enough data to analyse the dropouts separately, but it is planned to do so.

Three patients were unable to complete all aspects of the mobility programme (one had angina, one was involved in a car accident, and one slipped on a kerb thus producing a new, but short-lived injury).

With these exceptions the data set is virtually complete and with the exception of the dropouts, (14.7% of the patients), the missing data would not seem to contain any systematic bias.

9.4.8 *Salford PMP: outcome evaluation – results*

Changes in pain, mobility, distress and beliefs about pain are shown in Table 9.8. Data shown were obtained immediately at the beginning of the programme and at the seventh (last) session. The number of patients in each comparison is shown, as are means, standard deviations, a paired-*T* value and significance level.

It can be seen that although pain levels remained essentially unchanged (in fact a small non-significant decrease), mobility on each of the three measures was significantly increased (decrease in bike time represents an increase in speed). The reduction in somatic anxiety (MSPQ) failed to

Table 9.8 Changes occurring following Salford Pain Management Programme

	n	*Prior to PMP*	*Post PMP*	*t*
Pain now (VAS: mms)	27	55.8 (19.0)	54.7 (27.2)	0.27
Pain last week (VAS: mms)	27	59.8 (18.2)	51.4 (25.2)	1.17
Step-ups/min	28	19.4 (5.2)	27.3 (9.0)	−5.67 **
Bike time (min for 0.5 km)	28	1.40 (0.63)	0.96 (0.49)	4.32 **
Treadmill tolerance (min)	25	0.88 (0.40)	2.38 (1.30)	−6.88 **
Somatic anxiety (MSPQ)	27	9.22 (4.44)	7.93 (5.12)	1.50
Depressive symptoms (Modified Zung)	27	31.5 (7.35)	27.4 (6.58)	2.94 *
Cognitive control (PLC A27)	27	5.67 (5.04)	9.93 (5.62)	−4.06 **
Pain responsibility (PLC B18)	27	6.19 (2.80)	9.30 (3.29)	−4.44 **

Values are means (SD). Level of significance: $p <$: * 0.007; ** 0.001.

reach significance, but there was a significant decrease in depressive symptoms. Patients also became significantly more optimistic about being able to manage back pain, and were willing to take more responsibility themselves for managing it.

9.4.9 *Salford PMP outcome evaluation: self-evaluation questionnaire*
Following the PMP the patients were posted the self-evaluation questionnaire (SEQ) (previously described). Changes in the PMP necessitated changes in the SEQ which asks a number of fairly specific evaluations of parts of the programme. The questionnaire was sent only to those who completed the PMP. The overall ratings are presented in Table 9.9.

Overall, the response to the PMP was extremely favourable and most of the patients responded positively about most aspects of the programme. The PMP seems to have been particularly important for increasing understanding (and correcting misunderstanding) about back pain, and in identifying and reducing stress but the value of being part of a group was considered particularly important.

Table 9.9 Salford Pain Management Programme: self-evaluation questionnaire

	Min	*Max*	*Mean*	*SD*
1. Overall Worth of PMP	35	100	76.96	10.38
2. Understanding low back pain	50	100	74.57	14.11
3. Identifying/reducing stress	35	100	68.82	17.97
4. Reducing low back pain	14	90	56.55	21.08
5. Boosting confidence	23	100	60.35	23.05
6. Reducing need for medicine	13	93	56.57	25.48
7. Reducing practical problems	20	92	58.04	19.66
8. Being part of a group	45	100	75.22	15.12

9.4.10 *Salford PMP: further analysis of the outcome data*

Influences on the outcome measures were examined using multiple regression analyses separately on each of the major outcome variables. Initial levels were used as covariates and various predictors of change were then identified. A detailed statistical appraisal is not presented since the data set is small, the analyses are exploratory and the observations are preliminary.

Pain levels at the end of the PMP were predicted by initial pain level (16.4%) but this represented a weaker relationship than that found on some of the other measures. Pain at outcome was explained in part by age, initial inappropriate symptomatology and degree of work loss over the previous year, but levels of prediction were small. Since the change in pain level was not itself significant, these relationships will not be discussed further.

In contrast, initial levels on each of the mobility measures explained 30–40% of the variance of the corresponding outcome measure. Initial bodily impairment (OPC) was negatively related to improvement on step-ups, while initial disability level had a small effect on improvement on both step-ups and exercise bike. Patients with 'simple' back pain (i.e. without radiation or root involvement) improved more on the treadmill tolerance test and on the exercise bike. Patients taking NSAIDs improved more on both treadmill and step-ups. Magnified illness presentation and distress bore little relationship to improvement in mobility. The strongest predictors were degree of work loss and receipt of benefits of various sorts. Work loss in the previous 12 months had a strong negative relationship with change on step-ups even when initial levels of physical impairment and disability had been taken into account. Total work loss since beginning of the present episode was a strong (negative) predictor of bike change.

Relatively little change was evident on somatic anxiety (MSPQ), but men changed more than women, and patients with intermittent back pain improved more than those with unremitting continuous back pain. There was a tendency for patients with 'simple' back pain to improve more on depressive symptomatology, but improvement in depression was unrelated to initial level of total bodily impairment. Patients taking narcotics did not improve as much as those who were not.

Changes in beliefs about the possibility of controlling pain were predicted by total bodily impairment, chronicity, and work loss over the previous 12 months (all negative relationships which appeared to be relatively independent of each other). Change in pain responsibility was less marked (although statistically significant) but may be affected (negatively) by age, litigation status and total work loss.

No further interpretation is offered at this stage of what is clearly a complex set of interrelationships.

9.5 **Discussion**

In this chapter an attempt has been made to clarify and define a number of aspects of the psychological concomitants of low back pain. During the last three decades numerous psychological instruments have been devised, but very few have been properly validated. The uncritical adoption of complex personality tests such as the MMPI has confused as much as it has clarified the nature of psychological factors. Its dubious validity and insensitivity has led to widely discrepant research findings; although it has at least made clinicians aware that a simple physical model is insufficient to explain either levels of disability or outcome of treatment.

The IBQ and the MPQ have had an important influence on the conceptualisation of pain problems, but are inherently limited by the uncertain relationship of the instruments themselves to their underlying conceptual structures. The problems with the IBQ result from failure to understand the difference between conceptual structures devised from (essentially) psychiatric models of illness, and empirically derived classifications or taxonomies. Lack of appreciation of how patients actually use questionnaires explains some of the problems with the MPQ. Later revisions may resolve some of the methodological limitations of the earlier instrument, but any test relying entirely on patients' use of pain vocabulary is bound to be inherently limited. (It may be worth retaining as a 'first stage' screening instrument, or as a measure of change in the individual patient for selecting items which the patient normally uses.)

Simple measures of distress (assessing depressive symptomatology and somatic awareness) have been developed for use in the UK and proved sensitive as screening instruments and (particularly depressive symptoms) as a measure of change. Although theoretically much less elaborate, such concepts at least allow the beginnings of a descriptive system. (Indeed it is far from clear that the MMPI consistently identifies anything more of real clinical value than simple distress, and it fails singularly to differentiate general distress from specific distress about back pain and its effects.)

The identification of inappropriate illness behaviour has represented a theoretical advance and certain aspects of such behaviour occurring during doctor–patient communication have been quantified. These inappropriate signs and symptoms have been shown to influence levels of disability and outcome of treatment. Such facets of illness behaviour may be extremely specific aspects of a wider phenomenon but would seem to have a value nonetheless. Identification and description of more general aspects of illness behaviour, such as consulting behaviour and compliance with treatment, await clarification and integration into a general clinical model, but it seems likely that the role of social, economic and occupational factors will be shown to be of considerable importance.

The expansion of the behavioural model into the 'learned helplessness' model has had important implications. It has led to the development of new questionnaires (such as the Pain Locus of Control Questionnaire) investigating specific beliefs about pain and its treatment. The shift in emphasis from general personality structure to specific beliefs may lead to a much clearer initial classification of patients, better selection for treatment, and progressive refinement of treatment procedures in the light of experience. Careful work is needed, however, before such claims can be substantiated.

Differences in assessment procedures and poor initial description of patients have made the evaluations of PMPs extremely difficult. The need to offer a proportion of patients rehabilitation programmes specifically designed to reduce distress and minimise invalidism has long been recognised. Heterogeneity of patients and differing objectives have made comparison of PMPs even more difficult.

The Salford PMP is the first programme of its type specifically for low back pain in the UK. Its emphasis on detailed initial assessment and selection has made it possible to offer a preliminary evaluation of such an approach to treatment. Results suggest that such a programme is effective in changing levels of mobility quite considerably, despite little change in reported levels of pain. There are concomitant changes, particularly in depressive symptomatology, in optimism about being able to manage pain, and in accepting more responsibility for it. Preliminary data suggest little change in objective physical characteristics or in magnified illness presentation.

Such beliefs do not appear to change either with simple conservative treatment, with an 'educational' back school, or with the simple passage of time (unless their back pain resolves). A number of correlates of change have been identified, but further data will be amassed before these are interpreted more fully. It appears at this stage that occupational and financial factors may turn out to be important predictors of change in mobility.

9.6 **Conclusion**

On the basis of a decade of research into psychological and clinical assessment, and 5 years' experience with PMPs for low back pain the following conclusion can be drawn.

(1) It is necessary to consider physical, psychological and socioeconomic factors in assessment of the chronic low back pain patient.

(2) Physical assessment should incorporate standardised procedures based on careful physical examination, a detailed clinical history (including the patient's response to previous treatment), present level of disability and an evaluation of current drug usage.

(3) Psychological assessment should contain assessment of the patients' distress, beliefs about treatment and magnified illness behaviour, and a thorough understanding of the nature and use of the materials is necessary to prevent inappropriate conclusions.

(4) In planning treatment programmes, far too much emphasis has been placed on the self-report of pain.

(5) The role of benefits (such as disability awards, invalidity awards and mobility allowance) and medico-legal issues have to be considered, together with an evaluation of occupational factors.

(6) Selection for Pain Management Programmes must be on the basis of identified distress or unnecessary disability with a willingness to consider a self-help approach (once it has been carefully explained). Selection must never be made on the basis of tests alone. A robust 'no nonsense' approach has already been tried with many of these patients in an effort to get them to improve their mobility. The topic of assuming more responsibility in increasing their mobility must be handled with sensitivity.

(7) From the time the patient is first contacted with an offer of an appointment for assessment, a potential treatment contract has been established, although further negotiation will take place. Much of the distress evident in chronic back patients is a consequence of bad medical management in the form of poor doctor-patient communication, unnecessary assessment and ineffectual treatment which does not match the promises which the patients have been given.

(8) Pain Management Programmes are no more a 'miracle cure' than anything else. They have a place as part of an interdisciplinary treatment service which offers sensible physical treatment when indicated, good doctor-patient communication and considers the person who has the low-back problem and not just their back.

Acknowledgements

We acknowledge the contribution of Dr C. Spanswick in developing the Pain Management Programme and with preparation of this manuscript.

References

Anderson, K. O., Bradley, L. A., Mc Daniel L. K., Young, L. D., Turner, R. A., Agudelo, C. A., Keefe, F. J., Pisko, E. J., Snyder, R. M. & Semble E. L. (1987). The assessment of pain in rheumatoid arthritis, *Arthritis and Rheumatism*, **30**, 36–43.

Andersson, G. B. J. (1987). Back schools. In: *The Lumbar Spine and Back Pain* (3rd Edn.), ed. M. I. V. Jayson. Churchill Livingstone, Edinburgh.

Atkinson, J. H., Kremer, E. F. & Ignelzi, R. J. (1982). Diffusion of pain language with affective disturbance confounds differential diagnosis, *Pain*, **12**, 375–84.

Baker, R., Hall, J. N. & Hutchinson, K. (1974). A token economy project with chronic schizophrenic patients, *British Journal of Psychiatry*, **124**, 367–84.

Beck, A. T. (1976). *Cognitive Therapy and the Emotional Disorders*. International Universities Press, New York.

Bond, M. R. (1971). The relation of pain to the Eysenck Personality Inventory, Cornell Medical Index and Whitley Index of Hypochondriasis, *British Journal of Psychiatry*, **119**, 671–8.

Bond, M. R. (1973). Personality studies in patients with pain secondary to organic disease, *Journal of Psychosomatic Research*, **17**, 257–63.

Bonica, J. J. & Fordyce W. E. (1974). Operant conditioning for chronic pain. In: *Recent Advances in Pain: Pathophysiology and Clinical Aspects*, ed. J. J. Bonica *et al.*. C. C. Thomas, Springfield, Illinois.

Carlsson, A. M. (1984). Assessment of chronic pain. II Problems in the selection in relevant questionnaire items for classification of pain and evaluation and prediction of therapeutic effects, *Pain*, **19**, 173–84.

Coppola, R. & Gracely, R. H. (1983). Where is the noise in SDT pain assessment? *Pain*, **17**, 257–66.

Costello, R. M., Hulsey, T. L., Schoenfeld, L. S. & Ramamurthy, S. (1987). P-A-I-N: a four cluster MMPI typology for chronic pain, *Pain*, **30**, 199–209.

Cummings, C., Evanski, P. M., Debendetti, M. J., Anderson, E. A. & Waugh, T. R. (1979). Use of the MMPI to predict outcome of treatment for chronic pain. In: *Advances in Pain Research and Therapy*, Vol. 3., ed. J. J. Bonica *et al.*, pp. 667–70. Raven Press, New York.

Dahlstrom, W. G. & Welsh, G. S. (1960). *An MMPI Handbook: a Guide to Use in Clinical Practice and Research*. University of Minnesota Press, Minneapolis.

Derogatis, L. R. (1977). *SCL-90 Administration, Scoring and Procedures Manual*. Johns Hopkins Press, Baltimore.

Eysenck, H. J. & Eysenck, S. B. G. (1975). *The Manual of the Eysenck Personality*

Questionnaire. Hodder and Stoughton, Sevenoaks.

Follick, M. J., Smith, T. W. & Ahern, D. (1985). The Sickness Impact Profile: A global measure of disability in chronic low back pain, *Pain*, **21**, 67–76.

Fordyce, W. E. (1976). *Behavioral Methods for Chronic Pain and Illness*. C. V. Mosby, St Louis.

Fordyce, W. E., Lansky, D., Calsyn, D. A., Skelton, J. L., Stolov, W. C. & Rock, D. L. (1984). Pain measurement and pain behaviour, *Pain*, **18**, 53–69.

Grossberg, J. M. & Grant, B. F. (1978). Clinical psychophysics: applications of ratio scaling and signal detection methods to research on pain, fear, drugs and medical decision making, *Psychological Bulletin*, **85**, 1154–76.

Hanvik, L. J. (1951). MMPI profiles of patients with low back pain, *Journal of Consulting and Clinical Psychology*, **15**, 350–53.

Hoffman, N. G. & Butcher, J. N. (1975). Clinical limitations of three MMPI short forms, *Journal of Consulting and Clinical Psychology*, **43**, 32–39.

Jensen, M. P., Karoly, P. & Braver, S. (1986). The measurement of clinical pain intensity: a comparison of six methods, *Pain*, **27**, 117–26.

Keefe, F. J. & Block, A. R. (1982). Development of an observation method for assessing pain behavior in chronic low back pain patients, *Behavior Therapy*, **13**, 363–75.

Lynn, B. & Perl, E. R. (1977). A comparison of four tests for assessing the pain sensitivity of different subjects and test areas, *Pain*, **3**, 353–65.

Main, C. J. (1983). The Modified Somatic Perception Questionnaire, *Journal of Psychosomatic Research*, **27**, 503–14.

Main, C. J. (1984). *Psychological Factors in Low-Back Pain*. PhD Thesis, University of Glasgow.

Main, C. J. Spanswick, C. C., Berger, S. M. & Wood, P. L. R. (1985). Low back pain, psychological disturbance and the health-care system. Paper presented at *1st International Conference on Low Back Pain*, Vienna.

Main, C. J. & Waddell, G. (1982). Chronic pain, distress and illness behaviour. In: *Clinical Psychology & Medicine: a Behavioral Perspective*, ed. C. J. Main. Plenum Press, New York.

Main, C. J. & Waddell, G. (1984). The detection of psychological abnormality in chronic low-back pain using four simple scales, *Current Concepts in Pain*, **2**, 10–15.

Main, C. J. & Waddell, G. (1987). Psychometric construction and validity of the Pilowsky Illness Behaviour Questionnaire in British patients with chronic low-back pain, *Pain*, **28**, 13–25.

Margolis, R. B., Tait, R. C. & Krause, S. J. (1986). A rating system for use with pain drawings, *Pain*, **24**, 57–65.

Melzack, R. (1975). The McGill pain questionnaire: major properties and scoring methods, *Pain*, **1**, 277–99.

Melzack, R. (1987). The short form McGill pain questionnaire, *Pain*, **30**, 191–7.

Naliboff, B. D., Cohen, M. J. & Yellen, A. M. (1982). Does the MMPI differentiate chronic illness from chronic pain? *Pain*, **13**, 333–41.

Ng, L. K. Y. (1981). New approaches to the treatment of chronic pain: a review of multidisciplinary pain clinics and pain centers, *NIDA Research Monograph Series* 36, Rockville, Maryland.

Nordin, M. (1985). Back schools. Paper presented at *1st International Conference on Low Back Pain*, Vienna.

OHE (1985). *Back Pain*. Office of Health Economics.

Pavlov, I. P. (1927). *Conditioned Reflexes*. Oxford University Press, London.

Pilowsky, I. & Spence, N. D. (1975). Patterns of illness behaviour in patients with intractable pain, *Journal of Psychosomatic Research*, **19**, 279–87.

Ransford, A. O., Cairns, O. & Mooney, V. (1976). The pain drawing as an aid to the psychologic evaluation of patients with low-back pain, *Spine*, **1**, 127–34.

Reading, A. E. (1980). A comparison of pain rating scales. *Journal of Psychosomatic Research*, **24**, 119–24.

Reading, A. E., Everitt, B. S. & Sledmere, C. M. (1982). The McGill pain questionnaire: a replication of its construction. *British Journal of Clinical Psychology*, **21**, 339–49.

Reesor, K. A. & Craig, K. D. (1988). Medically incongruent back pain: physical limitations, suffering and ineffective coping, *Pain*, **32**, 35–45.

Seligman, M. (1975). *Helplessness: on Depression, Development and Death*. Freeman, San Francisco.

Shacham, S., Dar, R. & Cleeland, C. S. (1984). The relationship of mood state to the severity of clinical pain, *Pain*, **18**, 187–97.

Skinner, B. F. (1938). *The Behavior of Organisms: an Experimental Analysis*. Appleton-Century, New York.

Smith, G. M., Egbert, L. D., Markowitz, R. A., Mosteller, F. & Beecher, H. K. (1966). An experimental pain method sensitive to morphine in man: the submaximum effort tourniquet technique, *Journal of Pharmacology and Experimental Therapeutics*, **154**, 324–32.

Sternbach, R. A. (1974). *Pain Patients: Traits and Treatment*. Academic Press, New York.

Strassberg, D. S., Reimherr, F. Ward, M., Russell, S. & Cole, A. (1981). The MMPI and chronic pain, *Journal of Consulting and Clinical Psychology*, **49**, 220–26.

Thorndike, E. L. (1931). *Human Learning*. Macmillan, New York.

Turk, D. C., Meichenbaum, D. & Genest, M. (1983). *Pain and Behavioral Medicine: a Cognitive-Behavioral perspective*. The Guilford Press, New York.

Turner, J. A. & Romano, J. (1984). Self-report screening measures for depression in chronic pain patients, *Journal of Clinical Psychology*, **40**, 909–13.

Von Baeyer C. L., Bergstrom, K. J., Brodwin, M. G. & Brodwin, S. K. (1983). Invalid use of pain drawings in psychological screening of back pain patients, *Pain*, **16**, 103–7.

Von Graffenfried, B., Adler, R., Klaus, A., Nuesch, E. & Spiegel, R. (1978). The influence of anxiety and pain sensitivity on experimental pain in man, *Pain*, **4**, 253–63.

Waddell, G. (1987). A new clinical model for the treatment of low back pain, *Spine*, **12**, 632–44.

Waddell, G., Bircher, M., Finlayson, D. & Main, C. J. (1984b). Symptoms and signs: physical disease or illness behaviour? *British Medical Journal*, **289**, 739–41.

Waddell, G., Kummell, E., Lotto, W. N., Graham, J. D., Hall, H. & McCulloch, J. A. (1979). Failed lumbar disc surgery and repeat surgery following industrial injuries, *Journal of Bone and Joint Surgery*, **61A**, 201–7.

Waddell, G., McCulloch, J. A., Kummell, E. & Venner, R. M. (1980). Nonorganic signs in low-back pain, *Spine*, **5**, 117–25.

Waddell, G. & Main, C. J. (1984). Assessment of severity in low back disorders, *Spine*, **9**, 204–8.

Waddell, G., Main, C. J., Morris, E. W., DiPaola, M. & Gray, I. C. M. (1984a). Chronic low back pain, psychological distress and illness behaviour, *Spine*, **9**, 209–13.

Waddell, G. Morris, E. W., DiPaola, M., Bircher, M. & Finlayson, D. (1986). A concept of illness as an improved basis for surgical decisions in low back disorders, *Spine*, **11**, 712–9.

Walsh, T. D. (1984). Letter to the editor, re 'Practical problems in pain measurement', *Pain*, **19**, 96–98.

Weisenberg, M., Wolf, Y., Mittwoch, T., Mikulincer, M. & Aviram, O. (1985). Subject versus experimenter control in the reaction to pain, *Pain*, 23, 187–200.

Wolpe, J. (1958). *Psychotherapy by Reciprocal Inhibition*. Stanford University Press, Stanford, California.

Wood, P. L. R. & Main, C. J. (1985). Changing influence of physical and psychological factors on subjective disability in low back pain. Paper presented at *1st International Conference on Low Back Pain*, Vienna.

Zung, W. W. K. (1965). The Self-Rating Depression Scale, *Archives of General Psychiatry*, **12**, 63–70.

Discussion

Frank (Northwick Park): When we gained a psychologist at Northwick Park I was desperate for some insight and I sent my first ten problems to her. What was interesting was that they fell straight into two groups which I hadn't appreciated. The first group were those with acute back pain, virtually all of whom had had a traumatic onset, and the second group were the patients most of us recognise as chronic pain syndromes with a clear behaviour, fat files, a psychiatric past history. The question is, does your programme differentiate between different groups of people in terms of their aetiological cause of the distress and can that understanding help you in a group situation rather than individually?

Main: That's a complex question. I think that one of the problems is that in 60% of patients presenting, even when they are being investigated in hospital, they are not given a clear diagnosis. So that's the first problem. There are all sorts of predictors of outcome and predictors of change. The difficulty for us is that statistically when you are looking at a wide ranging database, it gets more and more difficult to partial out the effects. This is why we have set up the collaborative studies with Gloucester and indeed we are setting one up with the Rehabilitation Unit in Helsinki at the moment. I cannot give you a simple answer except to say we select patients positively. We don't just select them because there is nothing else to do. The patients have reached the end of sensible medical treatment. Firstly I think we shoud recognise that there is an end to sensible medical treatment and stop over-treating patients. Secondly, we don't take them unless they are showing signs of unnecessary disability and unnecessary distress and we can persuade them to make some effort towards their own rehabilitation. I am hopeful that this new questionnaire that we have got will help us just a little bit. It's not a magic answer but perhaps will help us a little better in selecting patients because I am not sure yet exactly which patients benefit. A significant number of them do benefit a bit but until we have got these controlled comparisons with other sorts of treatment it is going to be difficult to answer your question intelligently.

Porter (Doncaster): Have you looked at the effect of financial gain on your outcome?

Main: No but that is some of the data that we have got that we are looking at. It certainly is our impression that if a patient is consulting us and shows very little in the way of physical limitation, and very little in the way of distress, you have got to look at the financial reasons for consulting the doctor. I think it is very important generally but if you are thinking of people who are actively involved in compensation claims we tend to have few of those. We prefer if possible for the claims to have been settled. We do take people who are in receipt of all sorts of mobility awards and disability allowances, but they have to convince us that they are prepared to take the risk of that being affected if they improve.

Nelson (Leeds): You have perhaps rightly criticised doctors for the way in which we manage back pain. Are you perhaps suggesting that doctors shouldn't see back pain patients at all, or should confine their role simply to excluding those diseases which in a sense are not to do with mechanical or other factors for which we have specific treatments, and at that point send them to a non medical person?

Main: I think there are two aspects to that. First of all you have got to ask what skills the doctor has got, and there will be a lot of skills, but they are primarily diagnostic and treating treatable disease. There is another function of the doctor which has been eroded I think over the last couple of centuries and that is that they have become over-specialised and appalling at communicating with patients.

Johns (Hastings): If you sort out the low back pain in these patients with personality problems do you then find they get something else to take its place?

Main: We don't know, but my guess would be not because they themselves have set up a support group and interestingly there are a number of support groups for back pain in Britain. One of the Liverpool groups is called PIP (People in Pain), our group is called POP (People overcoming Pain) and I think there is a difference.

10 *R. W. Porter, C. Ellingworth, T. Hughes and F. Trailescu*

Assessment of a 'School for Bravery' – modification of abnormal back pain behaviour

10.1 **Introduction**

Our individual response to illness is unique. From the stoical acceptance of pain with a reluctance to let illness interfere with normal life, to an exhibition of marked distress and the adoption of an invalid role, there is a whole spectrum of illness behaviour. The clinician treating patients with back pain is aware that identical pathology can produce a variable response. This not only adds fascination to the unravelling of back pain diagnoses but, when managing patients, it makes appreciation of the size of the behavioural component essential.

Fortunately, most patients attending a hospital back pain clinic present their history in a factual manner, and their abnormal signs are quite appropriate to the organic problem in the lumbar spine. Perhaps for as many as one in four their history and examination suggest a non-organic element compounding their problem; they may have one or two inappropriate signs that cannot be explained in terms of an organic pathology and which suggest they are exhibiting a degree of distress. Occasionally, however, there is a gross exhibition of abnormal pain behaviour, with many symptoms and signs quite inappropriate to a mechanical disorder in the lower back, and these patients are the most difficult for the clinician to treat.

One inappropriate item, in the history of a patient presenting with back pain, is a consistent failure to respond to therapeutic measures. Corsets, drugs, physiotherapy, injections, and the whole armamentarium of the pain clinic may have been tried, even hospital admission, all to no benefit. Generally the natural history of back pain is for a spontaneous resolution of symptoms with time, but when many therapies have been found wanting, one suspects there is a non-organic problem, particularly when this is supported by a host of inappropriate signs.

Such a patient is difficult to treat. It is probable that further active therapy will not only fail but will also compound the abnormal pain behaviour. Surgery will carry a particularly poor prognosis. What can be done?

10.2 The 'School for Bravery'

We have been encouraged to see a number of patients who are grossly disabled with abnormal back pain behaviour make a sudden and dramatic recovery in a programme called 'School for Bravery'. This programme was developed in Doncaster by Mrs J. Williams in 1982. Within a few weeks the patients have abandoned their disability and adopted a healthy life style. The programme attempts to modify abnormal pain behaviour. It is conducted in the physiotherapy department gymnasium, using exercise and fitness as a means of change.

Patients are asked to attend daily on an out-patient basis, for a 3-week period, and are thereafter gradually weaned from the programme, attending monthly and at six monthly intervals for a 4-year period.

Many of the patients are obviously distressed and angered because they cannot understand why there is no organic explanation for their pain. They find it difficult to accept that the cause of the pain is not in the back, and are unimpressed by descriptions of the complex pain mechanism. They often refuse psychological help. The 'School for Bravery' however is deliberatly non-confrontational. The patient's version of pain and disability is accepted and not challenged.

Before being accepted, patients are told that the programme is not intended to cure their pain but will concentrate on improving their fitness and overall disability. They are told this improvement will be obtained only by 'blood, sweat and tears'. This concept is readily accepted in the physiotherapy gymnasium setting. Patients attend daily wearing a track-suit, or shorts and trainers, which confirms the idea that hard work will be required to achieve fitness. They are assured that pain in itself is unimportant, but living a better life is a higher goal. They are offered a place in the programme, and challenged to find the necessary courage.

Assessment includes very little physical examination. Rather it concentrates on exploring the poor quality of life, and on searching for fresh goals in relation to their family, discarding analgesic drugs and walking aids, rediscovering old hobbies, recreational and social activities and future work. These are identified and documented, and the patient is assured that they are within their grasp.

During the early stages of the assessment, the patient's gait, posture and activity are recorded on video. This provides a useful objective record, but can also be used as positive feedback for the patient. A second video is taken after 2 weeks for comparison and this is used as part of a reward system.

The rewards of praise, attention, fun, the satisfaction of success and increasing ability, the promise of promotion to more demanding team games, are all motivation to change.

Many patients make a relatively sudden transition from illness to 'wellness' behaviour over a few sessions. Their recovery is a stimulus and challenge to others in the group. They attend daily for 3 weeks, and are reviewed once a month, and at 6-monthly follow-up for 4 years.

10.3 **Method of assessment of the behaviour modification programme**

We have attempted to evaluate the 'School for Bravery' by randomising a group of patients with abnormal pain behaviour, either to be discharged from the hospital department or to enter the programme and both groups were assessed more than 1 year later.

Patients with abnormal back pain behaviour were interviewed in a multidisciplinary clinic. They had first presented at an orthopaedic back pain clinic and had been fully investigated to exclude any treatable organic pathology. This involved extensive review of the previous records and where necessary further myelography and CT scans.

Each patient had also been examined independently by the anaesthetist in the pain clinic and by the psychologist, confirming grossly abnormal pain behaviour. They were not included in the study if they had evidence of psychiatric illness nor if they were involved in any litigation procedures.

The patient and their spouse were invited to attend a multidisciplinary conference with the:

orthopaedic surgeon
anaesthetist
psychologist
superintendent physiotherapist
pharmacist
patient's general practitioner.

The multidisciplinary team first reviewed the usually generous records and X-rays from different specialties within the hospital and from other hospitals: then the general practitioner presented the patient's history from childhood, the orthopaedic surgeon, the anaesthetist and the psychologist their current assessment of the patient, and the pharmacist and medical staff reviewed the degree of drug dependency.

The patient and their spouse were then invited to join the team, express their views about the current disability and confirm the salient features of the past history. The discussions were held in a relaxed, unhurried and informal atmosphere. Notes were not taken during the conference but a comprehensive record was subsequently written of the patient's history and disability, the objectives they would like to achieve if they were fit, and a consensus view of any factors in the environment that could be considered gainful and supportive of the invalid role, particularly the influence of the spouse.

Patients were excluded if there was a psychotic component to their illness behaviour or if they appeared satisfied with their invalid role and were showing no evidence of a desire to change. In addition, spouses were occasionally reluctant to give up their supportive role. Some patients were found to be receiving distinct financial benefits from their illness behaviour and they too were not included in the study. These patients were discharged after receiving a frank and full explanation of the views of the team.

All the patients were asked to adopt a more active lifestyle, to discard props that enhanced their invalidism and slowly to reduce or discard their analgesic drugs at once.

The patient and their spouse were asked to retire and the team confirmed with the physiotherapist that the patient was a suitable candidate to be offered the programme for modification of abnormal pain behaviour. The patient was then randomised to be discharged or offered the 'School for Bravery'.

Twenty one patients seen in the multidisciplinary clinic were considered suitable for the programme to modify abnormal pain behaviour. None of them were seen again by the multidisciplinary team but 12 months or more after the multidisciplinary conference, the 21 patients in the study were asked to attend for reassessment by an independent examiner.

10.4 **Results**

Of the 21 patients considered suitable for the study, ten were enrolled in the 'School for Bravery' (Table 10.1) and eleven controls were discharged (Table 10.2). Twelve months or more after the conference seven patients from the 'School for Bravery' and ten controls who had been previously discharged were seen for review. Of the seven patients reviewed 12 months or more after the conference who had been in the 'School for Bravery', four were still well. The three who were still adopting the invalid role had originally failed to change from their illness behaviour during the 'School for Bravery' programme. Patients 2 and 5 both discharged themselves and the latter was found to have litigation pending. Patient 8 did not improve during the 'School for Bravery' programme and eventually she visited an orthopaedic surgeon in another district and had a private spinal fusion. She was bitterly disappointed that this operation was not successful.

Of the eleven control patients who had been originally discharged, ten

Table 10.1 Patients admitted to 'School for Bravery'

Patient no.	*Sex*	*Age (yrs)*	*On admission to the study*		*Immediately after leaving 'School for Bravery' comments by physiotherapist*	*Months after conference when patient was assessed*	*No. of symptoms*	*No. of inappropriate signs*	*Still adopting invalid role*
			No. of symptoms	*No. of inappropriate signs*					
1	M	37	15	5	Success	28	0	0	No
2	F	41	9	6	Discharged herself before completing course	19	2	3	Yes
3	M	57	17	7	Success	51	9	1	No
4	F	42	11	3	Success	34	2	0	No
5	M	41	16	8	Discharged himself Discovered to have litigation pending	17	13	8	Yes
6	M	43	12	8	Success	22	0	1	No
7	M	36	15	4	Partial response		Did not attend		
8	F	66	16	5	Did not improve	22	11	8	Yes
9	F	68	12	5	Partial response		Died		
10	M	42	12	3	Success		Did not attend		

Table 10.2 Controls (discharged)

Patient no.	*Sex*	*Age (yrs)*	*On admission to study*		*Follow-up (months)*	*Number of symptoms*	*Number of inappropriate signs*	*Still adopting invalid role*
			Number of symptoms	*Number of inappropriate signs*				
11	F	62	10	3	23	8	2	Yes
12	M	46	8	3	32	8	6	Yes
13	M	51	16	7	50	11	7	Yes
14	M	61	17	8	28	15	8	Yes
15	F	50	19	4	28	17	5	Yes
16	M	59	15	8	45	10	7	Yes
17	M	51	16	4	34	16	6	Yes
18	F	47	10	6	24	11	6	Yes
19	M	36	6	6	33	7	6	Yes
20	M	51	9	3	36	7	4	Yes
21	M	37	7	6		Did not attend		

attended for review and all ten were still adopting an invalid role over 23 months later.

We conclude that full assessment of the patients in the control group with a lengthy conference and advice about life-style and drug dependency was not enough to persuade those patients to modify their abnormal pain behaviour. Perhaps this was not surprising because patients were only accepted for this study who had thick medical files and a long history of invalidity. By contrast, however, the 'School for Bravery' was effective in the rehabilitation of some of the small groups of patients allocated to the programme and their recovery was maintained for at least a year.

10.5 **Conclusions**

Abnormal illness behaviour is notoriously difficult to modify. We can recognise it and postulate causative mechanisms, but it is not easy to correct. Patients who adopt an invalid role with back pain can be disabled for years and many may never regain a normal lifestyle. We suggest that a time-consuming review of the problem, a multidisciplinary approach, a frank explanation of what is meant by a pain behavioural problem with no organic basis and exhortation to change a lifestyle is not sufficient to produce rehabilitation.

We have found that a restoration of function is possible with a programme challenging the patient to ignore pain and use exercise as a means of achieving fitness. Both patient and spouse need to understand the new approach. The importance of pain is actively devalued. They are told that recovery lies in their hands alone. They are encouraged to take pride in their progress; improvement is rewarded by praise. Group activity is challenging and an incentive to recovery. A video before and after rehabilitation serves as an objective measure of progress, provides the reward of self-satisfaction, and is a strong incentive not to return to illness behaviour.

There is no therapeutic counselling, but a listening ear often proves helpful and, once function is restored, tensions, anxieties and family problems are often resolved.

We have evidence that this type of programme can be successful in modifying abnormal pain behaviour, producing sudden and dramatic rehabilitation which does not revert in the short term.

Discussion

Morrison (Swindon): You say initially that patients are assessed in a multidisciplinary clinic. Earlier you said they were individually assessed by an orthopod and an anaesthetist. When they come do they sit in front of this group of people?

Porter: These particular 21 patients were all seen in my clinic first of all. I then referred them to the Pain Clinic for a second medical opinion to see what the anaesthetist thought. He wasn't treating them, just assessing them, and then they went to a psychologist who had a look at them to make sure we were not missing a psychotic problem, then if the three of us agreed they were suitable for the programme, they then came up to a multidisciplinary clinic where there were the three of us, the physiotherapist, the pharmacist, the GP with all his notes, which were amazing sometimes, and the spouse, and we sat round for an hour and discussed the problem. Half of them we discharged, but that concentration on their problem made no difference to the 11 that were untreated.

Stanley (Sheffield): In the gym, is there more than one person with a back problem at the same time? Do they interact with each other?

Porter: Very much. Our patients come in at different stages, so someone who has responded is a challenge to someone who is just begining, so they do encourage one another a lot.

Nelson (Leeds): How do you decide who you are going to put on the programme?

Porter: Well, excluding this particular study of these 21 patients, they have to have the inappropriate symptoms and signs. They have to have been investigated very thoroughly to be sure that at least I don't think there is any organic problem to be treated. I mean, while I could possibly be missing something that could be treated, it is my view that I cannot do anything more for them. They haven't got a psychotic problem, they haven't got any litigation, and they haven't got any monetary gain by being ill.

Nelson (Leeds): So you are saying that at some stage in the management of a patient you decide that conventional methods of treatment are no longer relevant.

Porter: Yes.

Nelson (Leeds): How do you come to that sort of decision, is it emotional, or is it scientific?

Porter: It's a little bit emotional I suppose, but I try to make it as scientific as possible. I use Gordon Waddell's signs and I look for eight distinct inappropriate signs in back pain. If a patient has two, well then that doesn't excite me very much, but if they have got four or five I feel that is quite important. For this particular group I think they all had more than four.

Nelson (Leeds): So if you saw a patient for the first time with a 6-month history and he had eight of these signs you would put them into this programme?

Porter: Well yes, I probably would, but first I would send them to our pain clinic, then they would go to the psychologist, and then back to me, so that usually takes about 2 months and if we are not seeing any progress and we all agree, they would go into the programme.

Mulholland (Nottingham): The group that responded, but then dropped back, was there any difference between those and the group who remained good?

Porter: There is an unstable period after the initial response, there was an example when this chap looked 15 years younger and he went down to the pub and they said 'By jove, I wouldn't have recognised you' and the women started taking an interest in him and his wife got very upset and there was a great family squabble and he reverted very quickly. So they are very unstable for a while but once the physiotherapists have discharged them we see them 12 months and 2 years later and they haven't gone back. I think once they get through the unstable phase they vow that they will never be like that again. They can't really believe they got so bad.

Maddocks (Birmingham): How much freedom did the physiotherapists have in determining the programme?

Porter: They had complete freedom. It was nothing to do with me but it is not any physiotherapist who does it. They are sensible people and they use their own intelligence. The reward is very important. It is important to have a physiotherapist who can reward the patient by understanding and encouraging them. It is not treatment as such but is called fitness, exercise and reward.

11 *A. K. Burton and C. J. M. Getty,*

Differences between 'orthopaedic' and 'osteopathic' patients with low back trouble – implications for selecting patients for rehabilitation

11.1 Introduction

Musculoskeletal disorders of the lower back remain a major clinical challenge despite much recent research. These conditions generally are referred to under the term 'low back pain', but we prefer the use of the phrase 'low back trouble' to emphasise that the subject of concern is lumbar dysfunction rather than one of its symptoms. Management strategies for low back trouble (LBT) might be divided conveniently into 'therapeutic' and 'rehabilitation' categories; the former being generally concerned with alleviating the symptoms of an acute or sub-acute spell, whilst the latter is directed more to altering the natural history in the chronic or recurrent case. Ideally the two approaches should be employed in tandem, but because resources and time are frequently scarce there is a need to identify patients for whom additional rehabilitation measures are indicated.

The clinical diagnosis of LBT is frequently uncertain; however, it is commonly held that most episodes will resolve within 2 months. Against this background it has been shown that recurrence rates are high (Lloyd & Troup, 1983) and, furthermore, the question has been raised as to whether chronic cases are such from the beginning, or whether they result from inadequate management of a previous spell (Wood & Baddley, 1980). For some, LBT will be an isolated experience; others will suffer varying degrees of recurrence (Burton, 1987) and it is these patients for whom rehabilitation measures are needed if the socioeconomic impact of LBT is to be reduced. The importance of homogenous groups in clinical trials has been emphasised by Weber & Burton (1986) among others, and for this reason it is necessary to identify those subjects at risk of chronic/recurrent trouble in order to develop effective rehabilitation programmes.

Most clinical trials, whether of therapeutic or rehabilitation regimes, are reported from hospital departments which, whilst convenient for researchers, ignores that possibility that these patients may not be representative of LBT sufferers in general; those attending 'office'-based practices may display a different natural history and the findings from trials in one environment may not be applicable to the other.

This study was performed to test the hypothesis that there are significant clinical differences between LBT patients attending orthopaedic out-patients and those presenting to osteopaths, and that the two groups follow a dissimilar course over the following year.

An osteopathic practice, rather than a general practice, was used to represent the office-practice environment on the basis of availability; it has been shown previously that LBT patients attending osteopaths are similar in nature to those attending general medical practice (Burton, 1981).

11.2 **Method**

A sequential sample of LBT patients attending an orthopaedic out-patient department and an osteopathic practice were considered for the study. Those eligible had a primary complaint of back and/or sciatic pain, but those with inflammatory, neoplastic and metabolic disorders were excluded. Of the 113 patients eligible, four refused their consent (two orthopaedic two osteopathic), thus the results are based on 109 patients (54 orthopaedic, 55 osteopathic).

At consultation each patient completed a questionnaire concerning the history and nature of their current spell, and of any previous LBT. They were also required to provide pain drawings which were scored for psychological influences (Ransford *et al.*, 1976). A structured examination was performed which included assessment of 'inappropriate illness behaviour' (Waddell *et al.*, 1984), and a battery of pain-provoking clinical tests (PPCTs); all examinations were performed by the same person. The PPCTs (described in Table 11.1) comprised a number of procedures in general use which are thought to be related to the biomechanical function of the spine. There was no attempt in this study to ascribe diagnostic significance to these tests, rather they were used simply as indicators of spinal dysfunction. Follow-up was by self-administered questionnaires, completed at 1 month, 3 months and 1 year, to record the course of symptoms according to forced-choice check-lists.

Statistical analysis was by means of the chi-square test for 2 × 2 contingency tables; the null hypothesis was rejected at the 5% level of significance.

11.3 **Results**

The orthopaedic patients comprised 29 males and 25 females with a mean age of 41.1 years (standard deviation 11.7), whilst the osteopathic patients

Table 11.1 Pain-provoking clinical tests used in the clinical examination; production of pain in back or leg = positive

Name	*Description*
PSOAS	Passive resisted hip flexion (knee bent) with patient sitting [anterior lumbar muscle involvement]
FEMBAK	Passive flexion of both kness with patient prone [passive lumbar extension impaired]
TENDER	Mid-line or paraspinal tenderness on moderate digital pressure (prone) [posterior soft-tissue involvement]
SLR	Straight leg raise (supine) – only positive if pain provoked at less than 50°
SLRQUALT	Ankle dorsiflexion and medial hip rotation just below the point of pain on SLR [qualifying tests for SLR indicating increased root tension]
NOSITUP	Attempt to sit up from supine with knees and hips flexed [abdominal muscle function]
FLXADD	Passive flexion/adduction of hip (supine) [sacro-iliac joint involvement]

comprised 30 males and 25 females with a mean age of 42.5 years (standard deviation 11.5).

Thirty-four orthopaedic and 35 osteopathic patients claimed a previous history of LBT, and the orthopaedic patients were the more likely to have experienced a duration in excess of two months for that spell (Table 11.2). The mean age at onset of LBT was 33.5 years (standard deviation 11.5) for the orthopaedic, and 36.9 years (standard deviation 12.7) for the osteo-

Table 11.2 Duration of the first and current spell of LBT in orthopaedic and osteopathic patients

	Orthopaedic		*Osteopathic*
First spell:			
<2 months	16		28
>2 months	18		7
		(χ^2 = 6.7; p = <0.01)	
Current spell:			
<2 months	16		35
>2 months	38		20
		(χ^2 = 11.3; p = <0.001)	

Table 11.3 Psychological assessments of orthopaedic and osteopathic patients at consultation

	Orthopaedic (54)		*Osteopathic (55)*
Pain drawing score:			
Positive: 3+	10		2
Negative: <3	44		53
		($\chi^2 = 4.7$; $p = <0.05$)	
Inappropriate illness behaviour:			
Positive	7		0
Negative	47		55
		($\chi^2 = 5.6$; $p = <0.05$)	

A pain drawing score of 3 or more (positive) indicates poor psychometrics; a positive classification of inappropriate illness behaviour was determined by the presence of multiple signs.

pathic patients. When the presenting spell was considered, the orthopaedic patients were more likely to report a history of over 2 months (Table 11.2).

The psychological assessments showed significant differences between the two groups. Almost 20% of orthopaedic patients had a pain drawing score of three or more, compared with less than 5% of osteopathic patients. Multiple signs of inappropriate illness behaviour were recorded for 13% of orthopaedic patients, but none of the osteopathic patients showed more than one such sign. These differences were statistically significant (Table 11.3).

Virtually all patients in both groups reported back pain at consultation. However, a significantly greater proportion of orthopaedic patients reported sciatic radiation (70%, $n = 38$) compared with osteopathic patients (49%, $n = 27$); $\chi^2_1 = 4.3$, $p < 0.05$. There was no significant difference between the groups in respect of pain quality (constant or intermittent); 57% of orthopaedic and 51% of osteopathic patients reported constant pain. Most of the patients stated that the severity of their symptoms varied, either during each day (18 orthopaedic, 35 osteopathic) or from day or day (21 orthopaedic, 15 osteopathic). This difference between the groups was statistically significant ($\chi^2_1 = 4.2$, $p < 0.05$); the osteopathic patients were more likely to be able to find relief each day.

The results for the PPCTs are given in Table 11.4; for the sake of brevity, only the numbers with a positive (pain provocation) result are shown. All tests, with the exception of lumbar tenderness, were more frequently positive in the orthopaedic group, but only for FEMBAK, SLR and SLR-QUALT were the differences significant.

Figure 11.1 gives bar-charts for the proportion of patients in each of

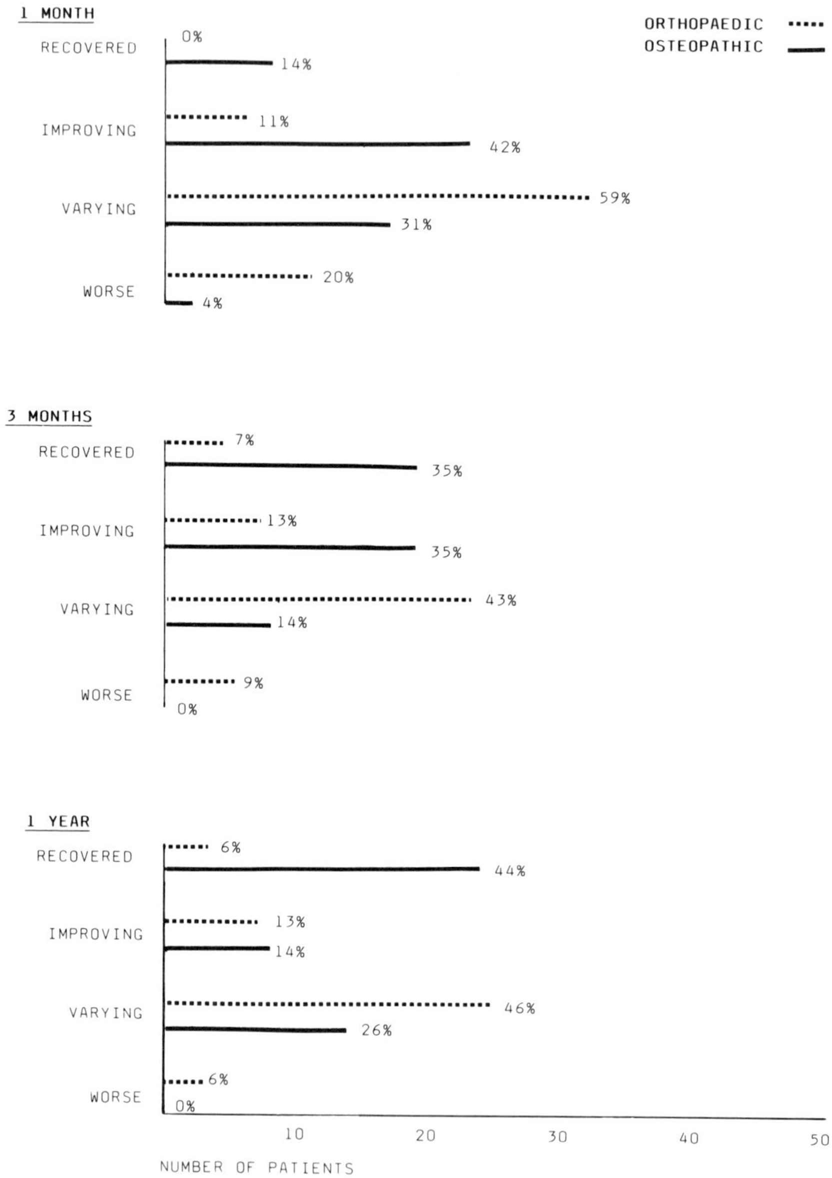

Fig 11.1 Bar charts for symptomatic status at three assessment points for (———) orthopaedic and (———) osteopathic patients

Table 11.4 Positive responses to pain-provoking clinical tests in orthopaedic and osteopathic patients

	Orthopaedic (n = 54)	*Osteopathic (n = 55)*	χ^2	*P*
PSOAS	11	9	0.3	n.s.
FEMBAK	35	25	4.1	<0.05
TENDER	39	44	0.9	n.s.
SLR	22	10	6.7	<0.01
SLRQUALT	20	8	7.5	<0.05
NOSITUP	34	28	1.6	n.s.
FLXADD	20	16	0.7	n.s.

χ^2 tests were performed on 2 × 2 contingency tables – the above figures are positive results, the remainder for each patient group were negative for each test.

four symptom groupings, at the three assessment points. These groups for symptomatic progress were defined from subjective responses as follows: *recovered* = symptom free, *improving* = progressive improvement, *varying* = fluctuating course, *worse* = symptoms increased. There was a consistent trend for the osteopathic patients to report improvement at each assessment point, whereas the orthopaedic patients more frequently reported a fluctuating or deteriorating course. Table 11.5 shows the results for outcome at 1 year, expressed as *recovered* or *persisting symptoms*; a significantly higher proportion of osteopathic patients were without symptoms; 44% compared with 6% of orthopaedic patients ($p < 0.001$).

11.4 **Discussion**

The two patient groups studied here were very similar in respect of age and sex. Because the precise diagnosis in LBT is difficult to determine objectively, no attempt was made to ascribe patients to diagnostic categories, rather the concern was whether there were clinically evident dif-

Table 11.5 Outcome at 1-year expressed as *recovered* or *persisting symptoms*

	Orthopaedic (n = 54)	*Osteopathic (n = 55)*
Recovered	3	24
Persisting symptoms	37	25
	$\chi_1^2 = 16.0$; d.f. = 1; $p < 0.001$	

ferences between the groups of patients (related to their natural histories) which might indicate differing management needs.

The results of this study have shown that patients attending the two types of practice were not homogenous in a number of respects. The orthopaedic patients had a slightly lower mean age for the first onset of LBT, more frequently reported a chronic history for their present spell, were more likely to display evidence of a psychological component, and had a greater likelihood of presenting with sciatic symptoms associated with signs of nerve root tension. This clinical profile might reasonably be expected to indicate chronicity, and indeed most of the orthopaedic patients fared considerably less well than the osteopathic patients during the follow-up year. A somewhat disappointing number of patients failed to return their 1-year assessment forms; these patients were not, however, significantly different from the others for any of the variables studied.

We do not conclude that these results demonstrate any superiority of osteopathic management of LBT, but rather that the patients attending the orthopaedic department fall into a different category in the sense that their complaints are generally more chronic, and as such they require more intensive rehabilitation. Whilst the hospital environment is probably the more suitable for development and testing of rehabilitation programmes, the measures which are successful there will not necessarily be referrable to 'office-practice' environments.

This study has indicated general associations between clinical presentation and the subsequent course of the disorders. Further work is required, in both hospital and office practice, to define specific selection criteria for those patients/conditions requiring rehabilitation measures in order to overcome a chronic natural history.

References

Burton, A. K. (1981). Back pain in osteopathic practice, *Rheumatology and Rehabilitation*, **20**, 239–46.

Burton, A. K. (1987). Patterns of lumbar sagittal mobility and their predictive value in the natural history of back and sciatic pain. PhD Thesis, CNAA/ Huddersfield Polytechnic.

Lloyd, D. C. E. F. & Troup, J. D. G. (1983). Recurrent back pain and its prediction, *Journal of the Society of Occupational Medicine*, **33**, 66–74.

Ransford, A. O. *et al.* (1976). The pain drawing as an aid to the psychologic evaluation of patients with low-back pain, *Spine*, **1**, 127–34.

Waddell, G. Bircher, M., Finlayson, G. & Main, C. J. (1984). Symptoms and signs: physical disease or illness behaviour? *British Medical Journal*, **289**, 739–41.

Weber, H. & Burton, K. (1986). Rational treatment of low back trouble? *Clinical Biomechanics*, **1**, 160–7.

Wood, P. H. N. & Baddley, E. M. (1980). Epidemiology of back pain. In: *The Lumbar Spine and Back Pain*, ed. M. I. V. Jayson, pp. 29–55. Pitman, London.

Discussion

Cook (Birmingham): Do you not feel that the pain provocation tests which you describe have any diagnostic value?

Burton: They may well do but that wasn't the point of including them in this particular study. The specific diagnostic value of the flexion and adduction test is that it stresses the sacro-iliac joint and some people think that it locates their problem in the sacro-iliac joint rather than the lumbo-sacral joint.

Cook (Birmingham): And the psoas test?

Burton: The psoas test is a test which again is positive if there is pain on resisted use of the psoas.

Nelson (Leeds): Are you saying that the trial supported by the MRC which compared hospital and chiropractic treatment is in fact invalid?

Burton: I suspect that the patients in the two groups are different types of people with different conditions who may respond differently over a period of time, so I have my concerns about the study you are talking about.

Frank (Northwick Park): Can I respond to that. The whole point of randomised allocation is that whatever your strengths or weaknesses when you present, you are randomly put into either group, so that becomes irrelevant. In the MRC study if you go to a chiropractor you have an even or equal chance of going to treatment from a chiropractor or for hospital treatment. If you presented to a hospital you would have an equal chance of being treated either in the hospital group or by the chiropractor, so your warts on presentation are equally distributed by either mode of practice.

12 *D. J. Baker, P. B. Pynsent and J. C. T. Fairbank*

The Oswestry Disability Index revisited: its reliability, repeatability and validity, and a comparison with the St Thomas's Disability Index

12.1 Introduction

The assessment of disability is an important component of the clinical evaluation of all musculoskeletal complaints. Back pain is no exception. A disability score can be used in the initial assessment of the patient, to monitor the response to treatment and to measure the effects of rehabilitation (Deyo & Diehl, 1983; Lehmann, 1983; Million *et al.*, 1982; Saunders; 1985). Waddell in his writing has made much of the psychological aspect of back pain disability and tried to distinguish disability due to organic disease from that perceived by the patient (e.g. Waddell & Main, 1984). In practice it is often difficult to make this distinction, and an overall disability assessment remains a very important component of clinical decision making.

The Oswestry Disability Index (ODI), described by one us (Fairbank *et al.*, 1980), has found favour both as a clinical and as a research tool. This paper presents some data concerning our experience with the questionnaire. A slight modification of the original questionnaire was made by the Medical Research Council (MRC) in their multicentre trial of chiropractic treatment of back pain (Meade *et al.*, 1986). We have adopted this modified version. Comparisons of the ODI with a computer-based version of the questionnaire and with the St Thomas's Back Pain Questionnaire, described by Roland & Morris (1983), are presented here. We also review the internal consistency of the questionnaire. The computer-based version is part of a detailed questionnaire which we have developed for patients with back pain (Pynsent & Fairbank, 1989). As a result of this study we suggest some minor modifications to the original version of the questionnaire, and confirm its repeatability and reliability in both paper and computer format.

12.2 **The Oswestry Disability Index**

The index is based on ten stem questions, each followed by six mutually exclusive items, covering aspects of daily living which may be affected by back pain. These are: (1) present pain; (2) washing and dressing; (3) lifting; (4) walking; (5) sitting; (6) standing; (7) sleeping; (8) sex life; (9) social life; (10) travelling. The questionnaire in its current form is shown in Appendix 12.1. This wording is the same as the original questionnaire (Fairbank *et al.*, 1980), except in Section 1, where 'pain' was originally assessed in terms of analgesic intake. This presented difficulties for patients who were not using analgesics, so the MRC version now uses items framed in terms of 'pain severity'. The version of the questionnaire used in the computer interview is identical with the paper interview, except in section 3, dealing with lifting, where the wording is too long to be fitted on a single screen. The adaptation is shown in Appendix 12.2.

In each section, the six mutually exclusive items are scored from 0–5, and expressed as a percentage:

$$\text{ODI} = \frac{\text{Sum of items scored}}{\text{Sum of sections answered}} \times 20\%$$

If all the questions are answered, the scores for each stem question may be added together (maximum 50), and expressed as a percentage by doubling this total. If any of the questions are omitted, then the percentage disability score is scaled appropriately out of the maximum possible score for the question groups that have been answered. If more than one answer is given in each question group, then the higher score is added to the total.

12.3 **Method**

The MRC modified ODI was given either on paper, or presented in the computer interview as 10 or 11 consecutive screens (a second screen may be used for section 3, depending on the answer given to the first screen). The St Thomas's questionnaire was also presented as part of the computer interview with no significant alteration to the original wording. A single screen was given to each of the 24 questions (which have a yes/no answer) and a single screen to the pain thermometer (a vertical linear analogue pain scale). The St Thomas' score was converted to a percentage to aid comparison with the ODI and included the answer to the pain thermometer. The patients were studied in three groups:

Group A: 104 patients completed the computer and paper versions of the ODI on the same attendance to the clinic. There was randomisation as to whether the patient completed the computer or paper version first. These patients presented as new referrals to an orthopaedic outpatient clinic.

Group B: A total of 250 patients completed the computer version of the ODI and the St Thomas's questionnaire (both presented on the computer) at a single interview. This group includes the 104 patients in Group A.

Group C: The paper interview was completed by 237 patients on each of their attendances at the clinic, a total of 673 questionnaires. This group includes the 104 patients in Group A.

12.4 **Results**

12.4.1 *Oswestry Disability Index – paper questionnaire vs Oswestry Disability Index computer questionnaire*

In Group A, there was a close correlation between the scores of the two methods of presenting the questionnaire ($r = 0.89$; $p < 0.0001$). There was no significant difference in the computer or written scores that could be ascribed to whether the paper or computer method was used first. The correlation serves to establish that the computer interview method of presenting the questionnaire does not materially alter the overall score ob-

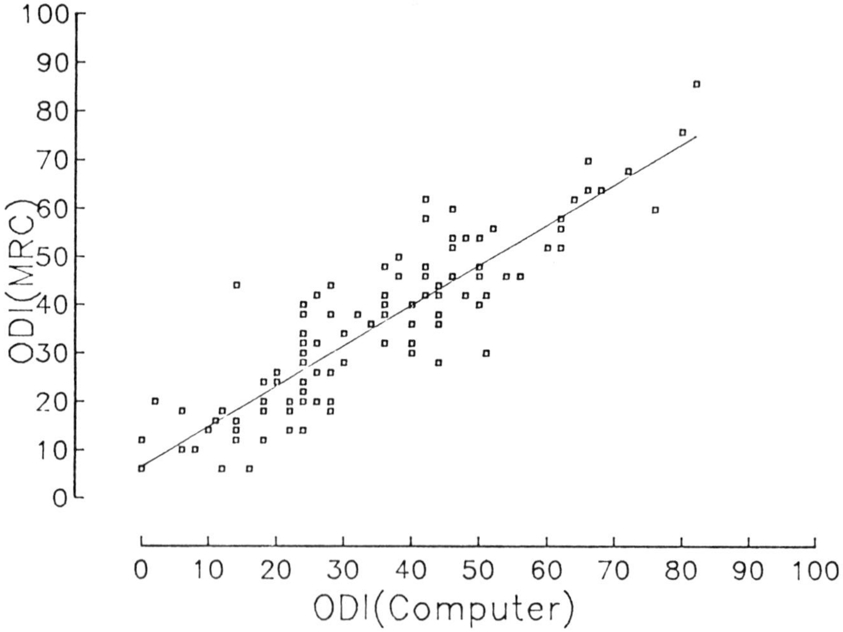

Fig 12.1 Scattergram of Oswestry Disability Index Scores obtained by the paper and computer methods on the same patients on the same day

tained by a conventional paper presentation of the questionnaire. It also confirms the high repeatability of the questionnaire, as was found in the original study. A scattergram of the scores can be seen in Figure 12.1.

12.4.2 *Oswestry Disability Index (computer questionnaire) vs St Thomas's questionnaire (computer questionnaire)*

In Group B, a scattergram of the ODI and St Thomas's score is shown in Figure 12.2. This shows that there is a non-linear relationship between the two scores. The St Thomas's score tends to score higher in the lower ranges of disability than the ODI, and thus reaches a maximum before the ODI.

12.4.3 *Internal consistency of Oswestry Disability Index*

The ODI is aimed at providing an opportunity for the patient to give personal assessment of the effect of their symptoms on their activities of daily living. The various syndromes of back pain may affect patients in different ways and, in general, it would be expected that the various components of the ODI would contribute to the overall score differently. The distribution of answers was analysed in group C. The mean score of each section

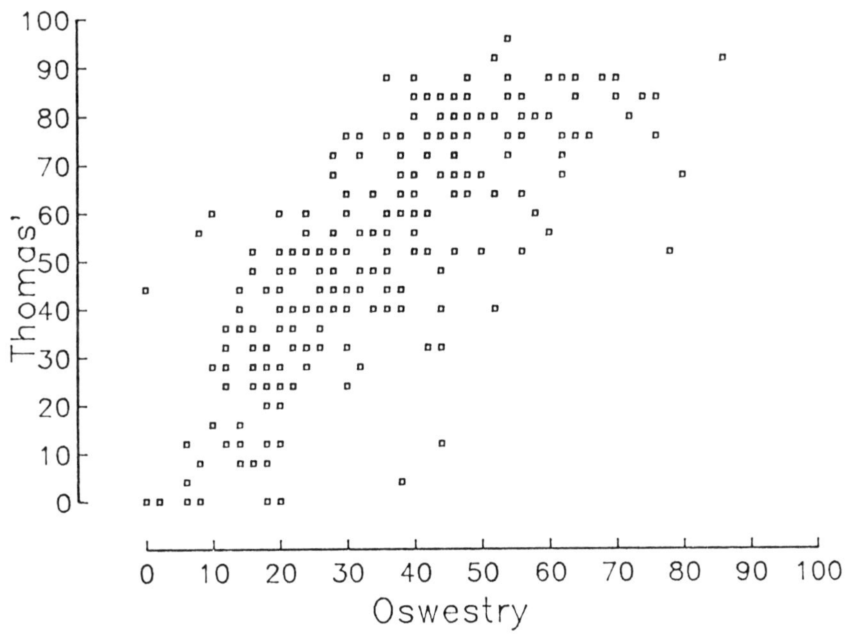

Fig 12.2 Scattergram of Oswestry Disability Index *versus* the St Thomas's questionnaire on the same day.

Table 12.1 Mean and standard deviation of the scores of each section in the paper and computer versions of the Oswestry Disability Index in Group A

Section	*Oswestry Disability Index*			
	MRC version		*Computer version*	
	Mean	*SD*	*Mean*	*SD*
1. Pain	1.93	1.19	2.03	1.04
2. Care	0.97	1.07	1.19	1.18
3. Lifting	2.74	1.33†	2.85	1.43
4. Walk	1.48	1.39	1.66	1.39
5. Sit	1.91	1.16	1.98	1.17
6. Stand	2.08	1.38	2.13	1.46
7. Sleep	1.21	0.96	1.31	1.13
8. Sex	1.42	1.49‡	1.37	1.52
9. Social	1.94	1.43	1.96	1.39
10. Travel	1.64	1.38	1.79	1.48
Total	1.73	0.91	1.77	0.86

n = 104 except: † n = 103; ‡ n = 91. In both these cases, some patients did not complete this section of the paper questionnaire.

is given for the paper and computer versions of the questionnaire in Table 12.1.

The way in which patients answered the ODI is illustrated by histograms in Figure 12.3. The distribution of how pain intensity was answered shows that there is a tendency for the patients to favour the mid-range of the available choice. The results illustrate that the computer interview shows a higher pain score than the paper interview. The personal care section shows a marked skew to the left suggesting that, in this sample of patients, the ability to maintain personal care themselves has not been unduly influenced by their back troubles.

Lifting is frequently painful in back pain patients; this is reflected by the highest mean score of all the sections. The paper version gives an even distribution but the computer version shows a sharp dip at the centre (Item 2), which reflects the change in wording necessary to adapt the question to the computer screen format. In spite of this, the mean paper score was 2.74, and the mean computer score was 2.85, an insignificant difference. It is clear that some modification of the computer version is needed, if it is to reflect the score derived from the paper version in the same patient.

The distribution of the answers to walking disability is irregular in both versions of the questionnaire. It seems that few patients are comfortable walking for ½ mile, whilst many can only manage ¼ mile. The questionnaire could probably be improved if Item 2 was changed to ¼ mile, and

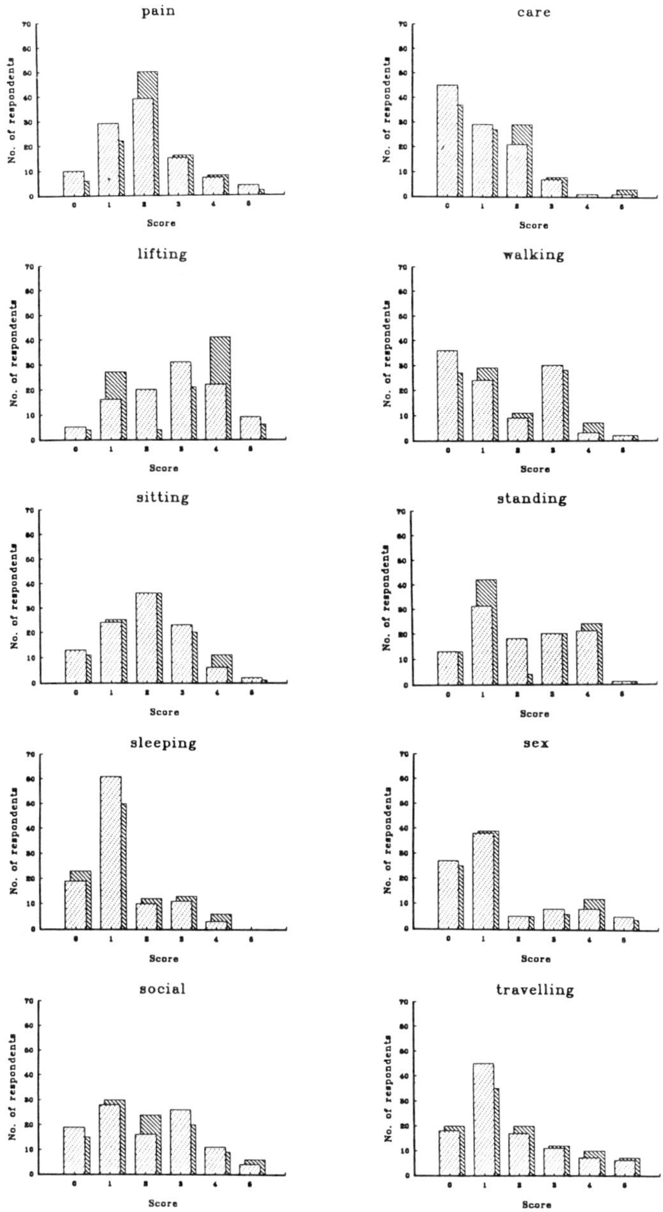

Fig 12.3 The histograms in this figure show the frequency of patient scoring for each section in the two versions of the Oswestry Disability Index. The bar charts are derived from data in group A. The ordinate refers to number of responses to each item, marked 0–5 along the abscissa. The results obtained from the 'paper' ODI is seen 'in front of' the results from the 'computer' ODI

Item 3 to 100 yards. The responses to sitting, standing and social life were reasonably distributed, whereas sleeping and travelling tended not to be important contributors to the final disability score of these patients.

Back pain affects sex life although patients may be unwilling to admit to this aspect of their disability; 13 patients were not prepared to complete the paper version of the sex section, but they were all prepared to answer the computer version (ten scored Item 0, two Item 1, and one Item 5). This may reflect the well-known tendency of patients to be prepared to answer personal questions in a computer format which they are not prepared to answer on a paper questionnaire or in response to direct questioning by a clinician.

12.5 **Discussion**

The St Thomas's questionnaire was designed originally for use in general practice, whilst the ODI was developed for the assessment of chronic back pain patients. It is of importance to realise that the scoring of these two questionnaires will be affected by the population being examined, this is clearly illustrated by Figure 12.2. The St Thomas's questionnaire is more sensitive than the ODI in detecting change when the patient has a minor disability but is less sensitive when there is severe self-rated disability. This should be taken into account when choosing which of these two questionnaires to use for monitoring patients with back pain.

The St Thomas's Questionnaire has transferred to the computer format without difficulty, although we have made no effort to validate this version against the original. Our experience with the ODI would suggest that there is unlikely to be any serious difference between the two versions. The patients found the format of this questionnaire very acceptable.

The ODI has transferred in abbreviated form to the computer well, although this study has revealed some difficulties in the assessment of lifting and walking (sections 3 and 4). The computer and paper versions produce comparable overall scores. The wording of Section 4 (walking) seems unsatisfactory, and will require modification in both forms, whereas the lifting section will require substantial rewording only in the computer version.

We have demonstrated that the Oswestry questionnaire remains a useful and reliable tool for the self-assessment of patients with back pain disability. It is to be expected that there will be a wide variation of self-assessed disability within each section, as different syndromes of back pain will affect different individuals in different ways. In fact it might be hoped that patterns of answers are related to recognisable syndromes. Also, because the patients represent a selected group of back-pain sufferers referred to a specialist's hospital clinic, the distributions may well differ from the total population of sufferers.

It is important to appreciate that whilst the outside observer may be surprised as to how an individual patient may assess their own disability (both too high or too low), its main value lies in its ability to detect change in self-rated disability. It is, after all, the patients' own assessment of their disability which will ultimately affect the result of any rehabilitation given for this enigmatic complaint.

Acknowledgements

We acknowledge the support of the Medical Research Council, the Health Promotion Research Trust and South Birmingham Health Authority in the preparation of this work.

References

Deyo, R. A. & Diehl, A. K. (1983). Measuring physical and psychosocial function in patients with low-back pain, *Spine*, **8**, 635–42.

Fairbank, J. C. T., Davies, J., Couper, J. & O'Brien, J. P. (1980). Oswestry disability questionnaire, *Physiotherapy*, **66**, 271–3.

Lehmann, T. R. (1983). A low-back rating scale, *Spine*, **8**, 308–15.

Meade, T. W. *et al.* (Report of a working group) (1986). Comparison of chiropractic and hospital outpatient management of low back pain: a feasibility study, *Journal of Epidemiology & Community Health*, **40**, 12–17.

Million, R., Hall, W., Haarvik Nilson, K., Baker, R. D. & Jayson, M. I. V. (1982). Assessment of the progress of the back pain patient, *Spine*, **7**, 204–12.

Pynsent, P. B. & Fairbank, J. C. T. (1989). Computer interview system for patients with back pain, *Journal of Biomedical Engineering*, **11**, 25–9.

Roland, M. O. & Morris, R. (1983). A study of the natural history of back pain 1. Development of a reliable and sensitive measure of disability in low back pain, *Spine*, **8**, 141–4.

Saunders, S. H. (1985). Cross-validation of the back pain classification scale with chronic, intractable pain patients, *Pain*, **22**, 271–7.

Waddell, G. & Main, C. J. (1984). Assessment of severity in low-back disorders, *Spine*, **9**, 204–8.

Discussion

Clarke (Bath): How long does it actually take to fill up the questionnaire?

Fairbank: A couple of minutes.

Troup (Liverpool): You said that in answer to one of your questions about sex, they had an opportunity on the computer to open up their hearts which means that you weren't asking 'yes/no' questions.

Fairbank: No, this is a stem with 6 alternative choices. Of the 50 patients we actually assessed in this particular way, I think 13 did not complete the paper questionnaire whereas all but one completed the computer version. They were identically worded, as it happened.

Roland (Cambridge): Can I ask you about your analysis when you relate the scores on the individual sub-scales to the overall score? I don't quite understand what you are looking for. Presumably if a question correlates 100 per cent with the total score you would throw it out, but equally if it didn't correlate at all, then what would that mean? How do you actually interpret all those figures?

Fairbank: Well, the idea of doing that was to see whether or not there were any of the sub-sections which were clearly not correlating at all with the overall score. In other words, if there was a question which a group of patients were answering quite differently in a way that they were answering the main body of the questions, then perhaps that question was misworded or inappropriate for this type of assessment. In fact, we had already been through this in Oswestry and had filtered out the questions which were inappropriate and I think really what we were saying was that looking at this data again, the fit between the individual sub-sections and the overall scores were really quite good.

Appendix 12.1 **Revised Oswestry Disability Questionnaire (with MRC modification)**

This questionnaire has been designed to give us information as to how your back or leg pain has affected your ability to manage in everyday life. Please answer every section and mark in in each section ONLY THE ONE BOX which applies to you. We realise you may consider that two of the statements in any one section relate to you, but PLEASE JUST MARK THE BOX WHICH MOST CLEARLY DESCRIBES YOUR PROBLEM.

•Section 1 - pain intensity

☐ I have no pain at the moment.
☐ The pain is very mild at the moment.
☐ The pain is moderate at the moment.
☐ The pain is fairly severe at the moment.
☐ The pain is very severe at the moment.
☐ The pain is the worst imaginable at the moment.

•Section 2 - Personal care (washing, dressing etc.)

☐ I can look after myself normally without causing extra pain.
☐ I can look after myself normally but it causes extra pain.
☐ It is painful to look after myself and I am slow and careful.
☐ need some help but manage most of my personal care.
☐ I need help every day in most aspects of self care.
☐ I do not get dressed, wash with difficulty and stay in bed.

•Section 3 - lifting

☐ I can lift heavy weights without extra pain.
☐ I can lift heavy weights but it gives extra pain.
☐ Pain prevents me from lifting heavy weights off the floor but I can manage if they are conveniently placed e.g. on a table.
☐ Pain prevents me from lifting heavy weights but I can manage light to medium weights if they are conveniently positioned.
☐ I can only lift only very light weights.
☐ I cannot lift or carry anything at all

•Section 4 - walking

☐ Pain does not prevent me walking any distance.
☐ Pain prevents me walking more than 1 mile.
☐ Pain prevents me walking more than 1/2 mile.
☐ Pain prevents me walking more than 1/4 mile.
☐ I can only walk using a stick or crutches.
☐ I am in bed most of the time and have to crawl to the toilet.

•Section 5 - Sitting

☐ I can sit in any chair as long as I like.
☐ I can sit in my favourite chair as long as I like.
☐ Pain prevents me from sitting for more than 1 hour.
☐ Pain prevents me from sitting for more than 1/2 hour.
☐ Pain prevents me from sitting for more than 10 minutes.
☐ Pain prevents me from sitting at all.

•Section 6 - Standing

☐ I can stand as long as like without extra pain.
☐ I can stand as long as I want but it gives me extra pain.
☐ Pain prevents me from standing for more than 1 hour.
☐ Pain prevents me from standing for more than 30 minutes.
☐ Pain prevents me from standing for more than 10 minutes.
☐ Pain prevents me from standing at all.

•Section 7 - Sleeping

☐ My sleep is never disturbed by pain.
☐ My sleep is occasionally disturbed by pain.
☐ Because of pain I have less than 6 hours sleep.
☐ Because of pain I have less than 4 hours sleep.
☐ Because of pain I have less than 2 hours sleep.
☐ Pain prevents me from sleeping at all.

•Section 8 - Sex life (if applicable)

☐ My sex life is normal and causes no extra pain.
☐ My sex life is normal and causes some extra pain.
☐ My sex life is nearly normal but is very painful.
☐ My sex life is severely restricted by pain.
☐ My sex life is nearly absent because of pain.
☐ Pain prevents any sex life at all.

•Section 9 - Social life

☐ My social life is normal and causes me no extra pain.
☐ My social life is normal but increases the degree of pain.
☐ Pain has no significant effect on my social life apart from limiting my more energetic interests e.g. sport, etc.

- ☐ Pain has restricted my social life and I do not go out as often.
- ☐ Pain has restricted my social life to home.
- ☐ I have no social life because of pain.

•Section 10 - Travelling

- ☐I can travel anywhere without pain.
- ☐I can travel anywhere but it gives me extra pain.
- ☐Pain is bad but I manage journeys over two hours.
- ☐Pain restricts me to journeys of less than 1 hour.
- ☐Pain restricts me to short journeys under 30 minutes.
- ☐Pain prevents me from travelling except to receive treatment.

Appendix 12.2 **Oswestry Disability Questionnaire adapted for computer-based interview**

On the computer screen there is a yellow box next to each item which can be " marked" with a light pen. The soft ware is arranged so that although a response can be altered, only one answer is stored when the patient moves on to the next screen of the questionnaire. The letter/number at the start of each section refers to the screen number of the computer questionnaire.

• Which box describes your pain at the moment?

- ☐ none
- ☐ very mild pain
- ☐ moderate pain
- ☐ fairly severe pain
- ☐ very severe pain
- ☐ worst imaginable pain

• Can you wash and dress yourself?

- ☐ normally
- ☐ normally but with extra pain
- ☐ I am slow and careful
- ☐ with help for some things
- ☐ with help for everything
- ☐ not at all

• Can you lift weights from the floor as follows

- ☐ heavy weights
- ☐ medium weights
- ☐ light weights
- ☐ none at all

- Can you lift weights if conveniently placed (e.g. on a table) as follows:

  ☐ heavy weights
  ☐ medium weights
  ☐ light weights
  ☐ none at all

- My back pain allows me to walk

  ☐ any distance
  ☐ about 1 mile
  ☐ about half a mile
  ☐ about a quarter of a mile
  ☐ only with a stick or crutches
  ☐ not at all

- My back pain allows me to sit

  ☐ as long as I like
  ☐ as long as I like in my best chair
  ☐ about 1 hour
  ☐ about half an hour
  ☐ only 10 minutes or so
  ☐ not at all

- My back pain allows me to stand

  ☐ as long as I like
  ☐ as long as I like,but causes pain
  ☐ for about 1 hour
  ☐ for about 30 minutes
  ☐ for about 10 minutes
  ☐ not at all

- My back pain allows me to sleep

  ☐ as much as I want
  ☐ wakes me sometimes
  ☐ only 6hrs or so
  ☐ only 4hrs or so
  ☐ only 2hrs or so
  ☐ not at all

- My back pain interferes with my sex life

  ☐ not at all
  ☐ with some extra pain
  ☐ with much extra pain

☐ and is severely restricted
☐ and is nearly absent
☐ and is totally absent

• My back pain interferes with my social life

☐ not at all
☐ not at all, but causes extra pain
☐ not at all, but stops my sports etc
☐ and often stops me going out
☐ and keeps me at home
☐ and has totally stopped it

• My back pain restricts my travelling

☐ not at all
☐ not at all, but causes extra pain
☐ to about 2 hour journeys
☐ to about 1 hour journeys
☐ to about 30 minute journeys
☐ to journeys for treatment only

13 *N. Hudson-Cook, K. Tomes-Nicholson and A. Breen*

A revised Oswestry Disability Questionnaire

13.1 Introduction

The ability of patients to describe their symptoms has not always been accepted as a useful vehicle for monitoring progress under treatment; nor indeed for establishing baselines. Traditionally, pain has been 'assessed' using words that describe intensity, frequency, duration, location and cause. (Beaver *et al.*, 1977; Kagan & Masheter, 1978; Storlite, 1978; Jacox, 1979). While useful for ascertaining the patient's perception of pain, the descriptions are difficult to quantify and are generally unreliable across patient populations. Yet there remains an overwhelming preference for patient verbalisation of pain intensity as the best measure of treatment success (Hilgard, 1969; Lee *et al.*, 1975; Campbell & Long 1976; Spoerel *et al.*, 1976; Evans & Kagan, 1986).

13.2 Literature review

Although attempts have been made to quantify verbalisation (Glover *et al.*, 1974; Toomey *et al.*, 1977), accepting a verbal report without question seems noticeably incomplete (Fordyce, 1976). Therefore, the investigation of pain mechanisms in a clinical setting is dependent upon the availability of reliable and sensitive methods of assessing the patient's pain experience. The objectives of these measurements include not only contributions towards a working diagnosis, but the wherewithal to monitor progress over time in the presence of controlling factors, including treatment (Reading, 1984). A number of scales for measuring patient function have recently been described and validated for use in low back pain (LBP) (Fairbank *et al.*, 1980; Deyo & Diehl, 1983; Lehmann *et al.*, 1983; Roland & Morris, 1983; Rock *et al.*, 1984; Waddell & Main, 1984; Follick *et al.*, 1985). Because therapy for LBP is directed towards restoring function as well as reducing pain, functional status is a crucial outcome to measure both for clinical care and therapeutic research. Unfortunately, there are few studies which compare the various scales currently available, and little to guide investigators in choosing suitable measures (Deyo, 1986). Two major forms of clinical measurement in existence are rating scales and questionnaire methods.

13.2.1 *Rating scales*

In one form or another, rating scales are the most commonly reported measure in clinical pain research. These vary according to the nature and number of the anchor points supplied – numbers, words or the presentation of visual analogue lines.

In a series of investigations of Visual Analogue Scales (VAS), patients ratings have been found to be highly reproducible (Scott & Huskisson, 1976). Revill *et al.* (1976) studied the reproducibility of VAS ratings and found that the subjects were able reliably to report a pain experience distant in time on different occasions and attributed this to memory, since further testing showed subjects were able to remember accurately the position of the mark over a 24-hour period. Using normal volunteers, Dixon & Bird (1981) found reproducibility to vary according to the position of the scale, with the most difficult region to produce being the centre of the line. Scott *et al.* (1977) reported the use of VAS to measure pain of children with chronic polyarthritis. However, there was substantial concern about the validity and practicality of this monodimensional approach in the out-patient clinical setting (Kagan & Evans, 1986).

Verbal ratings of pain were compared with VAS by Ohnhaus & Adler (1975) in a study of drug potency. The authors concluded that VAS 'reflected more precisely what a patient actually feels' than the Verbal Response Scales (VRS), even though their statistical analysis of the data supported the VRS. Joyce *et al.* (1975) also compared the two scales in a study of 74 patients, where VAS was found to be accurate, as reliable and more sensitive. The distribution of responses on VRS and VAS has been examined. Scott & Huskisson (1976) assumed that the tendency for VAS to yield more uniform distributions was a reflection of their superior sensitivity; Kremer *et al.* (1981) presented patients with visual analogue, numerical and verbal scales and found a consistent preference for the verbal scale. Leavitt (1987) used a recently introduced verbal pain measure which was accurate in differentiating patients with LBP from persons simulating pain. The results underscored the impression that people who have pain to build upon will be more difficult to identify when they simulate pain, than people who engage in the process when they are pain free. Although physiological function may be as important as physical function in understanding a patient's distress or monitoring therapeutic response, it is infrequently assessed.

Psychological tests such as the Minnesota Multiphasic Personality Inventory (MMPI) have some prognostic value (Dennis *et al.*, 1980), but its length makes it cumbersome for repeated or large scale use. The ability of the MMPI to predict or differentiate treatment outcome has been questioned (Sternbach *et al.*, 1973; Seres & Newman, 1976; Cladwell & Chase, 1977; Roberts & Reinhardt, 1980).

13.2.2 *Pain and disability questionnaires*

More sophisticated attempts to quantify patient's perception of pain have taken the form of a 'pain questionnaire' (Melzack, 1975; Fox & Melzack, 1976; Chen & Hwang, 1977; Devaul & Zisook, 1978; Hachen, 1978). While the data appear objective, the focus remains singly on the patient's verbalisation to the exclusion of other pain behaviours and physical status (Evans & Kagan, 1986).

Disability may be measured either by asking the patient to record his or her own (self-rated) disability, or by asking a professional (e.g. doctor or physiotherapist) to measure the disability on what may be deemed to be more objective criteria. In general, the scores of self-rated measures of disability have correlated more closely with other subjective measures than with objective criteria (Friedsam & Martin, 1963; Bergner *et al.*, 1976; Denniston & Jette, 1980). Unfortunately, however, it was shown that observers of different professional disciplines used different criteria for assessing performance (Kelman & Wilner, 1962). Moreover, perception of change in an individual's performance was related to the observer's role in the treatment and assessment situation (Tamerin, 1964). Garrad & Bennett (1971) also stated that when using an interview technique in research surveys, the problems of interviewer variation and interviewer drift arose. Cannell & Marquis (1967) and Cannell *et al.* (1969) have shown that the quantity and quality of data obtained in health surveys depended on the attitude and manner of the interviewer and the style of interviewing. Cochrane *et al.* (1951), Fletcher (1963) and Rose (1964) first stressed how difficult it was for a physician to ask clinical questions in a strictly standardised manner. This introduced individual bias which must be avoided if results of questions are to be used for comparative purposes. They emphasised the need to treat a medical question like any other test and evaluate its reproducibility, validity and discriminative power; they studied these attributes in administered questionnaires.

The self-administered questionnaire avoided any interviewer bias and ensured uniformity of presentation. The combination of 'closed' questions and self-administration gave a reliable format (Collen *et al.*, 1969). There was evidence to suggest that this type of questionnaire was comparable with data collected by an interviewer and was up to twice as effective in uncovering certain problems (Stouffer, 1950; Metzner & Mann, 1952; Young, 1972). Collen *et al.* (1969) also stated that in addition to being an economical way to record large amounts of historical information, self-administered questionnaires have the great advantage of permitting some standardisation, uniformity of administration, and minimal interviewer bias. Nevertheless, physicians are often wary of patient self-reports of function, and prefer more 'objective' measures of disease severity in their own evaluations (Deyo & Diehl, 1983). Some physicians were sceptical about the validity of questionnaire techniques in general (Petersdorf & Feinstein, 1981). Deyo & Diehl (1983) also stated that in other studies questionnaire reliability had often been somewhat lower for respondents of low educational status than for better educated respondents.

There have been other attempts to systematise the language of pain, in which language has been related to the seriousness of the condition (Agnew & Merskey, 1976), the location of pain (Klein & Brown, 1967) and whether or not of psychiatric origin (Devine & Merskey, 1965). The McGill Pain Questionnaire represented an attempt to systematise further verbal description by imposing an organisation on the pain adjectives, thereby achieving the objectives of quantifying the language of pain (Reading, 1984).

13.3 **The Oswestry low back pain Disability Questionnaire**

The Oswestry low back pain Disability Questionnaire (ODQ) was developed as a self-administered questionnaire (Fairbank *et al.*, 1980). The questionnaire was divided into ten sections selected from a series of experimental questionnaires designed for the assessment of limitations in various activities of daily living. The chosen sections were those found to be most relevant to the problems suffered by people with low back pain.

Each section contained six statements, with each statement describing a greater degree of difficulty in the activity than the preceding statement. The questionnaire was printed on pink paper, since it had been found that forms on coloured paper were more readily acceptable to patients (Eastwood, 1940). The disability score gleaned from the questionnaire was used as a guide to the patient's treatment programme, and ensured that the important aspects of the patient's disability were recorded on patient's notes. The authors also suggested that later changes in the score could be used in monitoring subsequent progress of the patient through treatment.

In February 1983, a feasibility study was conducted of a randomised controlled trial of chiropractic and hospital out-patient management, for low back pain of mechanical origin, by the working group of the MRC

Epidemiology and Medical Care Unit (Meade *et al.*, 1986). The feasibility study used the ODQ as a measure of progress. One of the questions raised in the study was the apparently low level of pain/disability indicated by the ODQ. It was suggested that a pain reflected by an ODQ score of 25% expressed over a long period of time, was of sufficient concern to the patient to justify seeking treatment.

Nevertheless, the low initial scores, (around 30%) observed both in chiropractic and hospital out-patients, low compliance in some sections and the inverse relationship between questionnaire sensitivity and the numbers required to detect small, but statistically significant differences between populations of such patients, suggested that a revision of this already useful questionnaire could be constructive.

13.4 **Method**

In the revised questionnaire, the structure remained the same, being a ten-section, one-page document with provision for recording personal details (name, age, duration of pain, etc.). The questionnaire retained a brief introduction designed to acquaint the patient with the study requirements (Appendix 13.1).

For this study, all of the sections were altered, and one section omitted entirely (Section 8: Sex life disability) due to poor compliance. A new section was created dealing with the patient's interpretation of their own changing pain pattern, entitled 'Changing Degree of Pain'. The criteria which had to be met before introduction of a patient to the study were the same as those used in the original Oswestry study; *viz*.

(1) The patient must not have been treated by the chiropractor on any previous occasion.

(2) The patient must present with a complaint of low back pain. This could be localised or radiating.

(3) The chiropractor must establish that the cause of the pain originates in the low back and be, as far as possible, judged to be of a mechanical nature. The low back was taken to include the lumbar spine and sacro-iliac joints.

(4) The patient must be judged by the chiropractor to be of sufficient intellectual ability to understand and complete the questionnaire without assistance.

13.4.1 *Classification of chronicity*

Once accepted into the study the patient was categorised as being acute or chronic at the time of presentation. If the complaint duration was less than

1 month, this classed the patient as being acute. More than this was classed as chronic. Once categorised, the patient received a package from the clinic receptionist. The procedure was explained, both by the receptionist and the introductory letter enclosed in the package, which also contained the questionnaires and stamp-addressed envelopes.

13.4.2 *Schedule for acute patients*

Twenty-four acute patients received a package containing four questionnaires with stamp-addressed envelopes. The first questionnaire was completed on the first day of treatment and thereafter at weekly intervals over the following 3 weeks.

13.4.3 *Schedule for chronic patients*

Twenty-two chronic patients received a package containing eight questionnaires with stamp-addressed envelopes. The first questionnaire was completed on the first day of treatment, and the second on the next day. Subsequent questionnaires were completed twice each week, on consecutive days. This was to record the changes in disability between 2 consecutive days, as in the original study.

The treatment schedule was not related to the dates of questionnaire completion – this was done to minimise disruption to the clinics. However, emphasis was placed on the questionnaire completion dates. These dates were indicated on the package envelope and agreed with the clinics before the patient received any documents. The patients were told in the introductory letter to post each questionnaire on the completion date so that they would not refer to previous questionnaires when filling in subsequent over.

13.4.4 *Statistical analysis*

Completed questionnaires were analysed using an Apple Macintosh microcomputer and the Statworks software. Analysis was similar to that carried out in the original study and included changes in mean disability scores for the acute patient group, test–retest reliability, and internal consistency for the chronic patient group. Both groups were included in the assessment of section-by-section compliance and sensitivity. In terms of scoring, there were ten sections each containing six statements describing increasing disability in one daily activity. The minimum score was 0, the maximum 5. By doubling the disability score it was possible to express the result as a percentage for example:

$$\frac{16 \text{ (total scored)}}{50 \text{ (total possible score)}} \times 100 = 32\%$$

13.5 **Results**

13.5.1 *Mean disability scores*

This test was performed on the acute patient group only. Figure 13.1 shows the percentage reduction in disability over a 3-week period which was significant at the 1% level. The initial mean disability score was 47.6%.

13.5.2 *Test-retest reliability*

The reliability of the questionnaire was determined using a test–retest reliability correlation. The scores of the sections in a questionnaire may be expected to remain equal if the level of disability has not changed. On a group of patients with chronic low back pain, where it is expected that their response to treatment will be slower than in the acute group, questionnaires were completed on 2 consecutive days. The correlation coefficient of paired

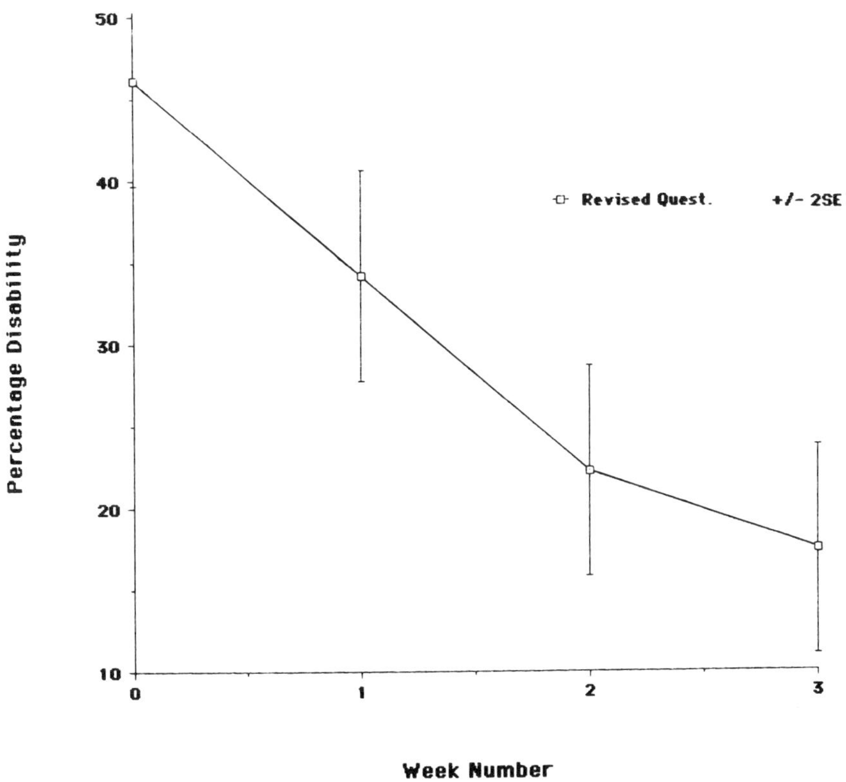

Fig 13.1 Mean disability score in 22 patients with acute low back pain (≤1 month's duration) measured over a 3-week period: scores on the revised Questionnaire, bars indicate ±2SE

forms was 0.88 which was statistically significant ($p < 0.001$, Wilcoxon Signed Rank Test).

13.5.3 *Internal consistency*

The Original Oswestry Questionnaire was tested for internal consistency (Fairbank *et al.*, 1980) to determine the consistency of the relationship between the pain section and the other sections grouped in threes. Revised questionnaires completed by the 22 chronic patients in this study were analysed similarly, for comparison. This involved dividing the patients into groups determined by their overall section scores. The results are shown in Figures 13.2 to 13.4.

It can be seen that in this population, two sections (Sleep and Social Life) did not closely relate to pain.

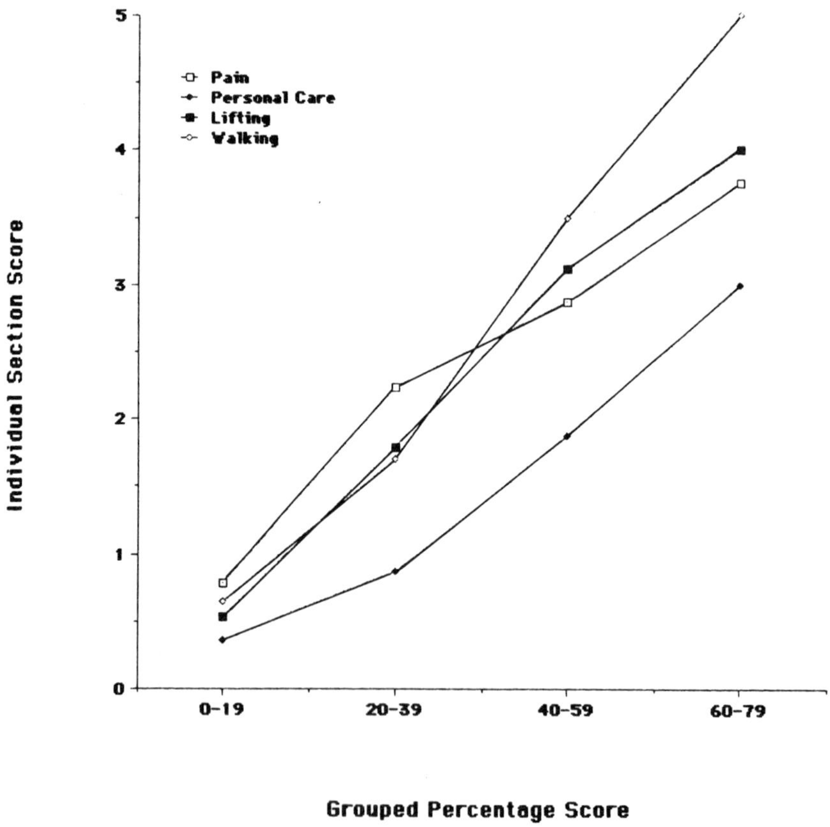

Fig 13.2 Comparison between and overall score (expressed as % of maximum possible score) and individual section scores: (□) pain; (■) lifting; (◆) personal care; (◇) walking

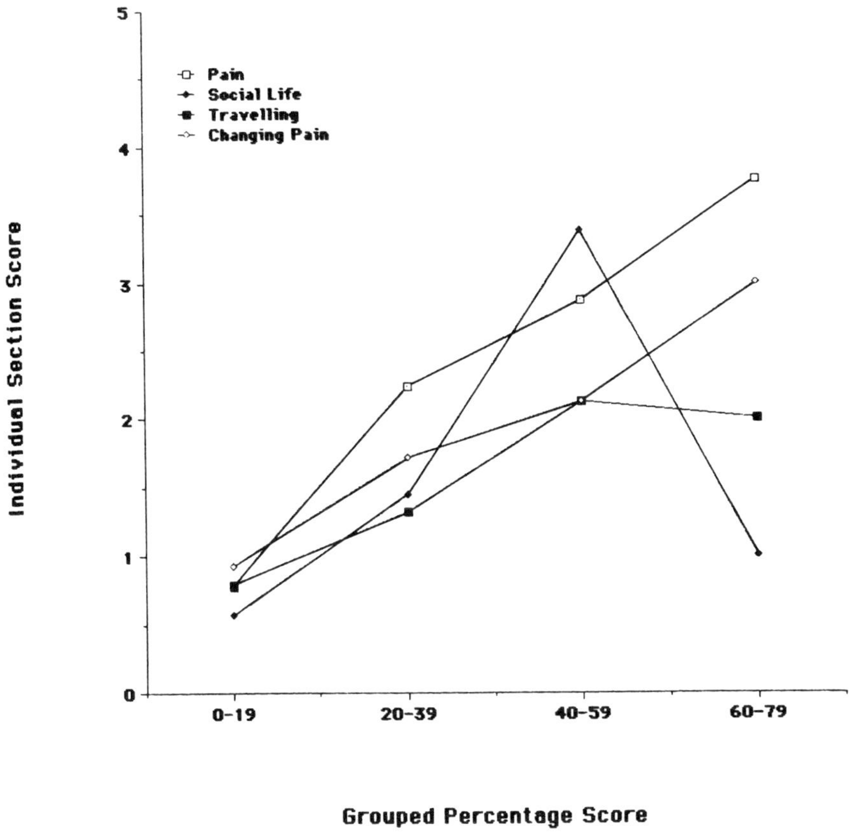

Fig 13.3 Comparison between overall score (expressed as % of maximum possible score) and individual section scores: (□) pain; (■) travelling; (◆) social life; (◇) changing pain

13.5.4 *Section-by-section compliance and sensitivity*

The individual section scores for the Revised Questionnaire recorded during the first 3 weeks after presentation were compared with those of the Original Questionnaire administered to a group of chiropractic and hospital outpatients (courtesy MRC Working Group) (Table 13.1). These patients had been selected as being suitable for either chiropractic or hospital outpatient management. All sections except one (Travel), show a wider dispersion of scores in the Revised Questionnaire and all except one (Sitting), higher mean scores. The section on Sex Life was replaced by Changing Degree of Pain to improve compliance.

In this study the onset scores were also examined section-by-section (Table 13.2). These show that the Revised Questionnaire can still accom-

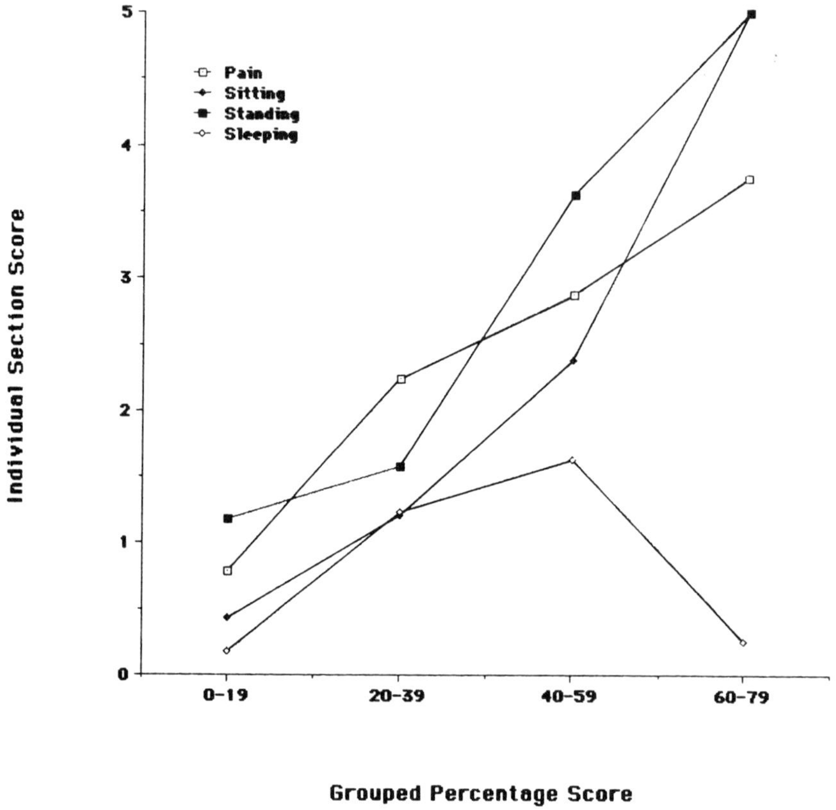

Fig 13.4 Comparison between overall score (expressed as % of maximum possible score) and individual section scores: (□) pain; (■) standing; (◆) sitting; (◇) sleeping

modate the highest scores which might be expected at initial presentation despite its increased sensitivity.

13.6 **Discussion and conclusion**

Although it is not possible to compare these results with those obtained in the original Oswestry study, comparison with the Original Questionnaire as it has been applied to chiropractic patients is reasonable. In this context the Revised Questionnaire as a whole produces higher mean disability scores and a wider representation of scores in each section. This is useful when monitoring changes in patients suffering from the less disabling forms of low back pain.

Table 13.1 Scores of each section in the revised and original versions of the Oswestry Questionnaire (averaged over the first 3 weeks after presentation)

	Oswestry Disability Index			
	Revised Questionnaire (n = 184)		*Original Questionnaire (n = 272)*	
Section	*Mean*	*SD*	*Mean*	*SD*
1. Pain	1.973	1.726	1.21[c]	1.55
2. Care	1.065	1.261	0.31	0.56
3. Lifting	1.734	1.630	1.81	1.33
4. Walk	1.560	1.655	0.64	0.92
5. Sit	1.380	1.525	1.59	1.19
6. Stand	1.663[a]	1.549	1.16	1.14
7. Sleep	0.880	0.915	0.45[d]	0.80
8. Changing pain/Sex	1.582[b]	1.194	0.51[e]	0.99
9. Social	1.500	1.343	1.37[f]	1.31
10. Travel	1.109[a]	0.975	1.06	1.07

n =: [a] 181; [b] 182; [c] 269; [d] 271; [e] 285; [f] 271.
Note: Section 8 was amended from Sex life to Changing degree of pain in the Revised Questionnaire.

Table 13.2 Mean and standard deviation of the scores of each section in the revised questionnaire at initial presentation

	Disability Index (n = 46)	
Section	*Mean*	*SD*
1. Pain	3.543	1.242
2. Care	1.761	1.303
3. Lifting	2.348	1.581
4. Walk	2.261	1.757
5. Sit	2.283	1.642
6. Stand	2.261	1.652
7. Sleep	1.326	0.944
8. Changing pain	2.609	0.954
9. Social	1.935	1.254
10. Travel	1.652	1.197

Two sections were not always consistent with the scores obtained from the pain section, namely Social Life and Sleeping. This highlights the heterogeneity of back pain patients and the ways in which sufferers adapt. Internal consistency should therefore not be rigidly sought in the production of back pain questionnaires.

At possible variance with current theory is the inclusion of more than one assessment criterion in a given section, for example, in Section 1 Question 3, degree of pain and its fluctuation appear together. The issue which this raises is whether or not any of the questions could be in incorrect order. The advantage is the placing of the questions in a context familiar to sufferers and thereby increasing sensitivity.

In this respect, the sections on Travel and Sitting do not represent an improvement over the Original Questionnaire. Nevertheless, the differences are small and the Revised version should be useful in future clinical trials where the numbers of patients needed to detect significant differences in outcome between two therapies can dramatically affect recruitment and costs.

Acknowledgements

The authors are grateful to the MRC Epidemiology and Medical Care Unit (Northwich Park Hospital, Harrow) for access to data obtained from their feasibility study, (Meade *et al.*, 1986) and to Sidney Hudson-Cook, Suzannah Ford, Michael Hutchinson, Michael Rufus, Michael Davidson, David Allen, and Ronald Keane: the chiropractors whose practices were the sources of patients for this study.

References

Agnew, D. C. & Merskey, H. (1976). Words of chronic pain, *Pain*, **3**, 73–81.

Beaver, W. T., Wallenstein, S. L., Houde, R. W. & Rogers, A. (1977). Comparisons of the analgesic effects of oral and intramuscular Oxomorphone in patients with cancer, *Journal of Clinical Pharmacology*, **17**, 186–98.

Beecher, H. K. (1972). The placebo effect as a non-specific force surrounding disease and the treatment of disease. In: *Pain: Basic Principles, Pharmacology and Therapy*, eds. R. Jongen, W. D. Keidel, A. Herz, C. Steichels, J. P. Payne & R. A. Burk. George Thieme, Stuttgart.

Beekman, C. E. & Axtell, L. (1985). Ambulation, activity level and pain. Outcomes of a programme for spinal pain, *Physical Therapy*, **65**, 1649–57.

Bergner, M., Bobbitt, R. A., Pollard, W. E., Martin, D. P. & Gilson, B. S. (1976). The sickness impact profile. Validation of a health status measure, *Medical Care*, **14**, 57–67.

Brand, R. A. & Lehmann, T. R. (1983), Low back impairment rating practices of orthopaedic surgeons, *Spine*, **8**, 75–78.

Breen, A. C. (1977). Chiropractors and the treatment of back pain, *Rheumatology and Rehabilitation*, **16**, 46–49.

Budzynski, T. H., Stoyva, J. M., Adler, C. S. & Mullaney, D. J. (1973). Electromyelographic biofeedback and tension headache: A controlled outcome study, *Psychosomatic Medicine*, **35**, 484–96.

Caldwell, A. B. & Chase, C. (1977). Diagnosis and treatment of personality factors with chronic low back pain, *Clinical Orthopaedics*, **129**, 141–9.

Campbell, J. N. & Long, D. M. (1976). Peripheral nerve stimulation in the treatment of intractable pain, *Journal of Neurosurgery*, **45**, 692–9.

Cannell, C. F. & Marquis, K. H. (1967). Effect of some experimental interviewing techniques on reporting in the health interview survey. Survey Research Centre, University of Michigan.
Cannell, C. F., Marquis, K. H. & Laurent, A. (1969). An experimental study of the effects of reinforcement, question length and re-interviews on reporting selected chronic conditions in household interviews. Survey Research Centre, University of Michigan.
Carter, W. B., Bobbitt, R. A. & Bergner, M. (1976). Validation of an interval scaling: The sickness impact profile, *Health Services Research*, **11**, 516–28.
Chen, G. S. & Hwang, Y. C. (1977). Therapeutic effect of acupuncture for chronic pain, *American Journal of Chinese Medicine*, **5**, 45–61.
Cochrane, A. L., Chapman, P. J. & Oldham, P. D. (1951). Observer's errors in taking medical histories, *Lancet*, **1**, 1007–9.
Collen, M. F., Cutler, J. L., Siegelaub, A. B. & Cella, R. L. (1969). Reliability of a self-administered medical questionnaire, *Archives of Internal Medicine*, **123**, 664–81.
Collins, F. L. & Martin, J. E. (1980). Assessing self-report of pain; A comparison of two recording procedures, *Journal of Behavioural Assessment*, **2**, 55–63.
Crockett, D. J., Prkachin, K. M. & Craig, K. D. (1977). Factors of the language of pain in patient and normal volunteer groups, *Pain*, **4**, 175–82.
Dennis, M. D., Greene, R. L., Farr, S. P. & Hartman, T. J. (1989). The Minnesota Multiphasic Personality Index: General guidelines to its use and interpretation in orthopaedics, *Clinical Orthopaedics*, **150**, 125–130.
Denniston, O. L. & Jette, A. (1980). A functional status assessment instrument: Validation in an elderly population, *Health Services Research*, **15**, 21–34.
Devaul, R. A. & Zisook, S. (1978). Chronic pain: The psychiatrists role, *Psychosomatics*, **19**, 417–21.
Devine, L. & Merskey, H. (1965). The description of pain in psychiatric and general medical patients, *Journal of Psychosomatic Research*, **9**, 311–16.
Deyo, R. A. (1984). Pitfalls in measuring the health status of Mexican-Americans: Comparative validity of the English and Spanish sickness impact profile, *American Journal of Public Health*, **74**, 569–73.
Deyo, R. A. (1986). Comparative validity of the sickness impact profile and shorter scales for functional assessment in low back pain, *Spine*, **11**, 951–4.
Deyo, R. A. & Diehl, A. K. (1983). Measuring physical and psychosocial function in patients with low back pain, *Spine*, **8**, 635–42.
Dixon, J. S. & Bird, H. A. (1981). Reproducibility along a ten centimetre vertical visual analogue scale, *Annals of Rheumatic Medicine*, **40**, 87–89.
Eastwood, R. P. (1940). In *Sales Control by Quantitative Methods*. Columbia University Press, New York.
Epstein, L. H. & Abel, G. G. (1977). Analysis of biofeedback training effects for tension headache patients, *Behavioural Therapy*, **8**, 37–47.
Evans, J. H. & Kagan, A. (1986). The development of functional rating scale to measure the treatment outcome of chronic spinal patients, *Spine*, **11**, 277–81.
Fairbank, J. C. T., Couper, J., Davies, J. B. & O'Brien, J. P. (1980). The Oswestry low back pain disability questionnaire, *Physiotherapy*, **66**, 271–3.
Fletcher, C. M. (1962). Some problems of diagnostic standardisation using clinical methods, with special reference to chronic bronchitis. In: *Epidemiology, Reports on Research and Teaching, London,* ed. J. Pemberton, pp. 253–60. Oxford University Press, Oxford.
Follick, M. J., Smith, T. W. & Ahern, D. K. (1985). The sickness impact profile; a global measure of disability in chronic low back pain, *Pain*, **21**, 67–76.

Fordyce, W. E. (1976). *Behavioural Methods for Chronic Pain and Illness*. C. V. Mosby, St Louis.

Fox, E. J. & Melzack, R. (1976). Transcutaneous electrical stimulation and acupuncture: comparison of treatment for low back pain, *Pain*, **2**, 141–8.

Friedsman, H. J. & Martin, H. W. (1963). A comparison of self and physician's health ratings in an older population, *Journal of Health and Human Behaviour*, **4**, 179–83.

Garrad, J. & Bennett, A. E. (1971). A validated interview schedule for use in population surveys of chronic diseases and disability, *British Journal of Preventative Social Medicine*, **25**, 97–104.

Gilson, B. S., Erickson, D. & Chavez, C. T. (1980). A Chicano version of the SIP, *Cultural Medicine and Psychiatry*, **4**, 137–50.

Glover, J. R. Morris, T. G. & Khosla, T. (1974). Assessing improvement of low back pain, *British Journal of Industrial Medicine*, **31**, 59–64.

Hachen, H. J. (1978). Psychological, neurophysiological and therapeutic effects of chronic pain: preliminary results with transcutaneous electrical stimulation proceedings, *Paraplegia*, **15**, 353–67.

Hadler, N. M., Curits, P., Gillings, D. B. & Stinnett, S. (1987). A benefit of spinal manipulation as adjunctive therapy for acute low back pain: A stratified controlled trial, *Spine*, **12**, 703–6.

Hilgard, E. (1969). Pain as a puzzle for psychology and physiology, *American Psychology*, **24**, 103–13.

Hunter, M. & Philips, C. (1981). The experience of headache – an assessment of the qualities of tension headache pain, *Pain*, **10**, 209–20.

Jacox, A. K. (1979). Assessing pain, *American Journal of Nursing*, **79**, 895–900.

Joyce, C. R. B., Zutshi, D. W., Hrubes, V. & Masion, R. M. (1975). Comparison of a fixed interval and visual analogue scales for rating chronic pain, *European Journal of Clinical Pharmacology*, **8**, 415–20.

Kagan, G. & Masheter, H. C. (1978). A controlled study of short-term treatment of tension headache, *Current Medical Research and Opinion*, **5**, 709–13.

Kelman, H. R. & Willner, A. (1962). Problems in measurement and evaluation of rehabilitation, *Archives of Physical Medicine*, **43**, 172.

Ketovuori, H., Kohvakka, A., Hurri, H. & Eskelinen, L. (1984). The Finnish pain questionnaire: comparisons of descriptions of pain in coronary heart disease and low back pain, *Scandanavian Journal of Rehabilitative Medicine*, **16**, 71–76.

Kirshner, B. & Guyatt, G. (1985). A methodological framework for assessing health indices, *Journal of Chronic Diseases*, **38**, 27–36.

Klepac, R. K., Dowling, J. & Hauge, G. (1981). Sensitivity of the McGill pain questionnaire to intensity and quality of laboratory pain, *Pain*, **10**, 199–207.

Kremer, E., Atkinson, J. H. & Ignelzi, R. J. (1981). Measurement of pain: patient preference does not confound pain measurement, *Pain*, **10**, 241–8.

Lawlis, G. F., Mooney, V., Selby, D. K. & McCoy, E. (1982). A motivational scoring system for outcome prediction with spinal pain rehabilitation patients, *Spine*, **7**, 163–7.

Leavitt, F. (1987). Detection of simulation among persons instructed to exaggerate symptoms of low back pain, *Journal of Occupational Medicine*, **29**, 229–33.

Lee, P. K., Anderson, T. W., Modell, J. H. & Saga, S. A. (1975). Treatment of chronic pain with acupuncture, *Journal of the American Medical Association*, **232**, 1133–5.

Lehmann, T. R., Brand, R. A., Thomas, W. O. & Gorman, M. S. (1983). A low back rating scale, *Spine*, **8**, 308–15.

Ljunggren, A. E. (1983). Descriptions of pain and other sensory modalities in patients with lumbago-sciatica and herniated intervertebral discs. Interview administration of an adapted McGill pain questionnaire, *Pain*, **16**, 265–76.

McNeill, T. W., Sinkora, G. & Leavitt, F. (1986). Psychologic classification of low back pain patients: a prognostic tool, *Spine*, **11**, 955–9.

Main, C. J. & Waddell, G. (1987). Psychometric construction and validity of the Pilowsky illness behaviour questionnaire in British patients with chronic low back pain, *Pain*, **28**, 13–25.

Meade, T. W. *et al.* (Report of a working group) (1986). Comparison of chiropractic and hospital outpatient management of low back pain: A feasibility study, *Journal of Epidemiology and Community Health*, **40**, 12–17.

Melzack, R. (1975). The McGill pain questionnaire: Major properties and scoring methods, *Pain*, **1**, 275–99.

Melzack, R., Katz, J & Jeans, M. E. (1985). The role of compensation in chronic pain: Analysis using a new method of scoring the McGill pain questionnaire, *Pain*, **23**, 101–12.

Melzack, R. & Torgerson, W. S. (1971). On the language of pain, *Anaesthesiology*, **34**, 50–59.

Melzack, R., Vetere, P. & Finch, L. (1983). Transcutaneous electrical nerve stimulation for low back pain. A comparison of TENS and massage for pain and range of motion, *Physical Therapy*, **63**, 489–93.

Metzner, H. & Mann, F. (1952). A limited comparison of two methods of data collection: The fixed alternative questionnaire and the open-ended interview, *American Sociological Review*, **17**, 486.

Million, R., Hall, W., Nilson, K. H. Baker, R. D. & Jayson, M. I. (1982). Assessment of the progress of the low back pain patient, *Spine*, **7**, 204–12.

Moroni, M., Cavalli, G. & Lodola, A. (1978). Viminol analgesic activity in elderly patients with chronic pain: A controlled evaluation, using self-grading questionnaires, *International Journal on Clinical Pharmacology and Biopharmaceuticals*, **6**, 513–5.

Morris, J. L. (1982). Radiologic evaluation. In: *Management of Low Back Pain*, eds. H. Carron, R. E. McLaughlin, Chapter 9, pp. 107–47. John Wright/PSG, Boston.

Ohnhaus, E. E. & Adler, R. (1975). Methodological problems in the meaurement of pain: A comparison between the VRS and the VAS, *Pain*, **1**, 379–84.

Petersdorf, R. & Feinstein, A. F. (1981). An informal appraisal of the current status of 'medical sociology'. In: *The Relevance of Social Science for Medicine*, eds. L. Eisenberg, L. & A. Kleinman, Chapter 2, pp. 27–28. D. Reidel, Boston.

Ransford, A. O., Cairns, D. & Mooney, V. (1976). The pain drawing as an aid to the psychologic evaluation of patients with low back pain, *Spine*, **1**, 127–34.

Reading, A. E. (1984). Testing pain mechanisms in persons in pain. In: *Textbook of Pain*, eds. P. D. Wall, P. D. & R. Melzack, p. 195. Longman, London.

Reading, A. E. & Newton, J. R. (1977). On a comparison of dysmenorrhoea and intrauterine device related pain, *Pain*, **3**, 265–76.

Revill, S. I., Robinson, J. O., Rosen, M. & Hogg, M. I. J. (1976). The reliability of a linear analogue for evaluating pain, *Anaesthesia*, **31**, 1191–8.

Roberts, A. H. & Reinhardt, L. (1980). The behavioural management of chronic pain: long term follow-up with comparison groups, *Pain*, **8**, 151–62.

Rock, D. L., Fordyce, W. E., Brockway, J. A., Bergman, J. J. & Spengler, D. M. (1984). Measuring functional impairment associated with pain: Psychometric analysis of an exploratory scoring protocol for activity pattern indicators,

Archives of Physical Medicine and Rehabilitation, **65**, 295–300.
Roland, M. & Morris, R. (1983). 1982 Volvo award in clinical sciences. A study of the natural history of back pain. Part I: Development of guidelines for trials of treatment in primary care, *Spine*, **8**, 141–4.
Roland, M. & Morris, R. (1983). 1982 Volvo award in clinical sciences. A study of the natural history of back pain. Part II: Development of a reliable and sensitive measure of disability in low back pain, *Spine*, **8**, 145–50.
Rose, G. (1964). Chest pain questionnaire. In: *Comparability in International Epidemiology*, ed. R. Acheson, R., pp. 32–39. Milbank Memorial Fund, New York.
Rybstein-Blinchik, E. (1979). Effects of different cognitive strategies on chronic pain experience, *Journal of Behavioural Medicine*, **2**, 93–101.
Scott, J. & Huskisson, E. C. (1976). Graphic representation of pain, *Pain*, **2**, 175–84.
Scott, P. J., Ansell, B. M. & Huskisson, E. C. (1977). Measurement of pain in juveniles with polyarthritis, *Annals of Rheumatic Diseases*, **36**, 186–7.
Seres, J. L. & Newman, R. I. (1976). The results of treatment of chronic low back pain at the Portland Pain Centre, *Journal of Neurosurgery*, **45**, 32–36.
Spoerel, W. E., Varkey, M & Leung, C. Y. (1976). Acupuncture and chronic pain, *American Journal of Chinese Medicine*, **4**, 267–79.
Sternbach, R. A., Wolf, S. R., Murphy, R. W. & Akeson, W. H. (1973). Traits of pain patients: The low back 'loser', *Psychosomatics*, **14**, 226.
Storlite, F. J. (1978). Pointers for assessing pain, *American Journal of Nursing*, **78**, 2071–2.
Stouffer, S. A. (1950). In: *Measurement and Prediction*, ed. S. A. Stouffer. Princeton University Press, Princeton, NJ.
Tamerin, J. S. (1964). The perception of progress in rehabilitation, *Archives of Physical Medicine*, **45**, 17.
Toomey, T. C., Ghia, J. N., Mao, W. & Gregg, J. M. (1977). Acupuncture in chronic pain mechanisms: The moderating effect of affect, personality and stress in response to treatment, *Pain*, **3**, 137–45.
Waddell, G. & Main, C. J. (1984). Assessment of severity in low back disorders, *Spine*, **9**, 204–8.
Young, D. W. (1972). Comparison of information collected by a questionary with that in a patient's hospital record, *Methods in Medical Research*, **10**, 222.

Appendix 13.1

The Revised Oswestry Pain Questionnaire.

Anglo-European College of Chiropractic.

Name: .... **Age:** .... **Date of Birth** ....
Address:.. **Occupation:** ....
....
....
How long have you had Low Back Pain?.............**YRS**..............**MONTHS**............**WEEKS.**
Is this your first episode of Low Back Pain? ☐ **YES** ☐ **NO**

Please Read: This Questionnaire is designed to enable us to understand how much your Low Back Pain has affected your ability to manage your every-day activities. Please answer each Section by marking in each Section the ONE BOX that most applies to you. We realise that you may feel that more than one statement may relate to you, but PLEASE JUST MARK THE ONE BOX WHICH MOST CLOSELY DESCRIBES YOUR PROBLEM. Thank You.

Please complete this Questionnaire on____/____/_____and return it to us in the Pre-Paid Envelope provided.

SECTION 1- Pain Intensity

- ☐ **The pain comes and goes and is very mild**
- ☐ **The pain is mild and does not vary much**
- ☐ **The pain comes and goes and is moderate**
- ☐ **The pain is moderate and does not vary much**
- ☐ **The pain comes and goes and is severe**
- ☐ **The pain is severe and does not vary much**

SECTION 2 - Personal Care

- ☐ I would not have to change my way of washing or dressing in order to avoid pain
- ☐ I do not normally change my way of washing or dressing even though it causes some pain.
- ☐ Washing and dressing increase the pain but I manage not to change my way of doing it
- ☐ Washing and dressing increase the pain and I find it neccessary to change my way of doing it
- ☐ Because of the pain I am unable to do some washing and dressing without help
- ☐ Because of the pain I am unable to do any washing or dressing without help

SECTION 3 - Lifting

- ☐ I can lift heavy weights without extra pain
- ☐ I can lift heavy weights but it causes extra pain
- ☐ Pain prevents me lifting heavy weights off the floor
- ☐ Pain prevents me lifting heavy weights off the floor but I can manage if they are conveniently positioned, e.g. on a table
- ☐ Pain prevents me from lifting heavy weights but I can manage light to medium weights if they are conveniently positioned
- ☐ I can only lift very light weights at the most

SECTION 4 - Walking

- ☐ I have no pain on walking
- ☐ I have some pain on walking but it does not increase with distance
- ☐ I cannot walk more than One Mile without increasing pain
- ☐ I cannot walk more than 1/2 Mile without increasing pain
- ☐ I cannot walk more than 1/4 Mile without increasing pain
- ☐ I cannot walk at all without increasing pain

SECTION 5 - Sitting

- ☐ I can sit in any chair as long as I like
- ☐ I can sit only in my favourite chair as long as I like
- ☐ Pain prevents me sitting more than one hour
- ☐ Pain prevents me from sitting more than 1/2 hour

□ Pain prevents me from sitting more than 10 minutes
□ I avoid sitting because it increases pain straight away

SECTION 6 - Standing
□ I can stand as long as I want without pain
□ I have some pain on standing but it does not increase with time
□ I cannot stand for longer than one hour without increasing pain
□ I cannot stand for longer than 1/2 hour without increasing pain
□ I cannot stand for longer than 10 minutes without increasing pain
□ I avoid standing because it increases the pain straight away

SECTION 7 - Sleeping
□ I get no pain in bed
□ I get pain in bed but it does not prevent me from sleeping well
□ Because of pain my normal nights sleep is reduced by less than 1/4
□ Because of pain my normal nights sleep is reduced by less than 1/2
□ Because of pain my normal nights sleep is reduced by less than 3/4
□ Pain prevents from sleeping at all

SECTION 8 - Social Life
□ My social life is normal and gives me no pain
□ My social life is normal but increases the degree of my pain
□ Pain has no significant effect on my social life apart from limiting my more energetic interests, e.g. dancing etc.
□ Pain has restricted my social life and I do not go out very often
□ Pain has restricted my social life to my home
□ I have hardly any social life because of the pain

SECTION 9 - Travelling
□ I get no pain whilst travelling
□ I get some pain whilst travelling but none of my usual forms of travel make it any worse
□ I get extra pain whilst travelling but it does not compel me to seek alternative forms of travel
□ I get extra pain whilst travelling which compels me to seek alternative forms of travel
□ Pain restricts all forms of travel
□ Pain prevents all forms of travel except that done lying down

SECTION 10 - Changing Degree of Pain
□ My pain is rapidly getting better
□ My pain fluctuates but overall is definitely getting better
□ My pain seems to be getting better but improvement is slow at present
□ My pain is neither getting better nor worse
□ My pain is gradually worsening
□ My pain is rapidly worsening

14 *S. J. Bulstrode, R. A. Harrison and A. K. Clarke*

Seating and low back pain

14.1 Seating and back pain

There is much evidence in the literature to suggest that sitting in chairs or car seats is a predisposing factor to low back pain. People with sedentary occupations have a higher incidence of all types of back pain than those whose jobs involve standing or walking around. In a survey conducted by Grandjean *et al.* (1962) of 261 men and 117 women who were employed in sedentary office work, 57% complained of back trouble when they were working.

A controlled survey of 233 hospital patients with probable or possible cases of herniated intervertebral disc conducted by Kelsey & Hardy (1975) revealed that men who spent more than half their working hours driving were three times more likely to develop a herniated lumbar disc than those who did not. In a survey of occupational back pain among a sample of 68 men, it was found that driving high mileages was a significant factor affecting both occurence and location of pain (Buckle *et al.*, 1980). People who drove more than 19 000 miles per year experienced right-sided symptoms and reported pain in the upper lumbar region, buttock and groin significantly more often than people who drove less then 19 000 miles per year.

The anatomical changes in the spine which occur when assuming the sitting position are well documented but their role in producing back pain remains a matter for speculation. Keegan (1953) stated that the most important postural factor in the causation of low back pain in sitting was the decrease of the trunk-thigh angle and consequent flattening of the lumbar curve. In his opinion the next most important factor was lack of primary back support over the vulnerable lower lumbar intervertebral discs. Sitting has been shown to have a profound effect on muscle activity and intradiscal pressure. Andersson *et al.* (1975) measured the myoelectric activity in several muscles of the back and the pressure within the third lumbar disc in various sitting and standing positions. Results showed that there was little difference in the myoelectric activity in standing and in relaxed unsupported sitting although the highest level of activity was found when leaning forward in the sitting position. The disc pressure was considerably higher in unsupported sitting than in standing. Both the myoelectric activity and the disc pressure decreased when the back was supported and showed further decrease as the back-rest inclination increased. The disc pressure was also considerably reduced when the lumbar support was increased and also when arm-rests were used. In the car-driver's seat, the intradiscal pressure increased when the gear lever was moved or the clutch pedal depressed. Gear lever shift was responsible for an increase in myoelectric activity.

When designing chairs and car seats, measurements of the physical characteristics of human beings, particularly their sizes and shapes (anthropometric data), are frequently used to select the most suitable chair dimensions. The next stage in the development is to conduct fitting trials to allow the subject to fit the chair to the body and workspace (Drury & Coury, 1982) but as Barkla (1961) stated 'good fit alone may not ensure comfort but bad fit will almost certainly ensure discomfort'. Finally, an evaluation of comfort should be made by potential users in their own environment. Several evaluations of chairs for the elderly have been conducted (Munton *et al.*, 1982; Research Institute for Consumer Affairs, 1970) but few have looked at comfort of chairs for people with low back pain. One of the main problems with this type of work is the large number of variables including anthropometric variations, requirements of the seating and behaviour of low back pain sufferers' symptoms. Consequently it is difficult to recommend individual chairs but specific design features which are thought to increase comfort can be identified.

14.2 **Easy chairs**

Atherton *et al.* (1980) conducted a study the aim of which was primarily to evaluate the relative comfort and acceptabilty of the various easy chairs which had been recommended to, or were commonly used by, arthritic patients. Patients with low back pain were however included in the trial as a separate group.

Ten chairs were selected for the study, some of which were chairs which were recommended or advertised as being of 'orthopaedic' value. A pilot study was carried out, one of the aims of which was to find out how much time would be needed in order to decide whether a chair was comfortable or not. Comfort was assessed at 10-min intervals over a period of 1 hour 50 min by the use of a visual analogue scale. This showed that low back pain patients who were 'uncomfortable' in a chair after 10 min found that particular chair was 'intolerable' after 30 min. These patients, in common with ankylosing spondylitis patients, recorded 'intolerable' on their visual analogue scales more often than patients in the other groups who were tested. The pilot study enabled a period of 15 min to be established as the minimum time in which the probable long-term comfort of a chair could be assessed. If the chair was uncomfortable during the first 15 min it was extremely unlikely that it would become more comfortable.

In the main study, the comfort of the chairs was evaluated by using the results obtained from a visual analogue scale and patient questionnaires.

The investigation did not produce any results from which it would be possible to match a particular patient to a chair which could be guaranteed to be comfortable. It did, however, indicate factors which are important for someone with back pain to take into account when selecting a chair. These factors are the rake of the back, the rake of the seat, the design of chair arms, the firmness of the padding and the covering.

14.2.1 *Rake of the back*

The rake of the back of the chair which was considered most comfortable by back pain patients was 105°. This was the greatest angle on any of the chairs which were tested. This may very well be explained by the findings of the electromyographic studies in people with back pain (Knutssen *et al.*, 1966), which showed that there was an appreciable decrease in the activity in the long back extensors when the rake of the seat back was changed from 100 to 110°. A study by Andersson *et al.* (1974) confirmed this and in addition found a decrease in the lumbar disc pressure as the angle of the back rest was increased.

14.2.2 *Rake of the seat*

The downward slope of the seat towards the back was more important to the back pain patients than to any of the other groups in the trial and the most comfortable chair for them had the greatest angle of seat slope which was 9°. This was 5° more than any of the other chairs tested.

14.2.3 *Arms*

The back pain groups were not the most critical when asked about chair arms. Where they were dissatisfied or uncomfortable, they complained of arms being 'too short' or 'too high'. It is not possible to give absolute heights or lengths for the arms because these measurements will vary with the patients' anthropometric measurements. However, when a patient is assessing a chair for comfort before purchasing, it should include a conscious rating of the chair arms both in the sitting position and when rising from the chair.

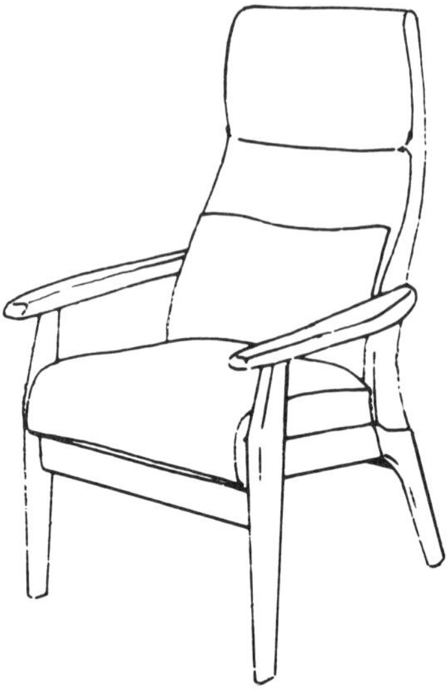

Fig 14.1 Easy chair found to be most comfortable by low back pain patients (Atherton *et al.*, 1980). Popular design features included a sloping seat-back, downward slope of the seat towards the back and firm upholstery. The preferred sitting position for most people was with a seat-back slope of 105° and a seat slope of 10°

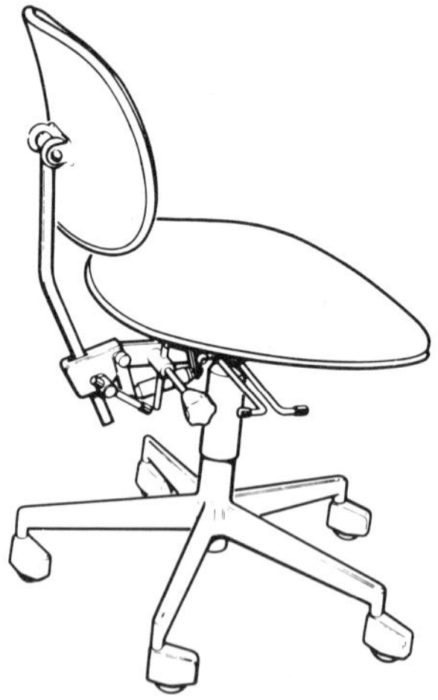

Fig 14.2 Office chair found to be most comfortable by low back pain patients (Atherton *et al.*, 1982). Popular design features included adjustable height and downward slope of the seat towards the waterfall front edge, adjustable height and angle of back-rest and firm upholstery. The preferred sitting position for most people was with a downward slope of 0–5° on the seat, a back-rest angle of 98° and an arm-rest length of less than 285 mm

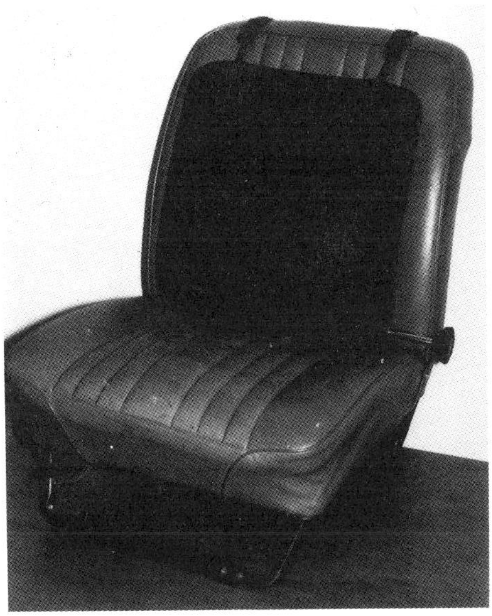

Fig 14.3 Back-rest found to be most comfortable by car drivers with low back pain (Bulstrode *et al.*, 1984). Popular design features included an adjustable lumbar support and a contoured shape to give support when cornering. The ability to alter the height of the back-rest was considered to be important

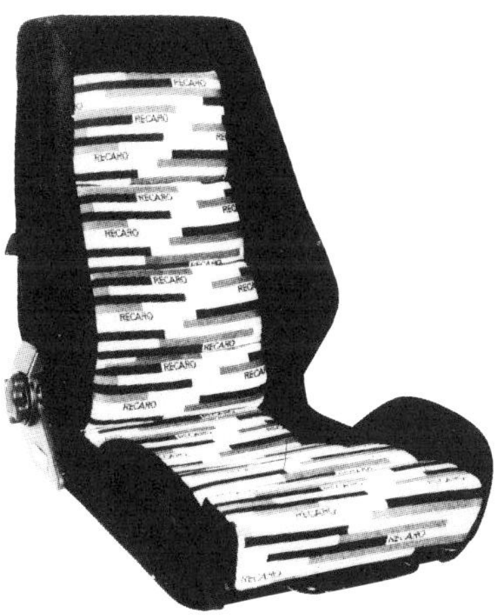

Fig 14.4 Replacement car-seat found to be most comfortable by drivers with low back pain (Bulstrode *et al.*, 1985). Firm support to the whole back including the upper thoracic region, a contoured shape and the ability to slide the seat forwards and backwards, alter the back-rest angle, seat tilt and squab length were considered to be important

14.2.4 *Padding*

Of the observations on the padding of the chairs, which were recorded by low back pain patients, 38% expressed dissatisfaction with the lack of firmness of the padding. This was at variance with the observations of the arthritic patients who, on the whole, found the softer seats more acceptable.

14.2.5 *Covering*

Eight out of the ten chairs which were tested, had vinyl covering and the majority of people in all four groups said that this type of covering 'felt sweaty'. A test for the preferred covering fabric was set up using the chair which had been felt to be most comfortable by most people. Four of these otherwise identical chairs, covered in four different fabrics, were tested by some of the patients from each of the four patient groups. People with low back pain preferred a tapestry fabric to any of the other three coverings and vinyl was the least popular. The reason which they gave for this was that in a vinyl covered seat they tended to slip from their position of comfort. This was contrary to two of the arthritic patients who found that the vinyl was more acceptable because it made it easier for them to slide forwards when getting out of the chair.

14.3 **Office chairs**

Since sedentary workers have been shown to be more vulnerable to low back pain than others (Grandjean *et al.*, 1962), selection of a suitable office chair is very important. Twelve standard office chairs, seven of which were advertised as being particularly suitable for those with back problems, were assessed for comfort when used by three different patient groups (Atherton *et al.*, 1982).

The groups which took part in the trial consisted of patients with rheumatoid arthritis, ankylosing spondylitis and back pain. The back pain patients were further divided into two sub-groups one containing those whose office work included typing and another whose work did not. The 'typists' group assessed eight chairs and the 'non-typists' group assessed nine.

A pilot study confirmed the work of Drury & Coury (1982) which showed that most people were only able to assess an office chair for comfort in their own work station. In addition it was found that a whole working day was necessary for them to be able to give a reliable assessment of comfort. In the trial, therefore, each patient used each chair for a full working day and completed a questionaire at the end of the day.

The assessment was in three parts, comfort in relation to the chairs' individual characteristics, overall rating of comfort and selection of the most comfortable of all the chairs used. This comparative judgement seems to be more reliable than an absolute judgement about an individual chair (Le Carpentier, 1969).

Although the trial described above was primarily intended to rate particular office chairs for comfort, certain factors were identified which are relevant to any office chair which is intended for use by back pain sufferers.

Patients in both back pain groups were more comfortable in chairs with back rests which pivoted and which also provided pronounced lumbar support. A fixed back which was set at 98° was found to be comfortable but these groups had a preference for a chair on which the angle of the back could be adjusted. This is also the case with office workers who do not suffer from back pain, for Burandt & Grandjean (1963) found that those whose chairs had adjustable back rests used them more frequently than those whose chair backs were fixed.

The preferred angle for the seat in this group, was between 0 and 5°. Of the non-typists, 60% chose a forward slope as being the most comfortable and the other 40% preferred a flat seat. In order that an individual may find his own particular position of optimum comfort, therefore, a facility for adjusting the angle of the seat between 0 and 5° forward tilt is essential. The back pain groups complained more often than the other two groups of discomfort behind the knees caused by pressure from the edge of the seat. Most office chairs consist of a moulded plastic or metal platform over which the padding and upholstery is layered. The front edge of the seating platform in some chairs has a pronounced curve in cross-section. Such chairs are said to have a 'waterfall' front. Seats with such a 'waterfall' front did not cause this problem for these groups.

The discomfort caused by pressure behind the knees is often a problem for short people who do not have a foot-rest on their chair. Such people find it necessary to sit towards the front of the seat and this causes the edge of the seat to press against the back of the thighs (Burandt & Grandjean, 1963). It is particularly important therefore that office workers of short stature who have back pain and who are not provided with the facility for lowering the desk height, should be provided with a chair which has a foot-rest.

The back pain groups in the office seating trial found, as did those in the easy chair study, that blended fabrics and wool coverings were more comfortable than leather or nylon. On nylon and leather coverings, they tended to slip from their comfortable position and also they found them 'sweaty'.

Most office chairs do not have arms but three chairs with arms were included in the trial by Atherton *et al.* (1982). It was found that the maximum practical length was 285 mm. If they were longer than this then the user could not get close enough to the desk for typing and had to lean away from the back-rest. The only patients who felt that padding of the arms was necessary were those with ankylosing spondylitis who took weight on the elbows regularly to adjust their position. The preferred arm-rest height differed from person to person according to their anthropometric measurements. Where arms are required on the office chair, and a suitable model cannot be found, a chair with adjustable arms may be considered.

Thick, firm upholstery was found to be most comfortable and the seat with the thickest padding, which was 70 mm in depth, was the only seat found to be comfortable by every individual in both back pain groups.

14.4 **Car back-rests**

Bulstrode *et al.* (1985) conducted an evaluation of eight back-rests for use in car-seats and also of three replacement car-seats. These had all been recommended for drivers whose symptoms were attributed to, or aggravated by, driving. Thirty drivers were asked to describe the factors associated with driving which they considered to be reponsible for aggravating their symptoms; the results are summarised in Table 14.1.

Preliminary studies revealed that it was not possible to form a true impression of the comfort of a car-seat by using a rig in the laboratory or by sitting in a stationary vehicle. Changes in comfort on unbroken long journeys were monitored by asking drivers to complete visual analogue scales at regular intervals. As expected there was a general trend towards decrease in comfort with time but people who were 'very comfortable' after 30 min remained 'very comfortable' for up to 2 hours. Anyone who experienced any discomfort within 30 min became 'intolerably uncomfortable' within 2 hours and had to stop driving and in most cases get out of the vehicle. It could be concluded that it is possible for drivers to predict their comfort on long journeys after 30 min. This has implications for drivers with back pain who are wanting to choose a new back-rest or car-seat.

Most drivers were able to improve comfort in their car seat by using a back-rest and in some cases symptoms were relieved; 80% of drivers preferred an adjustable back-rest, the shape of which could be altered to

Table 14.1 Factors considered by subjects to be responsible for aggravation of their symptoms when driving

93%	Sitting in an incorrect position
50%	Movements associated with reversing
47%	Sitting in one position for long periods of time
33%	Getting in and out of the vehicle
20%	Depressing the clutch pedal
10%	Inadequate lateral support provided by the car-seat

suit their individual requirements. People who attributed some of their symptoms to sitting in one position for long periods of time benefited from an adjustable back-rest. The ability to be able to alter the height of the back-rest was also found to be important.

Contouring of the car-seat was found to be important because it limited lateral trunk movement especially when cornering at speed. Where a car-seat lacked contouring a back-rest could provide the additional support required. In cases where the symptoms were aggravated by getting in and out of the vehicle, however, some people reported that the presence of the back-rest in the car-seat made this manoeuvre even more difficult.

14.5 **Replacement car-seats**

In cases where a back-rest is not suitable either because the seat is badly designed or worn, a replacement car-seat can be purchased. They can usually be supplied with a sub-frame to fit any make or model of car.

Although all seats which are fitted into new cars must satisfy strength tests in accordance with *EEC Regulation 17*, there are no such rulings for replacement car seats. Four replacement car seats tested by Bulstrode *et al.* (1985) were therefore subjected to a series of strength tests by the Automobile Association prior to evaluation. These tests included Seat Back Moment Tests and Seat Anchorage Tests. One seat failed to meet the test requirements because the permanent distortion of the seat following the Seat Back Moment Test exceeded the acceptable limit and it was therefore excluded from further testing.

Eighteen subjects took part in the trial. They all travelled in a car regularly and complained of discomfort when sitting in their car-seat. All the subjects travelled in a car fitted with each replacement car-seat in turn, on a 20-mile journey which included some driving in town and some driving on country roads. At the end of the journey subjects were asked to comment on ease of access to the vehicle, comfort, design, firmness, ease of adjustment and appearance of each seat.

The most popular seat provided firm support to the whole of the back including the upper thoracic region but the lumbar section was not adjustable. Two seats were fitted with adjustable lumbar sections but these were not considered to be useful, either because their shape was unsuitable or the adjusting mechanism was too difficult to use. Head restraints are always recommended to minimise the risk of whiplash injury.

Contouring of the car-seat was considered to be important providing its presence did not make it more difficult for the driver or passenger to get in and out of the car.

Most drivers felt that forward/backward (seat slide) and back-rest angle adjustments were essential but that squab angle (seat tilt) and adjustable squab length were also important. This was particulary the case for tall drivers who frequently complained that their seat did not provide adequate thigh support or that the front edge of the seat caused undue pressure behind the thigh.

14.6 **Conclusion**

In conclusion, it is not possible to recommend one chair, back-rest or car-seat which will suit all back pain sufferers but important design features which influence comfort can be identified.

The selection of a chair for use in the home or office for someone who experiences back pain when sitting should be based on careful comfort assessment. Atherton *et al.* (1980) reported that most of the subjects questioned in their study were strongly influenced by factors such as appearance or cost because they did not know how to assess comfort.

Many factors influence the choice of a car and frequently the comfort of the car-seat only forms a small part in the selection process. In recent years car manufacturers have become increasingly aware of the importance of well-designed car-seats but frequently only the models of cars at the top of a range will be fitted with the best seats. Hopefully this situation will change in the future.

Questioning of patients during the assessment of easy chairs (Atherton *et al.*, 1980) showed that chairs are often chosen for their appearance and their acceptablity in the home rather than for their comfort. The appearance of a very comfortable chair may be so displeasing that a patient or their spouse may feel that they do not wish to have it their home.

Cost is an important factor which must be taken into account, when choosing a chair, because the easy chairs and office chairs which were found to be most comfortable to back pain sufferers were also the most expensive (Atherton *et al.*, 1980, 1982).

Except for the severely disabled, people do not seem to consider chair comfort in any depth. If sitting for longer than half an hour is uncomfortable, then there is a tendency to modify their lifestyle so that it is not necessary to sit for this length of time, rather than to consider selecting a new chair.

Many people, however, modify their chairs by the addition of extra cushions and 69% of the patients on the trial stated that their own chair at home was more comfortable than any of the ones which they had tested.

Users of office chairs are not always aware of the adjustments which can be made to their chair or which adjustments may ease their discomfort. This is of particular importance where the same chair is used by different personnel (Atherton *et al.*, 1982).

As stated earlier, the provision of comfortable seating may conveniently be divided into three stages:

Assembly of anthropometric data
Fitting trials
Comfort evaluation.

The results of anthropometric and ergonomic research are gradually being applied by industry to the design and manufacture of all types of chair.

It is obvious, however, from some of the findings given above, that people with back problems are not always in possession of relevant information to enable them to select a comfortable chair from those which are available. They are not, therefore, aware of the necessity for carrying out comfort evaluations nor are they in possession of guidelines for doing so in satisfactory manner. This points to an obvious need for education not only of the back pain sufferer but also their advisors in the medical and related professions.

Acknowledgement

We would like to thank the DHSS for their support and funding for the evaluations of the easy chairs, office chairs, car back-rests and replacement car-seats under the Disability Equipment Assessment Programme.

References

Andersson, B. J. G., Ortengren, R., Nachemson, A. & Elfstrom, G. (1974). Lumbar disc pressure and myoelectric back muscle activity during sitting, *Scandinavian Journal of Rehabilitation*, **6**, 104–14.

Andersson, B. J. G., Ortengren, R., Nachemson, A. L., Elfstrom, G. & Broman, H. (1975). The sitting posture: an electromyographic and discometric study, *Orthopaedic Clinics in North America*, **6**, 105–20.

Atherton, J., Clarke, A. K., Chatfield, J. & Harrison, R. A. (1980). *Easy chairs for the arthritic*. DHSS Aids Assessment Programme, DHSS.

Atherton, J., Clarke, A. K., Harrison, R. A. (1983). *Office seating for low back pain and arthritic patients*. DHSS Aids Assessment Programme DHSS.

Barkla, D. (1961). The estimation of body measurements of British Population in relation to seat design, *Ergonomics*, **4**, 124–32.

Bulstrode, S. J., Clarke, A. K. & Harrison, R. A. (1983). *Evaluation of back rests for use in car seats*. DHSS Aids Assessment Programme, DHSS.

Bulstrode, S. J., Clarke, A. K. & Harrison, R. A. (1985). *Assessment of replacement car seats*. DHSS Aids Assessment Programme, DHSS.

Burandt, U. & Grandjean, E. (1963). Sitting habits of office employees, *Ergometrics*, **6**, 217–28.

Drury, C. G. & Coury, B. G. (1982). A methodology for chair evaluation, *Applied Ergonomics*, **13**, 195–202.

Grandjean, E. & Burandt, H. U. (1962). Das Sitzverhalten von Buroangestellten, *Ind. Organisation*, **31**, 243–50.

Keegan, J. J. (1953). Alterations of the lumbar curve related to posture and seating, *Journal of Bone and Joint Surgery*, **35A**, 589–603.

Kelsey, J. L. & Hardy, R. J. (1975). Driving motor vehicles as a risk factor for acute herniated lumbar intervertebral disc, *American Journal of Epidemiology*, **102**, 63–73.

Knutsson, B., Lindh, K. & Telhag, H. (1966). Sitting – an electromyographic and mechanical study, *Acta Orthopaedica Scandinavia*, 415–28.

Le Carpentier, E. F. (1969). Easy chair dimensions for comfort, *Ergonomics*, **12**, 238–337.

Munton, J. S. (1981). An overview of research on seating, *Engineering in Medicine*, **11**, 107–10.

Research Institute for Consumer Affairs (1970). *Comparative test report No. 6 – Easy Chairs*. National Fund for Research into Crippling Diseases.

Discussion

Nelson (Leeds): If you include in your questions to patients the position of comfort, many patients will say that sitting is more comfortable than standing and there is another group who say they can't sit they can only stand. I have yet to understand the significance of this in terms of their pathology but it is quite obvious that some people and some conditions are actually better in chairs so I don't share the view that chairs of any type are necessarily bad. It depends what the condition of your back is and how long you sit in them. I think even the best chairs, if you sit in them for a long time, are bad.

Bulstrode: I think that is absolutely right. When we were conducting the assessments we were looking for a population who defined our criteria for people with low back pain fairly carefully and we were looking at the reported problems when sitting, the reported discomfort when sitting in an easy chair, office chair or car-seat. So we were actually looking at that specific population. I appreciate there are people who come in who say they are better off sitting and we weren't specifically looking at that group.

Loebl (London): Any ergonomist will tell you that the design of a seat or chair doesn't rest solely with that. It depends very much what people are doing. If they are working levers, pressing pedals, looking into screens, and so on, the visual and manual requirements are really the basic things in the design. The seat itself is secondary. How do you control that?

Bulstrode: When we were looking at the office chairs, for example, we appreciated that problem and particularly looked at two groups of people. We looked at people who were doing typing as one task, and people who were not doing typing but working at a desk, and their requirements were slightly different. It also becomes very relevant with car-seats and I know you have done work on this yourself. It depends very much on the design of the compartment of the car, and the position of the controls. Quite often you find people come to us and they actually say that their symptoms are aggravated by depressing the clutch pedal or whatever and these are the people we would advise not to change their car immediately, but when they next consider it to think of an automatic. We find that one approach which is quite necessary is to actually make people consider what specific aspect of sitting, whether it is in a car-seat or an ordinary chair, they think is responsible for the aggravation of their symptoms. Although perhaps when you first mention it people cannot identify it, when you actually give them some ideas, such as 'Is it actually the position you are in?' or, 'Is it sitting in one position for a long period of time?', they start to think about it and perhaps they can analyse their problem a little bit better themselves and take some course of action to remedy it.

Breen (Bournemouth): Have you looked at or heard about designing car chairs for very young children who are supposedly not back pain sufferers?

Bulstrode: I think some work has been done on this. I think they have actually under the same scheme looked at furniture for children. Whether they have actually looked at it in terms of comfort for the occupants of the chair or whether they have looked at it from the satisfaction of the mother who keeps having to lift the child back up the chair, I don't know.

Shepperd (Hastings): Surely the problem of desk-bound office workers is that people need to get up and down from chairs and is it not chair-arms that they really need for this?

Bulstrode: I would question that because some people cannot have arms on the chair, some typists find that the arms actually get in the way, or certain tasks that are being performed would mean that arms would be a disadvantage. So I think that is one question to make people aware of but I don't think it is necessarily the answer.

Clarke (Bath): Can I add a side comment to that. In easy chairs, it wasn't just comfort we were looking at it was a whole range of things and, for instance, when you compare our work with the Leeds work of Ann Chamberlain's department, they come up with different results to us in that getting in and out of chairs was said to be the most important thing. The slight difference between our work and their work was the length of time that people were actually asked to sit in the chairs. We tried more to simulate what one would normally do, like sitting down watching the television and then comfort does become more important. So the important thing is to relate it to the task you are doing, and getting in and out becomes important if you are getting in and out lots of times, but if your back is sedentary for a long period of time then comfortability is the important thing.

Fairbank (Birmingham): Can I ask you about office furniture and the forward tilting chairs. Did your study group find that a good thing?

Bulstrode: We found that most of the people with low back pain preferred a chair which either sloped forward 5° or was flat. We tend to recommend people to try chairs with a forward slope because we feel it perhaps encourages a more healthy posture but we never stipulate that you must have a chair with a forward tilt because it depends on the individual and what task they are performing. The only think we do often recommend is a slope downwards on the desk top as well, as this encourages a slightly better posture.

Fairbank (Birmingham): With our computer questions we have actually had people on kneeling chairs which they found very uncomfortable and they were abandoned very rapidly indeed.

Bulstrode: We find the kneeling chairs suit a very specific population and there is certainly a novelty factor.

Carpenter (Reading): I have had these kneeler chairs for the patients to sit on in my clinic for a number of years now. It does seem that it is the time factor on the chair that seems to bring on the pain. I wondered whether you knew if any work has been done on solo assisted chairs that actually change position, run by computers, constantly moving.

Bulstrode: Car-seats, yes, somebody is actually designing a car-seat which keeps changing position, but I haven't come across office chairs like that.

15 *E. O. Otun, C. R. Daniels, D. C. Gardiner and J. A. D. Anderson*

The evaluation of job heaviness using ambulatory monitoring

15.1 Introduction

Low back pain (LBP) is responsible for considerable subjective discomfort in the general population and is claimed to affect up to 80% of all people in the industrialised world at some time during their lives (Kelsey & White, 1980). It also results in substantial expense to medical services (Wood & Badley, 1980), and in sickness benefit payments (Bonde, 1981).

It is, perhaps, axiomatic that mechanical factors contribute to the development of LBP. These factors may result from hazardous occupational activities which hasten the onset of degenerative changes in the musculoskeletal system. However, the extent to which this occurs, and the risk factors responsible, have proved difficult to evaluate despite many extensive studies into the association between occupation and back pain (Magora, 1970; Andersson, 1981; Anderson, 1987).

The epidemiological approach has inherent limitations of diagnosis and classification. In addition, the variability in measurement techniques, coupled with the inability objectively to quantify risk factors, does little to clarify the situation. Findings are often confused and open to criticism with regard to their true relationship to back pain. However, they do confirm the widespread prevalence of LBP in industry and imply an increased risk in heavy industrial occupations (Anderson, 1987).

If back pain risk factors associated with occupation could be assessed reliably, primary prevention might be possible. This could be achieved by establishing guidelines for work practice and design in order to minimise the more risk-bearing components.

Evidence of high levels of morbidity due to back pain in association with physically heavy work (Frymoyer *et al.*, 1980) suggests a need for tools which can accurately and objectively assess the heaviness of jobs and the tasks which these jobs comprise. As job heaviness can be considered to be a complex function of postural, physiological and environmental components, continuous monitoring of many parameters is needed if such an accurate and objective assessment of heaviness is to be achieved.

In addition, in individuals suffering from chronic non-specific low back pain, where the emphasis is on improving function, rehabilitation could be monitored by evaluating functional status over long periods. Information obtained relating to activities performed both at work and in the home, and the individuals' responses to those activities, could be used to evaluate the overall effectiveness of rehabilitation brought about by health education or the redesign of jobs and work-stations.

Such considerations have led to the development of equipment and a technique based on non-invasive, continuous monitoring of job heaviness. This is attained by measuring four physiological parameters relating to spinal stress:

(1) The electromyogram (EMG) of the erector spinae muscles of the back; this gives a general measure of muscular activity and effort.

(2) Intra-abdominal pressure (IAP) which gives an indication of weight lifted; the reflex action of an individual when lifting a weight is to tense the muscles of the abdomen, this leads to increased IAP with concomitant support to the lumbar spine.

(3) Anterior spinal flexion.

(4) Posterior spinal flexion. Together (3) and (4) give an indication of the angular movement of the spine.

In the past, measurement of each of these physiological responses individually has enabled only an incomplete assessment of spinal stress to be made. Their combination in a single system allows the complex relationships between them to be investigated.

The following sections in this chapter describe how the above-mentioned measures of back stress may be obtained and analysed and how, in combination, they have been used to assess job heaviness in the motor industry.

15.2 **Measures of spinal stress**

15.2.1 *Surface electromyography*

Left and right lumbar muscular activity (at the level of the fourth and fifth lumbar vertebrae: L4 and L5) may be monitored by recording the surface electromyogram using two pairs of silver/silver chloride cup electrodes. These are located vertically 3.5 cm apart along the main masses of the erector spinae muscles.

Many methods of analysis of EMG exist with each having its merits and demerits. Techniques such as integration and calculation of the average amplitude (Fuglsang-Frederiksen, 1981), frequency analysis (Lindstrom & Peterson, 1983), calculation of the zero crossing rate and negative wave duration (Willison, 1964; Fitch, 1967; Licht, 1971; Fusfeld, 1978) and turns analysis (Willison, 1963) have been used. The technique of turning point (spike) counting was adopted in preference to any other because of artifacts caused by movement of the electrodes across the surface of the skin during exertion and the inherent limitations of direct recording, for ease of analysis and because only a general measure of muscular activity was required.

15.2.2 *Intra-abdominal pressure*

The techniques for measurement of intra-abdominal pressure (IAP) have been fully described by Davis (1981). Currently, we monitor IAP along similar lines, by telemetry, using a Rigel miniature pressure-sensitive radio transmitter and a portable receiver which was developed at the Department of Surgery and Medical Physics, University of Nottingham.

The subject swallows the pressure 'pill' after it has been calibrated using a manometer. The 'pill' emits a signal with a frequency proportional to the pressure exerted upon a copper membrane within it. This signal may be processed and a measure of IAP in kPa obtained.

15.2.3 *Spinal flexion*

Flexion of the lumbar spine may be measured using opto-electronic devices known as inclinometers. These have been developed specifically to measure angular movement of the spine whilst an individual carries out his work (Otun & Anderson, 1988). They are small, light and unobtrusive and by attaching one over the spinous process at the level of the twelfth thoracic vertebra (T12) and another at the level of the first sacral vertebra (S1) the degree of anterior or posterior flexion of the lumbar spine may be calculated. Measurement at these two sites enables the contribution of hip-rotation to the degree of spinal flexion to be eliminated.

15.3 **The ambulatory monitoring system**

The elements described above were incorporated into a monitoring system named PADAS – Physiological Ambulatory Data Acquisition System. This was designed to be worn unobtrusively on a belt around the waist of a worker (Figure 15.1), beneath or on top of work clothing, and to operate both continuously and remotely for up to 8 hours, recording parameters as described above and in Otun *et al.* (1984, 1988).

Whilst monitoring a subject, data was recorded on two standard TDK

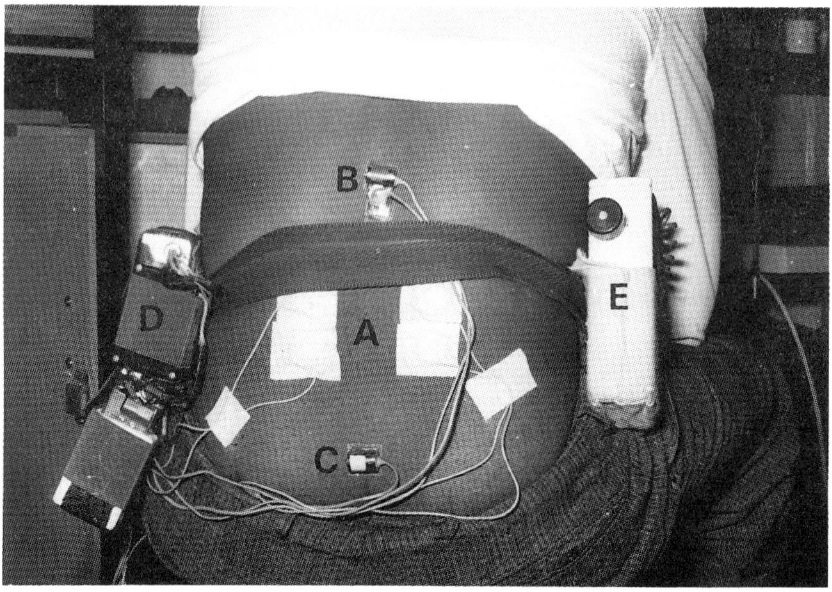

Fig 15.1 The Ambulatory Monitoring System: (A) surface electrodes to record the electromyogram of the erector spinae muscles of the back at L4 and L5; (B) inclinometer to measure anterior and posterior flexion of the spine at T12 (The lower inclinometer at position B may be used to measure lateral flexion); (C) inclinometer to measure anterior and posterior spinal flexion at S1; (D) Medilog recorders with associated timer/event marker and power supplies; (E) receiver for signals from the intra-abdominal pressure 'pill'. An aerial connected to this is positioned over the stomach of the individual and is therefore not visible in the photograph

C120 audio cassettes in two 4-channel, battery-powered, Medilog MR14 recorders. These recorders were connected, via the fourth channel of each, by a timer and event switch which were used for tape synchronisation and event marking. Six channels remained for recording physiological data. Each recorder was powered independently by a nickel/cadmium 6 volt rechargeable battery, and the complete system was worn in three pouches on the belt.

A custom-built Motorola 6800 microcomputer running the FLEX operating system was used to digitise, process and store the recorded data. The system and its associated software provided primary compression of the recorded data and produced ASCII (American Standard Code for Information Interchange) -coded datafiles.

15.4 Evaluation of job heaviness

The monitoring system was used to measure physiological responses in workers on the assembly lines of a car factory. In such an environment there is a broad spectrum of jobs, some of which may be considered subjectively to be 'light' whilst others may be thought of as being 'heavy'. Some workers' jobs involve little movement or apparent effort when, for example, operating a piece of machinery to assemble steering-columns, or when affixing hoses to an engine. However, other jobs appear to involve a great deal of lifting and many awkward movements as, for example, when operating an engine hoist and lifting exhaust-pipes from a bin to the assembly-line or when fitting a crash-pad (dashboard) to a car.

In order objectively to assess job heaviness the experimental procedure briefly outlined below was adopted. Twenty-nine individuals performing 27 different jobs were studied.

(1) Each individual's lifting capability in a number of different postures was evaluated. This enabled standardisation of their responses and, as a result of this, a comparison between jobs could be made.

(2) The component tasks comprising each job were evaluated. Whilst each worker performed his usual duties, each separate activity/job task was marked electronically on the recording tapes by an observer. This produced a series of 'events' defining the job being performed.

(3) The worker was allowed to continue working unobserved whilst his physiological responses were monitored for the remainder of his shift, usually for a period of up to 6 hours.

15.5 Statistical analysis

The analogue data recorded on the Medilog tapes were processed to generate files containing large amounts of digitised data. Following transference of these datafiles to a mainframe computer, the Statistical Analysis System (SAS Institute, 1985a and b) was used to create and analyse a multidimensional database.

Cluster analysis (Everitt, 1980; Gorden, 1981) grouped the 925 observed job tasks – see section 15.4(2) – from the 29 workers, according to the magnitudes of the four physiological variables, following their normalisation on a 0–100 scale. The analysis procedure was optimised when 40 job task groups (JTGs) were produced.

Within any JTG, the magnitude of a given variable lies in a range which itself may be positioned at any point on the 0 to 100 scale. Thus, in some cases, a JTG may contain job tasks with large measures of anterior flexion and, say, no measures of IAP, or *vice versa*. In addition, a given job task may appear in more than one JTG since measures of the four response variables may differ between repetitions of the same job task if, for example, a worker is inconsistent in the execution of his job.

To obtain an overall measure of heaviness for a group of job tasks the mean value of each variable in the group was calculated and the four means were totalled. These totalled JTG means were then ranked in order of magnitude, to produce a job task group heaviness scale (Figure 15.2).

During the period of work when no observer was present – (see section 15.4(3) – no events were marked on the recording tapes. Therefore, in order to analyse data from this period in a manner similar to that from the

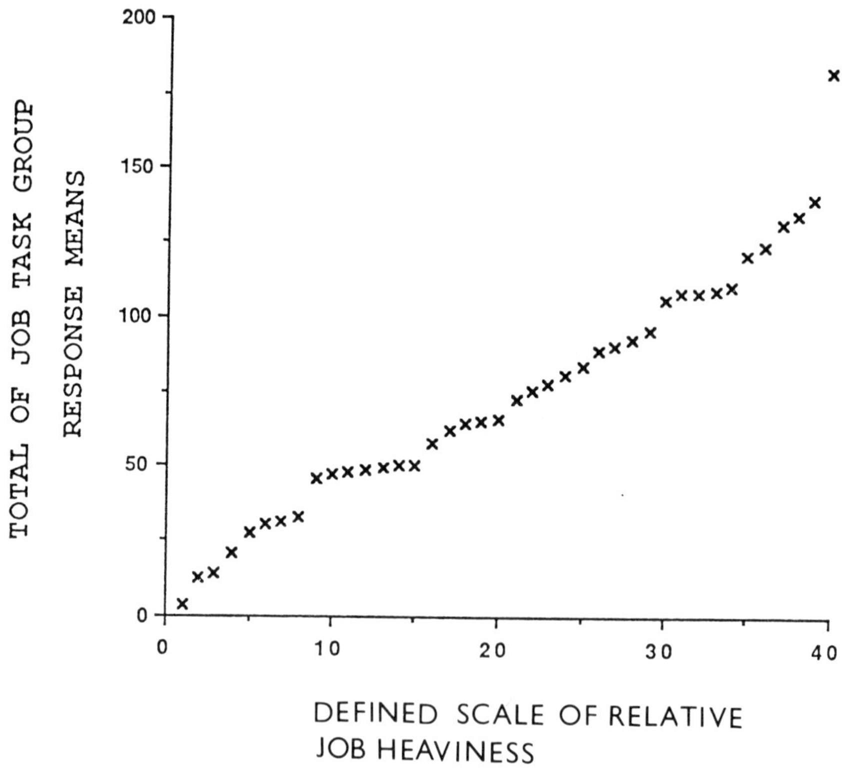

Fig 15.2 Job task group (JTG) heaviness scale: Normalised EMG, IAP, anterior and posterior spinal flexion responses from 925 observed job tasks were clustered into 40 job task groups. Within each group the mean values for each of these parameters were summed. The totals were ranked to produce a scale of relative heaviness. The figure shows the total for each job task group plotted against it's position on the scale

earlier period of observed work – section 15.4(2) – it was necessary to generate events artificially. These events could then be regarded as job tasks.

To generate the events the sums of EMG spike-counts per second (in the raw EMG datafiles) were calculated and plotted against time. Visual inspection detected the cyclical nature of the data and, when compared with data from the observed work period, suggested that peaks of EMG activity coincided with peaks of physical activity by the worker. After selecting a threshold value for EMG spike-counts per second (equivalent to a resting level) software was developed to mark events in the datafiles each time the sum of the spike-counts crossed this threshold. An algorithm matched the statistically summarised responses from the generated events to the JTGs described earlier.

Each worker's job contained events with responses matching several different JTGs. For a given worker, the percentage of events matching each JTG was calculated and plotted against the JTG's position on the JTG heaviness scale to produce a job profile. Weighting factors were calculated by multiplying each percentage by the corresponding JTG's position on the heaviness scale. Summation of these weighting factors produced a heaviness rating for each job.

15.6 **Job heaviness on a car assembly-line**

As an example of the type of data obtained using PADAS, Figure 15.3 shows the analogue signals recorded in a laboratory simulation where a

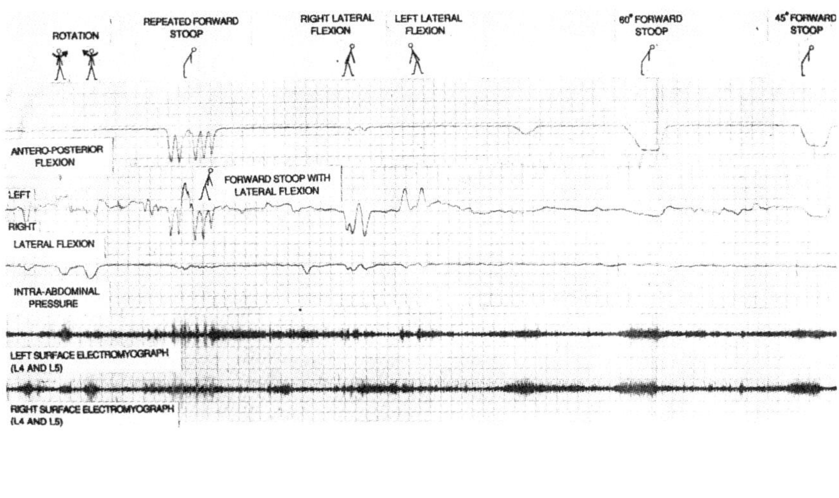

subject performed a number of formalised movements. In the industrial situation each of these could be regarded as an 'event' (though normally an event would comprise several movements) and descriptive statistics for each would be calculated. A measure of lateral flexion was included in the simulation but was not used in the study of the assembly-line workers.

Table 15.1 is the job heaviness rating scale for 29 workers on the assembly-lines of a car factory. It is a representation of the relative heaviness of their jobs and ranks them in decreasing order. Below, some of the jobs studied are described in more detail.

The heaviest job was found to be that of hose fitting. This activity took place on an engine-line and involved picking up bolts, collecting hoses, reaching for a pneumatic spanner, fixing hoses, tightening Jubilee clips and tightening bolts. The subject was working continually in a stooped position

Table 15.1 Job heaviness rating scale for 29 jobs performed on the assembly-lines of a car factory. The jobs are presented in decreasing order of heaviness

Position on scale	*Job description*
1	Hose fitting
2	Crash-pad (dashboard) fitting
3	Door-panel sub-assembly
4	Operation of engine hoist
5	Front brake assembly
6	Crash-pad (dashboard) fitting
7	Switch fitting
8	Panel/sound insulation fitting
9	Repairman
10	Windscreen assembly
11	Carpet fitting
12	Servo fitting
13	Repairman (garage)
14	Brackets/jack fitting
15	Choke-cable assembly
16	Brake-pipe fitting
17	Door-panel sub-assembly
18	Rubber/door-handle fitting
19	Wiring checking
20	Wiper fitting
21	Door setting
22	Starter-motor fitting
23	Front strut fitting
24	Wiper motor fitting
25	Production line supervision
26	Production line supervision
27	Specification checking
28	Panard rod fitting
29	Steering-column assembly

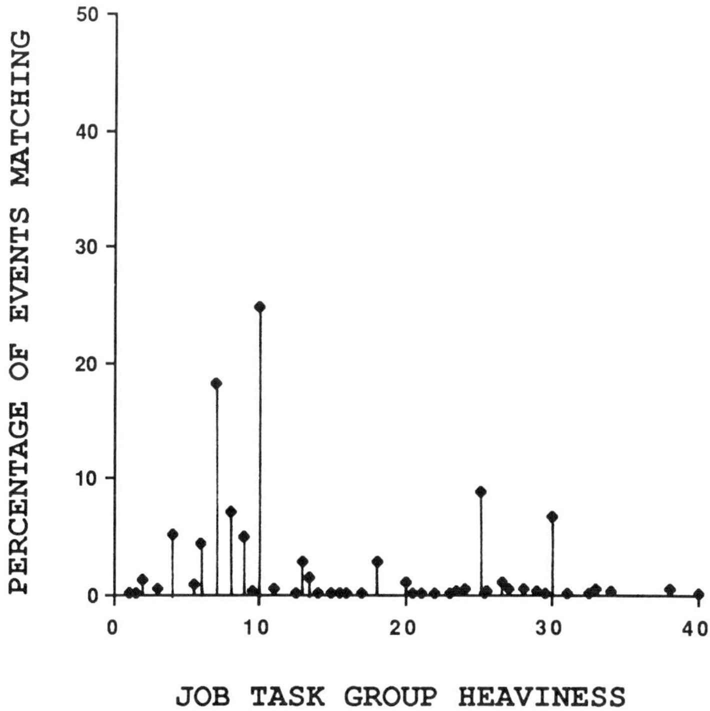

Fig 15.4 Job profile from the job at position one on the job heaviness rating scale, hose fitting. The percentage of generated events (tasks) from the unobserved work period with parameters matching each of the 40 job task groups is plotted against job task group heaviness

and often had to adopt awkward postures as he leant over the engine and applied lateral pressure to attach and secure heater-hoses and starter-motors. In addition, in reaching for the pneumatic spanner he had to stretch up, often across his body. Though ostensibly a job of medium heaviness, the analysis revealed high and varied levels of the measured responses which combined to produce the highest job-heaviness rating.

On examinating of the job profile for this worker (Figure 15.4) it is evident that a very low proportion of events appear in position 1. This JTG is characterised by no measures of IAP or antero-posterior flexion and only minimal EMG activity. It is usually associated with events with activity levels similar to those found during periods of rest. It could be inferred that the subject took few rests between working on different engines, a possible contributory factor to the heaviness of the job. However, it is clear that his responses matched JTGs positioned at most points along the JTG heaviness scale. Notwithstanding this, the subject did have a high resting

EMG level which, despite the standardisation procedure, may have influenced unduly the overall job heaviness rating.

Nevertheless, in the light of these results, it would seem advisable to reduce some of the hazardous elements which appear to contribute to the heaviness of this job. One way of achieving this might be to incorporate into the track carrying the engine a device which the worker could see effortlessly to rotate the engine into a position where he could apply pressure 'square on' to secure the hoses and bolts. As work is performed on both sides of the line by different workers an alternative suggestion would be to ensure that tasks associated with one side of the engine were performed only by the worker on the appropriate side.

The next two heaviest jobs were found to be crash-pad (dashboard) fitting and door-panel sub-assembly (Figures 15.5 and 15.6). The crash-pad fitter's job involved collecting nuts and bolts, checking wiring, collecting a crash-pad, carrying the crash-pad to the car, positioning and fixing the crash-pad, positioning wires, using a pneumatic spanner, collecting ducts for attachment to the heater and manipulating screws. A number of his responses for EMG and IAP matched those JTGs positioned at the upper end of the JTG heaviness scale. This, along with some antero-posterior flexion responses matching JTGs at the highest points on the heaviness scale, resulted in a high job heaviness rating.

At the start of the study, concern was expressed regarding the tasks associated with this job and their possible hazardous nature in terms of back pain. The job entailed working in limited space which restricted movement. This, coupled with the lifting and manipulation of unwieldy crash-pads, climbing in and out of the car and the fitting of awkward components (such as the ducting for the heater system) was thought to constitute a considerable risk. The results obtained support this.

Some modification of job design may be effective in reducing the magnitude of responses such as those recorded in this worker. A suggestion which would be simple (and cheap) to implement would be to have the crash-pad placed on the floor of the car before it reaches the fitter. This would mean that he need only position and secure it, rather than having first to collect it then climb into the car carrying it. In addition, it may help if the use of a stool over the propeller-shaft tunnel in the car became mandatory instead of being only occasionally used. The stool provides a steady and comfortable base upon which to work and could be used to advantage not only in this job but in all other jobs involving in-car assembly.

A second worker performing the job of crash-pad fitting produced responses which, when analysed, placed the job at position 6 on the job heaviness rating scale. The small difference in position is probably attributable to the fact that the same job was performed slightly differently

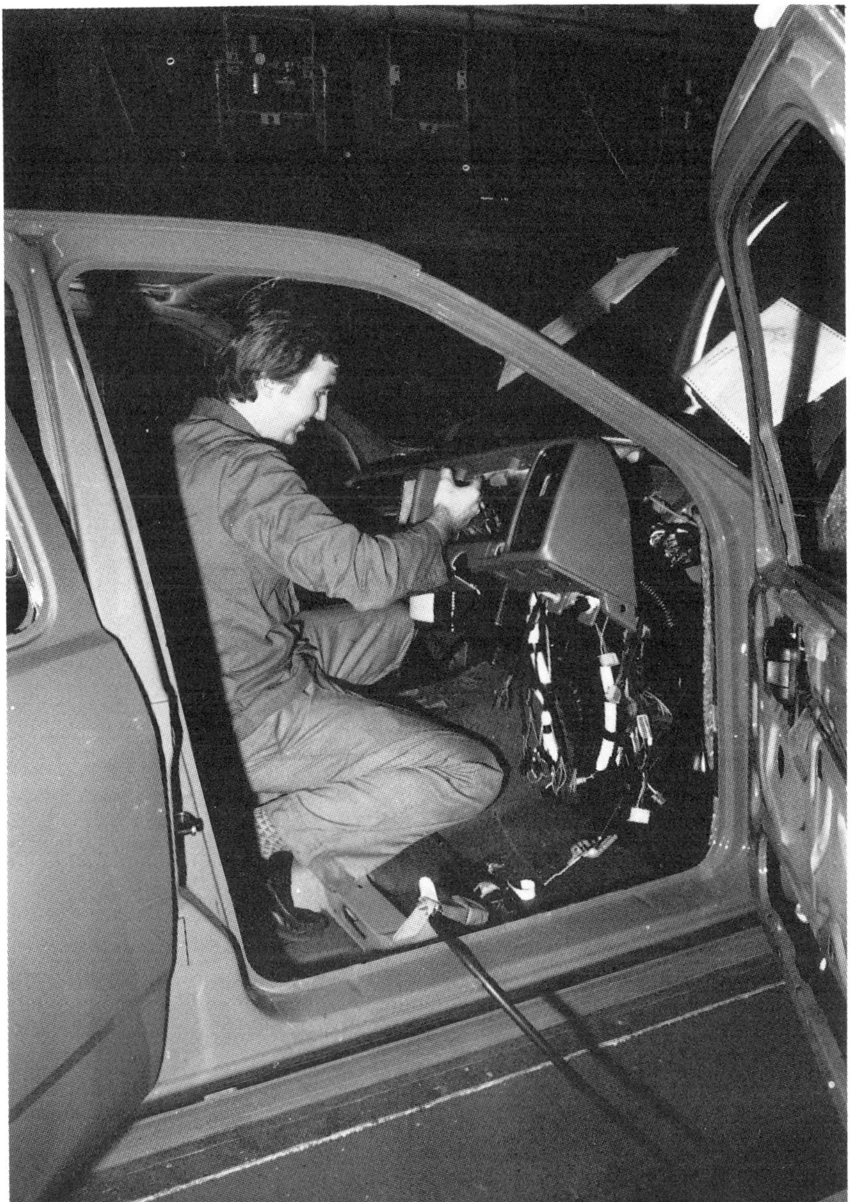

Fig 15.5 The job of crash-pad (dashboard) fitting. Note the subject's position straddling the propeller-shaft tunnel and the handling of the unwieldy crash-pad

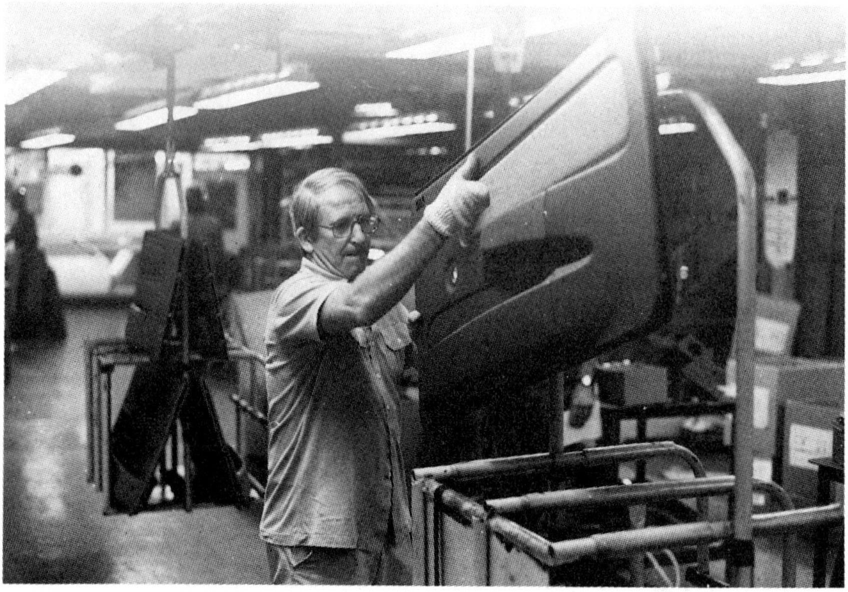

Fig 15.6 The job of door-panel sub-assembly. The panels are light but the necessity to lift them in awkward positions and to drag boxes of components to the work-bench produced responses which placed this job at position three on the job heaviness rating scale

by the two workers. In addition, anthropometric differences may have affected the way the two individuals worked. Job profiles for the individuals are presented for comparison (Figures 15.7a and b).

The job of door-panel sub-assembly involved stacking, dragging and positioning boxes of components, collecting and then positioning door-panels on a bench, fixing screws and studs to door-panels, fixing a door pocket and stamping holes in door-panels.

This job was considered, by those responsible for job allocation, to be one of the lighter jobs in the factory. However, the worker produced responses which placed his job at position 3 on the job heaviness rating scale. This was due mainly to his responses matching JTGs at most positions on the JTG heaviness scale and especially those characterised by high EMG. A worker performing a similar job appears at position 17 on the job heaviness rating scale. His responses matched JTGs at many positions on the JTG heaviness scale but the relative proportions at the upper end of the scale were lower. The latter did not have to drag boxes to his bench, a fact which may explain some of the difference. It would, perhaps, be advisable for the factory management not to consider the

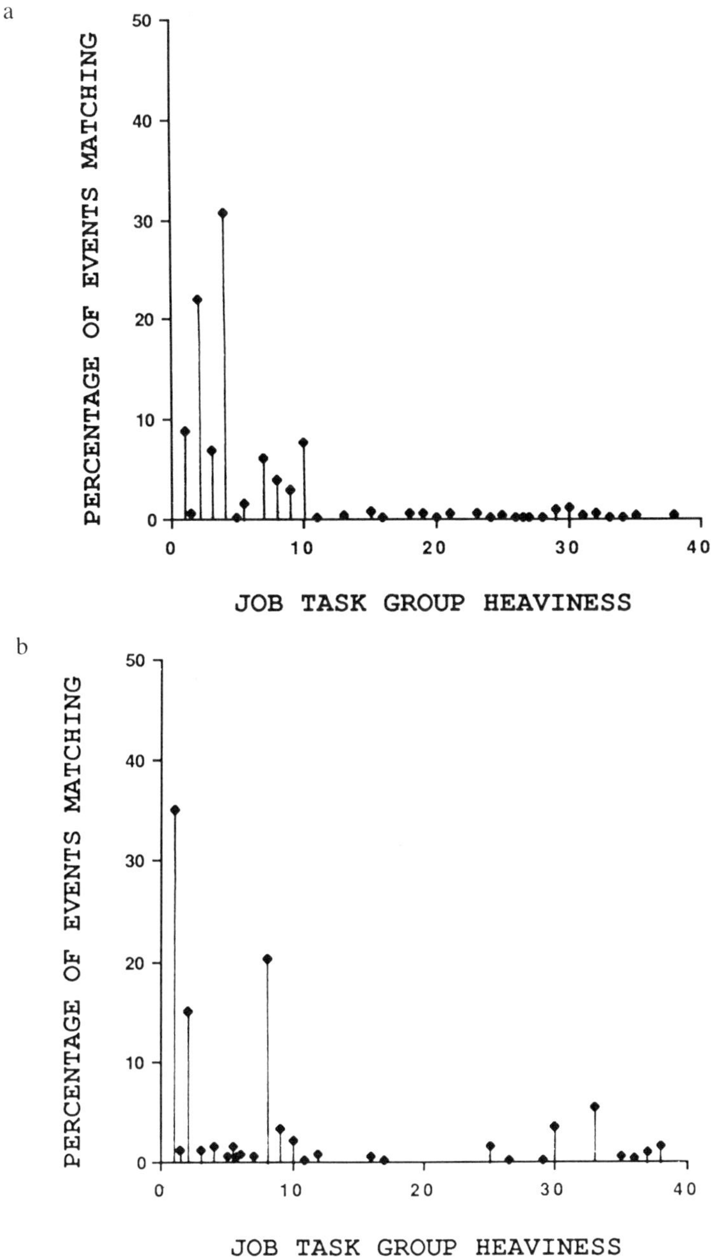

Fig 15.7 (a) Job profile for the crash-pad fitter at position two on the job heaviness rating scale. (b) Job profile for the crash-pad fitter at position six on the job heaviness rating scale

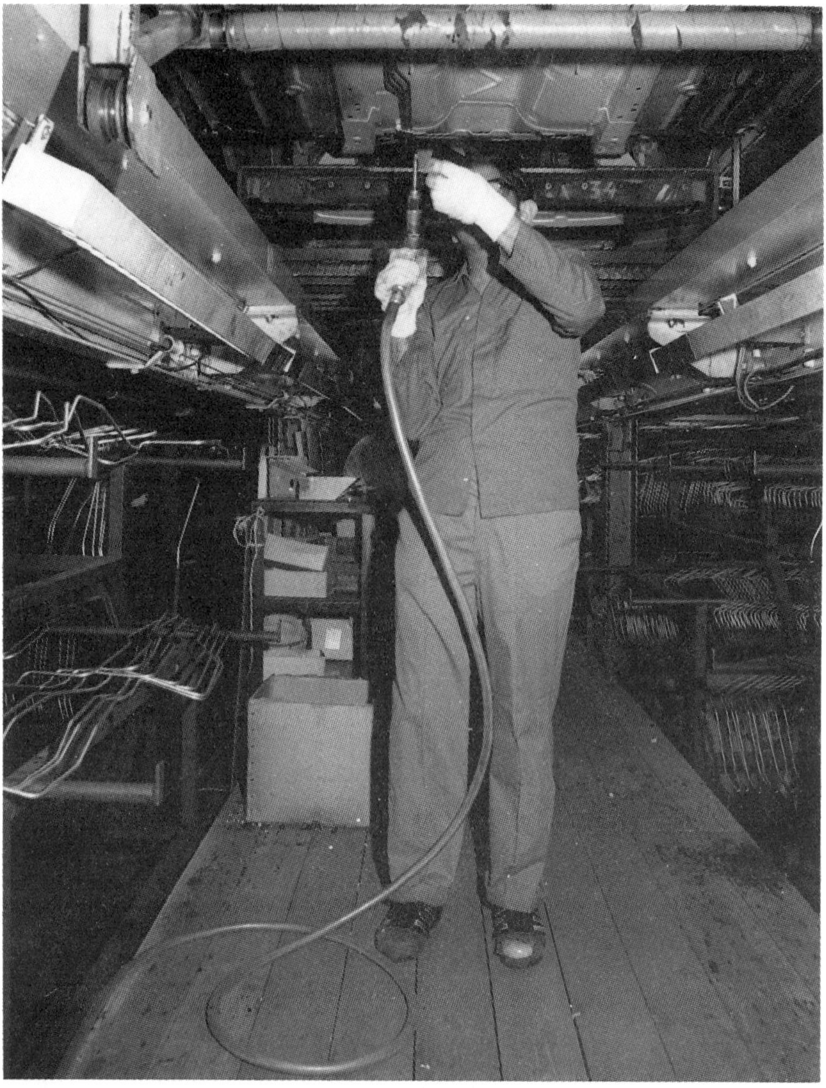

Fig 15.8 A fitter securing brake-pipes to the underside of a car. Note the platform which reduces the need for excessive stretching which would be necessary if the subject worked at ground-level

handling of heavy loads to be the only criterion when categorising a job as being light or heavy. Awkward postures and their sequelae would appear to be important.

A job which appears in the middle of the range of relative job heaviness is that involving the fitting of brake-pipes (Figure 15.8). In the job the subject worked beneath the cars which passed on a track approximately six feet above ground level. The job involved picking up and positioning brake-pipes and securing brackets to hold them in position. Although this job was observed to contain a great deal of left and right rotation and reaching upwards to exert pressure when securing the brake-pipes, the recordings obtained showed a predominance of events matching JTGs at the lower end of the JTG heaviness scale.

A very similar job was that at position 28 on the job heaviness rating scale, fitting Panard rods. Again, the subject worked beneath the cars and had to reach up to secure cables and bolts. However, in the main, the levels of his recorded responses were similar to those found during periods of rest and account for the low position of the job on the job heaviness rating scale.

The job in last position on the job heaviness rating scale was that of steering-column assembly (Figure 15.9). The subject worked a machine from a standing position and merely had to rotate right and left to collect and then place components in the machine before reaching up to pull a lever which operated it. His job profile is shown in Figure 15.10; 96% of his events matched JTGs at positions 1 to 4 on the JTG heaviness scale.

The results from two production-line supervisors whose jobs involved

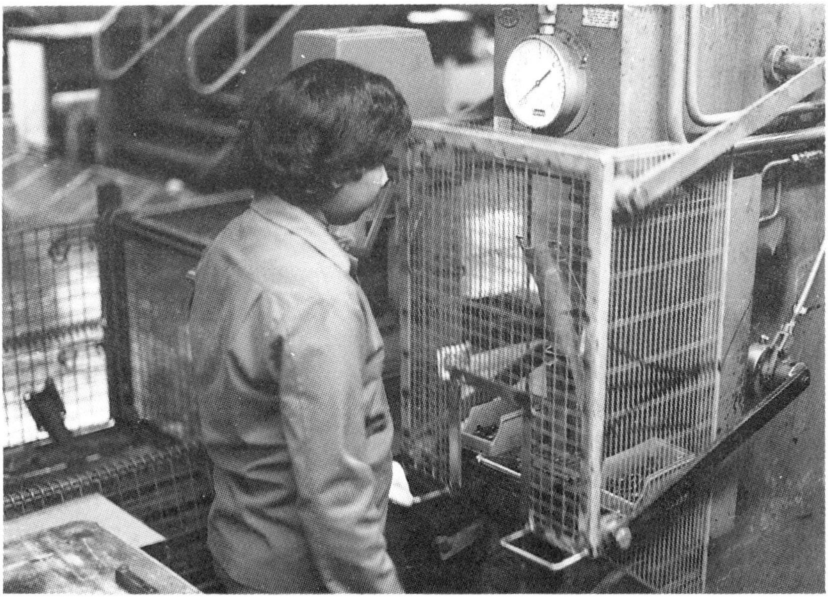

Fig 15.9 The job in last position on the job heaviness rating scale, steering-column assembly

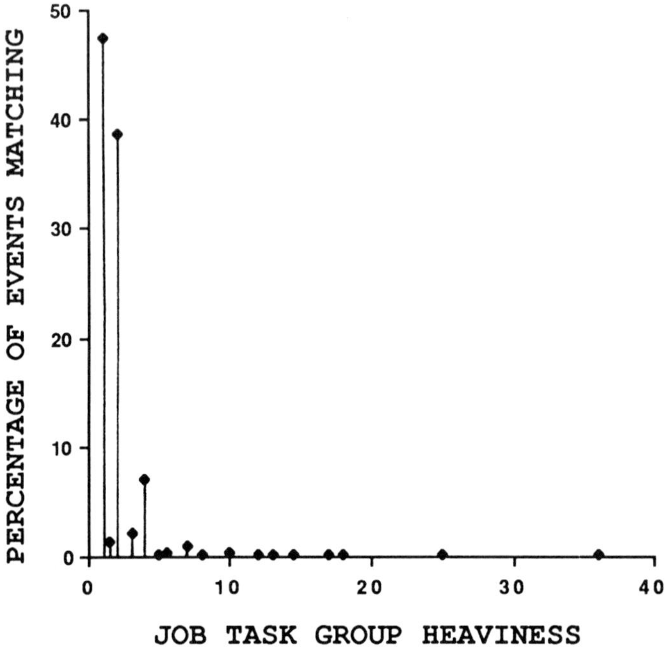

Fig 15.10 The job profile for the steering-column assembler

inspection of work (which entailed little physical effort) placed their jobs at positions 25 and 26 on the job heaviness rating scale.

15.7 **Discussion**

The examples given illustrate how the use of PADAS, and the associated analysis of data recorded in the workplace, enables the heaviness of jobs to be assessed objectively. Though difficult to prove in a study such as that described, we postulate that any job which produces levels of EMG, IAP and spinal flexion which categorise the job as heavy (according to our criteria), will, in the long-term, be injurious to the back.

Our equipment and techniques enable us to distinguish between heavy and light jobs with their positioning on the job heaviness rating scale generally supporting the subjective view. However, some results have highlighted aspects of job design and performance which, subjectively, were not thought to constitute a risk to the back.

Of the three heaviest jobs (all described above) only that of crash-pad fitting was deemed to be heavy. The worker assembling door-panels was assigned to his job as it was specifically designated as light (the man himself suffered from severe back pain). Clearly, the general view that the heaviness of a job is a direct function of the necessity to lift heavy weights is in error. Postural considerations (in the case of the door-panel assembler, the requirement to drag and manoeuvre boxes of components – with the resultant spinal flexion and increase in EMG activity) are important.

As previously stated, we are assuming that jobs which persistently produce responses which categories them as heavy will, in the long term, cause back problems. A sickness absence survey is currently being carried out and will attempt to correlate spells of absence due to back pain with estimated job heaviness.

The equipment and techniques described were developed to evaluate, objectively, job heaviness in terms of physiological and postural criteria. The relative importance of each of the response measures used to prepare the heaviness model is yet to be established. For the purposes of this study, equal importance was assumed.

Due to the complex relationships between the four response measures and the necessity to quantify these in order to gain a useful measure of spinal stress and job heaviness, we feel that the monitoring and analysis system, though elaborate, is uniquely suited for use in occupational studies. For example, the measurement of spinal flexion alone could indicate risk-bearing aspects of a job. By measuring EMG in addition, in the case of the door-panel assembler, we have been able to show that even greater strain is placed upon the spine than would otherwise have been indicated.

The only major problems encountered with the system have been the reluctance of volunteers to swallow and later to recover the pressure 'pill' and the logistics of managing and analysing the large quantities of data recorded for each worker. We are currently investigating other methods for measurement of IAP, and many adopt a device based on strain gauges (Dales *et al.*, 1987). In addition, we are attempting to develop the recording system so that much of the initial analogue-to-digital conversion and preliminary analysis will be accomplished by a microprocessor built into the body-borne apparatus.

The technique described frees the subject from the constraints of the laboratory and from cumbersome equipment, and allows for the evaluation of the individual's response to his work environment. It is our belief that the investigative strategy which this technique encompasses may be applied to many of the problem areas encountered in occupational studies, particularly those relating to low back pain.

Acknowledgements

The authors wish to thank Dr R. D. Kaye and H. Denyer for their help and advice in the development of the monitoring system. Thanks are also due to the management, medical staff and assembly-line workers at the Ford Motor Company, Dagenham, Essex, whose co-operation enabled this occupational study to be carried out.

This work is supported by the Arthritis and Rheumatism Council for Research.

References

Anderson, J. A. D. (1987). Dorsopathies. In: *Clinical Rheumatology*, ed. J. A. D. Anderson, Balliere Tindall, London.

Andersson, G. B. J. (1981). Epidemiologic aspects on low back pain in industry, *Spine*, **6**, 53–60.

Bonde, J. P. (1981). Maintenance allowance cases lasting for more than five weeks, *Ugeskar Laeger*, **143**, 43–49. (English summary)

Dales, J. L., Macdonald, E. B. & Anderson, J. A. D. (1987). Truncal stress measurement during manual handling, *Ergonomics*, **30**, 89–102.

Davis, P. R. (1981). The use of intra-abdominal pressure in evaluating stresses on the lumbar spine, *Spine*, **6**, 90–92.

Everitt, B. (1968) *Cluster Analysis*, 2nd Edn., pp. 31–34. Heinemann Educational Books, Halsted Press, London.

Fitch, P. (1967). An analyser for use in human EMG, *Electronic Engineering*, **39**, 240–3.

Frymoyer, J. W., Pope, M. H., Costanza, M. C., Rosen, J. C., Goggin, J. E. & Wilder, D. G. (1980). Epidemiological studies of low back pain, *Spine*, **5**, 419–23.

Fuglsang-Frederiksen, A. (1981). Electrical activity and force furing voluntary contraction of normal and diseased muscle, *Acta Neurologica Scandinavica*, **63**, Supplement 83.

Fusfeld, R. D. (1978). Instrument for quantitative analysis of the electromyogram, *Medical and Biological Engineering and Computing*, **16**, 290–5.

Gorden A. D. (1981). *Monographs on Applied Probability and Statistics: Classification*, pp. 41–44. Chapman and Hall, London.

Kelsey, J. L. & White, A. A. (1980). Epidemiology and impact of low back pain, *Spine*, **5**, 133–42.

Licht, S. (ed.) (1971). *Electrodiagnosis and Electromyography*, 3rd Edn., Licht E. New Haven, Connecticut.

Lindstrom, K. & Peterson, I. (1983). Power spectrum analysis of EMG signals and its application. Computer-Aided Electromyography. In: *Progress in Clinical Neurophysiology*, 10, ed. J. E. Desmedt. Karger, Basel.

Magora, A. (1970). Investigation of the relation between low back pain and occupation, *Industrial Medicine*, **39**, 31–37.

Otun, E. O. & Anderson, J. A. D. (1988). An inclinometric method for continuous measurement of sagittal movement of the lumbar spine, *Ergonomics*, **31**, 303–15.

Otun, E. O., Daniels, C. R., Gardiner, D. C. & Anderson, J. A. D. (1988). An assessment of job heaviness related to assembly-line work in the motor industry using EMG, intra-abdominal pressure and spinal flexion. In: *Contemporary Ergonomics*, ed. E. G. Megaw. Taylor and Francis, London.

Otun, E. O., Heinrich, I., Anderson, J. A. D. & Crooks, J. (1984). 'PADAS' – An ambulatory electronic system to monitor and evaluate factors relating to back pain at work, *Ergonomics*, 27, Supplement 1, 268–71.

Statistical Analysis System (1985a). *SAS Users Guide: Basics*, Version 5 Edition. SAS Institute.
Statistical Analysis System (1985b). *SAS Users Guide: Statistics*, Version 5 Edition. SAS Institute.
Willison, R. G. (1963). A method of measuring motor unit activity in human muscle, *Journal of Physiology*, **168**, 35–38.
Willison, R. G. (1964). Analysis of electrical activity in healthy and dystrophic muscle in man, *Journal of Neurology, Neurosurgery & Psychiatry*, **27**, 386–94.
Wood, P. & Badley, E. (1980). Back pain in the community. In: *Clinics in Rheumatic Diseases – Low Back Pain*, 6, ed. R. Grahame. Saunders, London.

Discussion

Mulholland (Nottingham): Have you any figures of the actual experience of back pain disability in those groups which we can then identify as heavy jobs?

Otun: Yes, at the moment we have just completed the first stage of the project and it has taken us 6 years to get this far. What we have done is to evaluate most of the jobs on the shop floor of the factory and what we are trying to do now is to look at sickness absence attributable to those jobs and to also look at that over the next couple of years to see whether the jobs we have actually identified are in fact the jobs which are responsible for sickness absence due to back pain. As regards to the actual figures regarding the incidence of back pain in the individuals who took part in the study, yes we do have those but you must bear in mind that most of the individuals who came forward were volunteers and they did not have back pain or have not suffered from any incidences of back pain. We had to screen them in this way. We did not want the fact of them having a back pain incident or having one in the past to influence our results.

Troup (Liverpool): The difficulty with your three methods of measurement is that no one of them relates directly to spinal loading and I wonder if, in the absence of subjects with susceptible back pain or in the absence of patients with back pain, have you considered relating your data and results to one direct biomechanical measure, the changes in stature, and the other to perception of loading, using scientific methodology.

Otun: Yes, we have considered this. At present the main emphasis has been on industrial problems. We found a considerable problem in industry in trying to get the management and the unions to agree to a performance study and secondly to pass the equipment used. What we tried to make sure of was that we did not take an individual out of his work place. The whole system is designed so that the responses were recorded in the work place, unobserved, unsupervised by any researcher, so that we could really get a good estimation of what exactly was happening to produce these responses in his back.

Troup (Liverpool): Yes, but the problem is to do the validation in the laboratory before you take it to the workplace.

Otun: I wouldn't say the validation. I don't quite understand what you mean. Perhaps it is standardisation procedures which you are referring to. They are done in a laboratory situation. The work I am actually referring to takes place in one's place of work.

Oldham (Chichester): You say that you didn't find much correlation between what the management thought were heavy jobs and what you decided were heavy jobs. Can I ask you were the jobs that were found to be heavy high status or low status jobs in relation to pay? So was there any correlation between grading and effort?

Otun: I'm afraid I don't have any data on that. Our observations as to what the management thought and what we observed was purely because of the experimentation that we had done and observing the personnel and their placements. I haven't got actual figures. What really did occur was that it was a general feeling that jobs that did not involve lifting heavy loads or working on the actual assembly line were considered as light jobs. By these I mean jobs such as sub-assembly jobs, putting screws into holes and then letting somebody else bolt them up, that kind of job was considered as light, but in fact based on the magnitude of the individual actually performing that job, we found them to be heavy. Now whether this has any implications for back pain I cannot say at this stage. The instrumentation is designed to evaluate relative job heaviness, the next stage is to find out whether the jobs we have actually identified are associated with increased sickness due to back pain.

16 *V. J. Markley and J. A. N. Shepperd*

Corset supply and the Hastings Corset Shop

16.1 Introduction

This chapter compares traditional made-to-measure corset prescription with the provision of ready-made corsets by self-selection under the guidance of a qualified occupational therapist. A survey of 100 patients suggests that the ready-made versions are preferred by patients and also carry substantial cost advantages.

The provision of external braces for back pain is far from new. Evidence of such devices exists in the fifth Egyptian Dynasty (2750–2625 BC). Many of the principles appear to stem from Hippocrates or possibly armourers in the middle ages (Smith, 1908). Despite wide use of corsets, surprisingly little information exists in the literature regarding their benefit (Perry, 1970; Million *et al.*, 1981; Sypert, 1987). Publications on the subject appear to be decreasing in frequency.

Controversy exists over the objectives of the corset which include:

(1) Immobilisation of the lumbar spine which may not be possible by external means (Norton & Brown, 1957; Perry, 1970; Fidler & Plasmans, 1983; Morris, 1960). Restriction of movement is always modest. Maximum flexion of the lumbo-sacral region takes place in the first 30° of forward flexion, and some argue this can only be properly controlled by a spica.

(2) Imposing a posture. This may be by three-point fixation, deterring inappropriate posture by discomfort, or by the reining in of a protruding abdomen (Rose, 1981).

(3) Enhancement of intra-abdominal pressure. This seems to be the most convincing biomechanical virtue of these appliances. It has been calculated that compressive force at the lumbo-sacral junction

is reduced by a third as a result of the inflatable support of intra-abdominal pressure (Davis, 1959; Davis & Troup, 1964).

(4) Warmth. It has been suggested that this is the most important function of a belt, particularly in the elderly (Rose, 1981).

(5) Placebo. The act of administering treatment to a patient may have a placebo effect on either the prescribing doctor or the patient or both (Selby, 1982).

Estimates vary concerning the number of corsets supplied in the United Kingdom because no accurate figures are maintained. It seems that anything from 200 000 (Van Der Rijt & Seal, 1982) to 1 200 000 (Rose, 1981) are used annually. The national expenditure can, therefore, only be guessed at but the figure of £7.2 million given by Van Der Rijt & Seal is likely to be conservative. They also reported a 26% non-compliance rate, indicating immediate wastage of at least £1.8 million.

Faced with a confusing array of devices, the traditional method of corset prescription was scrutinised at this Centre. A new method of supply involving the Occupational Therapy Department was established and christened the Occupational Therapy Corset Shop. The two methods of corset supply will now be described.

16.2 **Traditional method**

This is illustrated in Figure 16.1. Corsets are prescribed by the Rheumatology or Orthopaedic Department. The patient is referred to a corset fitter, measured and, after a period varying from 2–6 weeks, provided with a made-to-measure device and instructed in its use. This method may be used according to the preference of the individual practitioner.

16.3 **Occupational Therapy Corset Shop**

This method is illustrated in Figure 16.2. The Occupational Therapy Department obtained a wide range and variety of ready-to-wear corsets from standard manufacturers. These are mainly elasticated and without rigid steels. Patients are referred to the Corset Shop from the back clinic. An experienced member of staff demonstrates the range of devices in the department, guiding the patient over the key points. Patients are encouraged to become actively involved in choosing their own device, and it is hoped that this achieves a shift in emphasis of responsibility. If the patient's choice appears unsatisfactory, he or she is invited to return and change it. If no satisfactory device can be found the patient is referred back to the

a

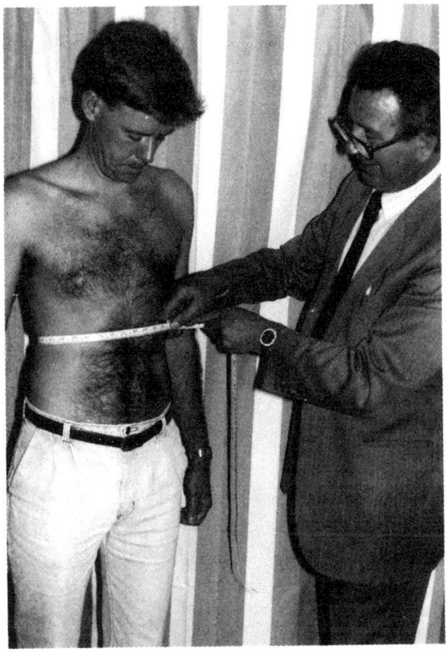

b

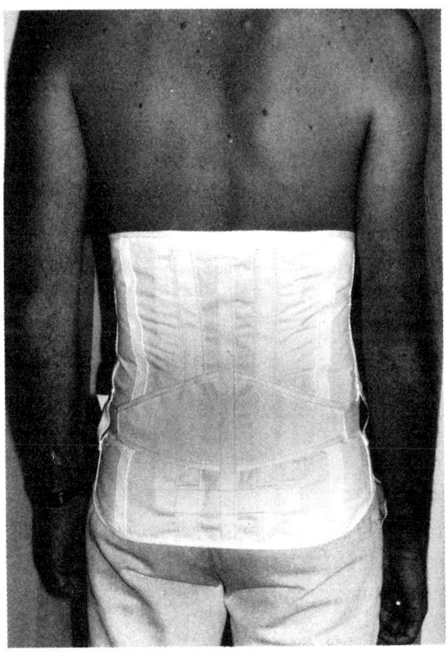

Fig 16.1 (a) Traditional corset prescription involves referral to a brace maker where the patient is measured. (b) 2–6 weeks later the patient is provided with the made-to-measure device and instructed in its use

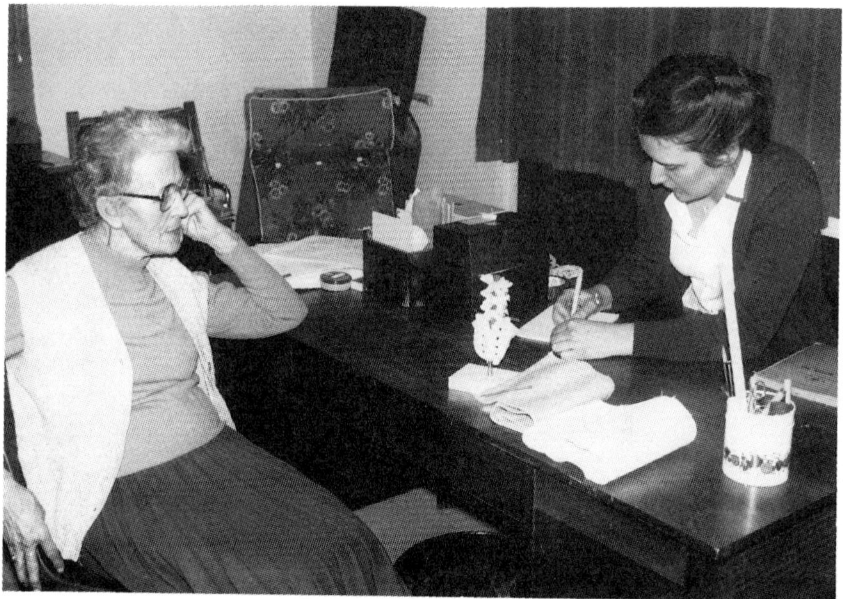

a

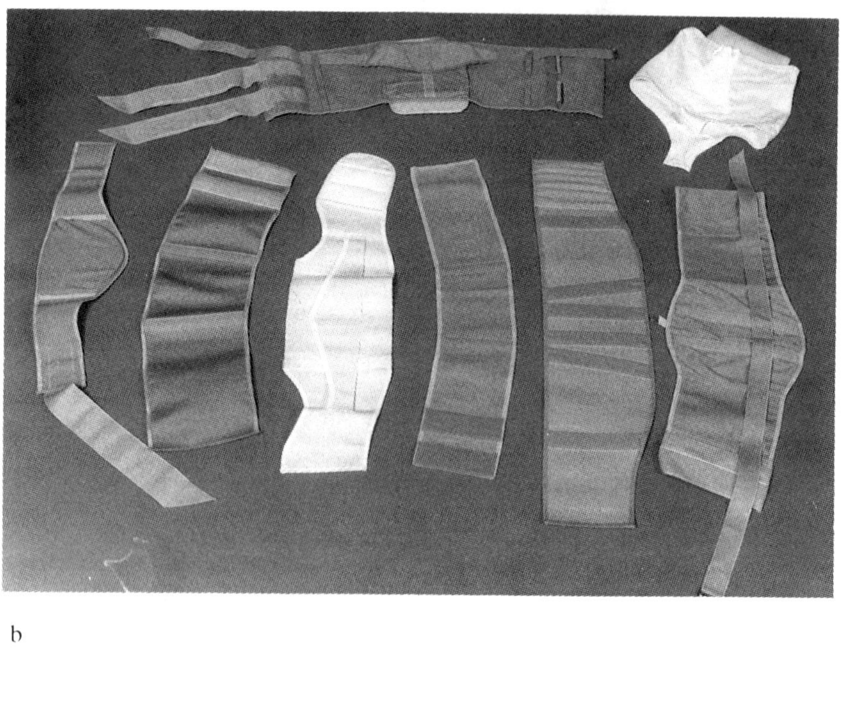

b

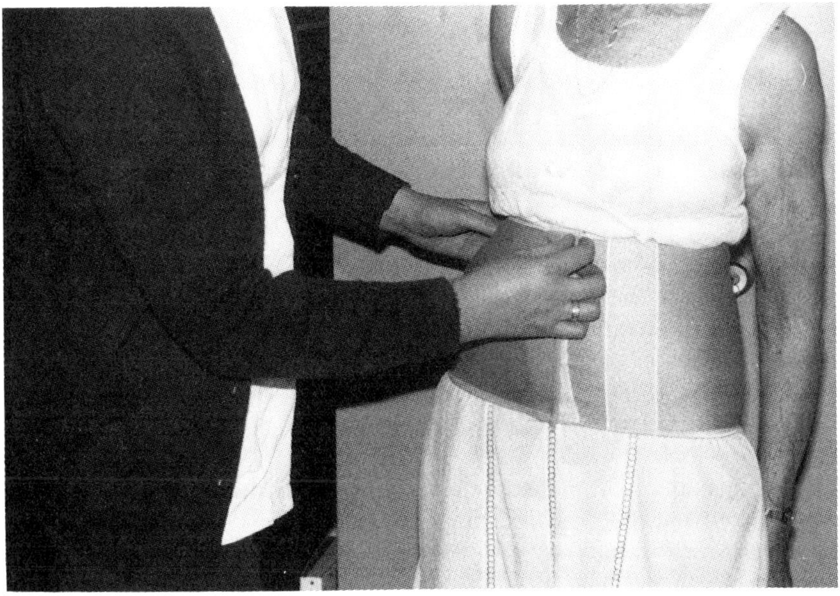

c

Fig 16.2 (a) The patient is referred to the Occupational Therapy Corset Shop where the Occupational Therapists arranges an interview and discusses general back care, advice and other details of life style. (b) The patient is shown a range of made-to-measure supports and invited to choose one that is comfortable, being guided by the Occupational Therapist. (c) The patient is usually provided immediately with the chosen support, and asked to return if it appears unsatisfactory

prescribing doctor and then either follows the traditional method, or the corset is abandoned. At the same interview, the patient receives other advice on aspects of daily living in connection with the back problem.

16.4 **Method**

In 1986–87, 252 traditional corsets and 349 Occupational Therapy Corset Shop corsets were supplied at the Hastings Orthopaedic Centre. Both systems are available to consultant rheumatologists and orthopaedic surgeons in this centre. The specific referral is at the discretion of the referring doctor. The survey was carried out using a postal questionnaire to a random sample of 100 of these patients (Appendix 16.1). Fifty of the patients had received corsets by the traditional method and 50 from the Occupational Therapy Corset Shop. The questionnaire considered compliance, symptom improvement and comfort of the device.

16.5 **Results**

Of the Occupational Therapy Corset Shop patients, 78% replied compared to 72% of the traditional method patients; 78% claimed to have gained benefit from the Occupational Therapy Corset Shop compared to only 68% from the traditional method; and 50% found the traditional corset uncomfortable compared with 22% for the Occupational Therapy Corset Shop (Table 16.1).

There is a striking difference in cost between the made-to-measure corsets and ready-made varieties (Table 16.2); as a result a substantial cost saving occurred. In 1986–87 this had a potential of £29 000 in the Hastings District. Extrapolating the figures of Van Der Rijt & Seal produces a nationwide annual saving in the order of £5.5 million.

16.6 **Discussion**

Inviting a patient to choose or reject the ready-made corset would be expected to improve the acceptance rate and this is borne out by the findings from this survey. We believe also that the psychological effect upon the patients may be important in implying that the patients have responsibility for their own backs. The occupational therapist reinforces this aspect by further back care advice at the same interview. This provides a different atmosphere from the collection of a corset from a manufacturer, where the onus of satisfaction lies as much with the prescribing doctor as the individual patient.

Compliance in both groups appears high compared with other reports for a traditional prescription. The age difference between the groups may reflect the referring doctor's decision in choosing one or the other method.

Traditionally made-to-measure corsets are clearly expensive. The cost analysis on wastage has to incorporate both non-compliance and lack of satisfaction. In the case of the traditional method these two figures amount

Table 16.1 Results of patient survey

	Occupational therapy corset shop (n = 50)	*Traditional (n = 50)*
Replied	78%	72%
Average age (range)	54 (21–86) yrs	69 (17–92) yrs
Compliance	96%	90%
Symptoms helped	78%	68%
Corset uncomfortable	22%	50%
Corset as expected	52%	82%

Table 16.2 Comparison cost of occupational therapy Corset Shop and the traditional method (estimates for financial year 1986–87)

	Traditional	*Occupational therapy Corset Shop*
Number of corsets supplied, 1986–87	252	349
Total cost of corsets fitted	£15 496.60	£3 693.94
Average cost of each corset including staff time	£61.49	£13.18
Cost of 601 corsets	£36 955.49	£7 921.18
Potential saving at Royal East Sussex Hospital, using Corset Shop system		£29 034.31

Note: Potential saving in England and Wales on estimated 200 000 corsets, costing £7.2 × 10^6 = £5 539 631.70 (Van Der Rijt & Seal, 1982).

to 42% of the patients questioned compared with only 22% for the Corset Shop patients. As well as the waste of resources that arise from such ineffective treatment, patient confidence in the prescribing physician may be undermined.

This report is limited both by numbers and lack of independent assessment. Nevertheless, there appear to be advantages attached to the Corset Shop method and we would value further reports from other centres.

References

Ahlgren, S. A. & Hansen, T (1978). The use of lumbosacral corsets prescribed for low back pain, *Prosthetics and Orthotics International*, **2**, 101–104.

Davis, P. R. (1959). Posture of the trunk during the lifting of weights, *British Medical Journal*, **1**, 87–89.

Davis, P. R. & Troup, J. D. G. (1964). Pressures in the trunk cavities when pulling, pushing and lifting, *Ergonomics*, **7**, 466–73.

Fidler, M. W. & Plasmans, C. M. T. (1983). The effect of four types of support on the segmental mobility of the lumbo-sacral spine, *The Journal of Bone and Joint Surgery*, **65A**, 943–7.

Lumsden, R. M. & Morris, J. M. (1968). An *in vivo* study of axial and immobilization at the lumbosacral joint, *The Journal of Bone and Joint Surgery*, **50A**, 1591–602.

Million, R., Haavik Nilsen, K. & Baker, R. D. (1981). Evaluation of low back pain and assessment of lumbar corsets with and without back support, *Annals of Rheumatic Diseases*, **40**, 449–54.

Morris, J. M. (1957). Spinal bracing. In: *Neurosurgery*, eds. R. H. Withins & S. S. Perganchez, pp. 2300–5. McGraw-Hill, New York.

Norton, P. L. & Brown, T. (1957). The immobilizing efficiency of back braces, *The Journal of Bone and Joint Surgery*, **39A**, 111–39.

Perry, J. (1970). The use of external support in the treatment of low back pain, *The*

Journal of Bone and Joint Surgery, **52A**, 1440–42.
Rose, G. K. (1981). Lumbo-sacral belts. Guest Lecture, Robert Jones and Agnes Hunt Orthopaedic Hospital.
Smith G. E. (1908). The most ancient splints, *British Medical Journal*, 732–5.
Selby, D. K. (1982). Conservative care of non-specific low back pain, *Orthopaedic Clinics of North America*, **13**, 427–35.
Sypert G. W. (1987). External spinal orthotics, *Neurosurgery*, **20**, 642–9.
Van Der Rijt, A. J. & Seal, P. V. (1982). The lumbar corset – A subjective analysis. Paper read to the Society for Back Pain Research.

Discussion

Loebl (London): Do you charge different prescription charges because the corsets from the Corset Shop are cheaper?

Markley: No.

Fairbank (Birmingham): Can I ask two questions. Firstly, what proportion of patients going through the Back Clinic in Hastings are fitted with corsets? Secondly in your follow up questionnaire you found that 96% of corsets were worn. I must say that that doesn't tie in with any other studies I have read about corset wearing. Do you think this is just people saying this to please you, or did you have any checking up on whether they were actually wearing them.

Markley: To answer your first question first. In the year 1986–87 the number of corsets fitted traditionally was 252 and by the corset shop was 349. I haven't got the figures regarding the proportion of back pain clinic attenders who were fitted with a corset. Secondly, we took what was answered on the questionnaire. I wonder in fact if the compliance is high because the patient is actively involved in their management as far as the corset fitting is concerned. They actually choose the corset they will wear and the emphasis is put back onto the patient to look at the corset and their life style.

Nelson (Leeds): Can you tell us whether the corset you provided had a specific name?

Markley: We use Flexifit, Spencer and Hallam posture belts. In fact we have a very large range.

Nelson (Leeds): What is the range of cost of the ones in the Corset Shop as opposed to the others.

Markley (Hastings): The cheapest corset fitted by the traditional method was £28 which is a ready-made corset. It is interesting to note that it if it goes via the fitters they actually charge a £5 fitting fee. If you go to the occupational therapist she will do it for you for nothing. The cheapest corset fitted in the Corset Shop was actually £8.70 and is called the Spencer 225. These are figures for 1986–87. The most expensive corset was £102 by the fitters and the Corset Shop was £14.97 which was the Paramount.

Roberts (Nottingham): Does that mean that when we write a prescription for a corset in the clinic whoever receives that prescription at the other end is giving the patient a Rolls-Royce when in fact something a little less substantial is required?

Markley: Well I think we are beginning to believe that, yes.

Roberts (Nottingham): In other words we should actually specify what we want on our prescriptions.

Clarke (Bath): One of the answers to this is to actually change our method of prescriptions and employ orthotists in the Health Service who will perform this role for us in the same way as the physiotherapists perform the role about what form of treatment is given in the physiotherapy department, but I don't want to particularly open that can of worms at this stage.

Hoskin (Nottingham): I would like to congratulate you on saving this sort of money for the Health Service and do you see any other areas where you might be able to save us some more?

Markley: When I actually gathered the figures for the traditional method the only way that I could get the costings was to go through every single appliance form in the Appliance Department for the financial year 1986/87, and I came across a multitude of sins. Things like hand splints which are obviously asked for which could be made for a fraction of the cost in the occupational therapy department, this sort of thing, and I think that it is certainly an area that people should start looking into.

Appendix 16.1 Questionnaire sent to patients supplied with corsets

Age . . . .
Occupation . . . .
Symptoms of leg pain and/or back pain . . . .
. . . .
Are your symptoms (a) continuous? . . . .
(b) intermittent? . . . .
(c) related to activity? . . . .
Have you found the corset (a) comfortable? . . . .
(b) acceptable? . . . .
(c) unacceptable? . . . .
Was the corset what you expected? (a) yes . . . . (b) no . . . .
Have you been able to wear the corset as directed? (a) yes . . . .
(b) no . . . .
(c) sometimes . . . .
Has your corset helped? (a) yes . . . . (b) no . . . .
(c) less than you had hoped . . . .
Any general comments about the corset?
. . . .

17 *J. P. O'Brien*

The role of fusion for chronic disabling low back pain

17.1 **Introduction**

The aim of this chapter is to outline briefly the role of surgical treatment for the patient disabled with low back pain. It must be clear from the outset that surgery in low back and leg pain syndromes is reserved solely for those patients where a thorough trial of conservative treatment has been tried and has failed. In a small percentage of patients with persistent sciatica, the indication for surgical intervention will be a ruptured disc with significant and/or deteriorating neurological function.

Lumbar discectomy has been shown, in a prospective randomised trial, to be superior to conservative treatment in these patients at a 1-year follow-up but this difference is lost by 10 years (Weber, 1983). Young *et al.* (1955) have suggested that 35% of patients undergoing discectomy for a herniated disc would benefit from a fusion at the same procedure. More conservative surgeons might reserve fusion for patients who have persistent disabling backache following a discectomy and who also have evidence of segmental instability (Frymoyer, 1981; Wright, 1981).

In the present context we are concerned with the much more common problem of chronic low back pain. In these patients removal of the disc alone will rarely improve the pain and lumbar fusion must be considered. Unfortunately no prospective trial of fusion exists but long-term follow-up of patients undergoing posterior fusion is disappointing with as many as 44% of patients still complaining of persistent back pain over 20 years after the original operation (Lehmann *et al.*, 1987).

In view of the controversies and apparently indifferent results that exist for the treatment of back pain by surgery, a new approach to the problem is presented below.

17.2 **Controversies in low back pain**

17.2.1 *The psychological background*

There is a significant number of medical practitioners who believe that there is a large psychological element in most low back pain sufferers. Doctors tend not to give the patient the benefit of the doubt and readily refer them for a psychiatric opinion. The psychologist is also frequently involved and in many centres around the world he is brought in at the time of the first consultation for a 'psychological profile'.

There are several structural features of a disc which makes it prone to injury and to recurrent episodes of breakdown. For example, take the L4–5 disc – it is the largest avascular structure in the body. The outer half of its annulus has a rich sensory nerve supply and is therefore sensitive (Yoshizawa *et al.*, 1980). A significant twisting injury will separate the outer fibres of the annulus; this is analogous to twisting a large onion and separating its outer layers. This tear of the annulus is liable to recur and there is inevitably poor healing potential in tissue which is avascular. Hence the frustration with the patient whose backache seems to be a constant source of complaint.

Faced with a patient with disabling low back pain, the doctor should not assume that the patient's problem is psychological. There are sound anatomical reasons why the patient's recurring pain may have resisted previous attempts at treatment.

17.2.2 *Referred pain*

The correct surgery for relief of pain originating in the vertebral column requires a working knowledge of the basic pain mechanisms involved. Irritation of any deep part of a low lumbar motion segment may produce an aching pain with referral distally into a limb, as demonstrated by Kellgren (1977) who injected irritant solutions into the motion segments of volunteers at various depths and could distinguish superficial from deep pain. Deep pain in the lower lumbar segments was associated with referral of pain, often as far as the foot. It should be noted that this irritant was injected some distance from the nerve root of the same segment (Figure 17.1).

One of the great diagnostic problems in low back disorders is failure to differentiate this pattern of deep pain referral to a limb from the typical pain of nerve root compression. This confusion accounts for a very high incidence of laminectomy and negative disc exploration.

It may be argued that these distinct types of pain may be clarified by myelography. However, severe back and leg pain may be accompanied by a negative myelogram and, conversely, the lumbar spines of asymptomatic individuals often reveal filling defects. In the whole spectrum of back and

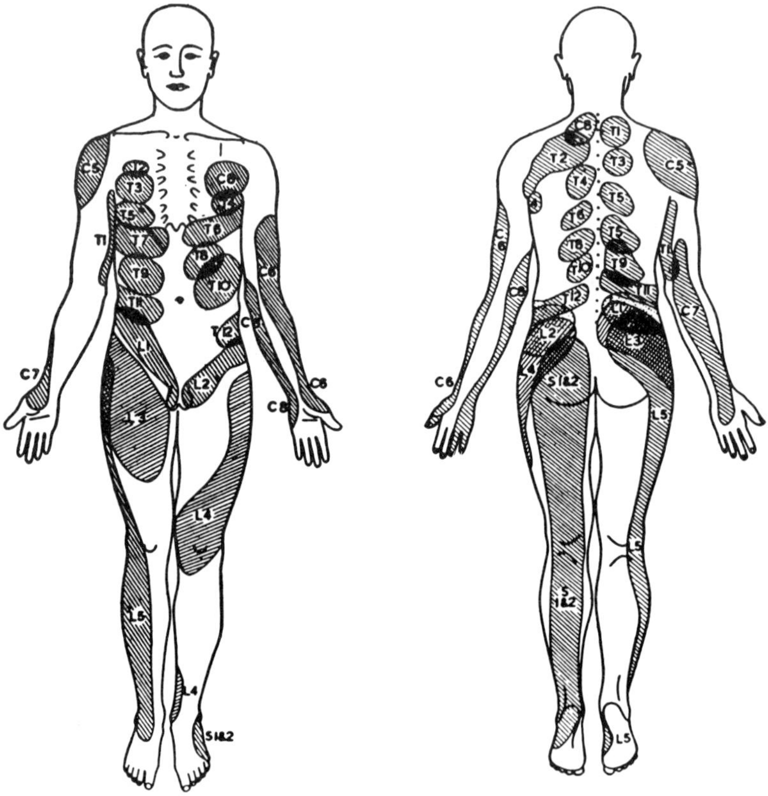

Fig. 17.1 The segmental areas of deep pain developed by the injection of the corresponding interspinous ligaments; diagrams constructed from Kellgren's material. Referred pain, for example L5 segment, is very easily confused with 'sciatica'

leg pain syndromes, nerve root compression accounts for less than 10% of the total problem. The so-called 'tumour theory' (the filling defect) is obviously not the answer in every case (Farfan & Kirkaldy-Willis, 1981).

The incidence of laminectomy varies from 8 to 88.8 per 100,000 per annum in different areas of the world (Kane, 1980); this discrepancy reflects the confusion in the field and is probably to a large extent explained by confusion concerning referred pain patterns in the limbs.

17.2.3 *Discopathies*

When one palpates the front of the low lumbar spine, there is occasionally exquisite local tenderness in patients suffering from low back pain. It was this unusual sign that prompted us to look for and fine nerve fibres in the outer half of the annulus fibrosus.

It was then approprate to undertake a pathological study of disc tissue and vertebral rim removed at the time of anterior fusion. We have been able to demonstrate a surprising incidence of chronic inflammatory reaction in the outer fibres of the annulus fibrosus that has not been previously described. Vascular ingrowth into the outer part of the disc is more common, and both of these lesions are likely causes of pain and disability (O'Brien, 1984).

'We are seeing many cases who have an unquestionably solid fusion yet persist in experiencing severe pain', wrote Wiltse (1977). It is possible that if the disc tissue is left intact and is the source of pain, symptoms will persist in the presence of solid posterior and lateral fusions.

17.2.4 *Discography*

Discography has been discredited for more than 20 years on the basis of unconvincing evidence (Holt, 1968). The proper use of discography and its correct interpretation are essential if one is to identify pathological changes in the disc. These lesions will not be demonstrated by myelography, and it is to be re-emphasised that the outer half of the annulus where these tears will often occur has a rich nerve supply. Discography and its exact interpretation is essential for spinal surgery in the 1980s. The use of this investigation has enabled us, for example, to identify the posterior annular tear syndrome (Park *et al.*, 1979) which produces disabling back and often leg pain following significant injury to the low back and in which the myelogram is negative.

17.3 **The role of fusion**

The role of surgery is to rehabilitate a disabled patient. The role of fusion in chronic low back pain is to stabilise the spine and so to make rehabilitation possible.

The key to the problem of whether one should fuse the spine of a patient with chronic low back pain and, if so, which fusion should be employed, depends entirely on finding the anatomical source of pain and the pathological mechanisms involved. There may be failure of various tissues in the same motion segment.

Precise radiological tests, including discography, radiculography and others, will yield accurate information upon which a decision can be made. These identify the abnormal motion segment(s) and in many cases the particular part of the motion segment responsible. This intensive preliminary work-up may define several lesions in one or several motion segments.

Failures in fusion will occur because of inadequate preliminary work-up, failure to identify the abnormal segment, or failure to identify that part of the motion segment responsible for the disabling back pain. Continuing, crippling back pain, despite radiologically intact posterior or lateral fusion, exists commonly and occurs when the source of pain is the nerve-sensitive disc that has not been adequately immobilised by the posterior fusion mass.

17.3.1 *Principles involved in selecting surgery*

The principles involved in the surgical technique are twofold:

(1) remove the anatomical source of pain;

(2) if in removing the pain source, the spine has been destabilised, then stability must be restored.

According to the principles above, in many situations in chronic sufferers a painful torn disc is the anatomical pain source. This is best removed through an anterior approach; although a posterior approach can be performed, it is technically difficult and takes a great deal of time.

Removal of the disc, leaving only part of the posterior annulus, through an anterior approach renders the spine unstable. This stability must be restored by blocks of bone removed from the left iliac crest and impacted between the vertebral bodies, thus replacing the disc with the patient's own bone.

This operation was first described more than 50 years ago in this country; Capener (1932), Burns (1933) and Mercer (1936) being amongst the pioneers of the operation. It is likely that it did not maintain its popularity, like many major surgical procedures in the mid 1930s, because of the lack of antibiotics and sophisticated blood transfusion techniques.

17.3.2 *Basic description of the operation*

A left sympathectomy-like incision is performed and a retroperitoneal approach is used. The lumbo-sacral disc can be approached between the bifurcation of the vessels, the L4–5 disc is most easily approached to the left side of the common iliac vessles. More than 90% of chronic back-pain sufferers have pain sources at one or both of these segments.

Control of bleeding is of fundamental importance. The discs are completely cleared out (one often observes inflammatory changes in the anterior annulus). Bone graft is removed from the left iliac crest, cut carefully into blocks and three or four such blocks at each level are used to replace the disc which has been excised.

The patient has an ileus for one to two days after surgery and is then allowed to mobilise with a light brace. Check X-rays 3 and 6 months after surgery has been performed. When fusion is demonstrated by lateral tomography, the patient is allowed to increase his activities.

17.3.3 *Advantages of the anterior approach*
Firstly, the whole of the torn painful disc is excised. Secondly, stability is completely restored to the motion segment. Thirdly, the nerve roots are not tampered with. Nerve root scarring is a notorious cause of persisting disabling low back pain and leg pain.

A comparison of the literature of postero-lateral fusion and anterior fusion confirms that fusion rates for these are similar. Say, for one-level postero-lateral fusion, the mean fusion rate in the literature is 81.5%. For one-level anterior lumbar fusion, the mean rate is 82.5% (Kozak & O'Brien, 1988).

Fusion of the transverse processes (postero-lateral fusion) is the commonest technique in use today. However, it is biomechanically inferior to the interbody fusion which has the distinct advantage of complete excision of the torn and painful disc.

17.3.4 *Indications for surgery in the disabled low back pain group*
It was mentioned earlier in this chapter that all conservative treatment should have failed before surgery is considered. This cannot be overemphasised. Many of the patients treated surgically will have had chronic relapsing low back pain for 5 or 10 years, in which all conceivable forms of conservative treatment have been tried and been shown to have failed. The patient's disability is best assessed by the Oswestry Disability Questionnaire (Fairbank *et al.*, 1980). This provides a numerical assessment of the limitations of the patient's daily living activities.

Detailed neurological assessment is often misleading, in fact, in many disabled patients, there are few, if any, physical signs to elicit. This is particularly so with discogenic lesions. It is common to have limited or misleading neurological signs in addition to a negative myelogram. It is at this stage that one would tend to proceed with discography to define the anatomical pain source. Magnetic resonance imaging, CT scans and other sophisticated studies all have their place but they have a single drawback in that they do not define the pain source, so essential in planning surgery of this magnitude.

17.3.5 *The post-laminectomy syndrome*
Failure of spinal surgery in relieving patients crippled with back and leg pain is common on a world-wide basis. This failure has usually accounted for increased disability, intense referred pain and nearly two-thirds of the paients in this category who are disabled have attempted suicide or certainly have suicidal tendencies.

The *simultaneous combined anterior and posterior fusion* technique has been developed over the past years for this specific group of patients with post-laminectomy syndrome (O'Brien *et al.*, 1986). The anterior fusion, as basically described above, is combined with exploration of the spinal canal and decompression of the nerve roots, together with instrumentation of the posterior segments and a lateral fusion.

A recent series of 69 patients treated by a simultaneous combined anterior and posterior fusion, in whom the average number of previous back operations was almost two, had the following results: fusion rates in excess of 90% were seen in patients who had undergone one- or two-level fusions, whilst the fusion for three-level procedures dropped to 78% (Kozak & O'Brien, 1988). These figures are at variance with Nachemson's (Nachemson, 1982) who pointed out that with a third operation, there is only a 5% chance of success.

Whilst it is agreed that this technique is major surgery, the evidence to date, with several years of follow-up, indicates that it is a sure way of gaining early fusion and in the large majority of patients a return to a reasonable lifestyle.

17.4 **Summary**

This chapter has outlined the surgical alternatives in the disabled low back pain sufferer. Anterior lumbar fusion with removal of the discs and their replacement with the patient's own bone graft, whilst being major spinal surgery, provides a very real chance of rehabilitation for this difficult patient group.

The commonest difficulty in diagnosing this group is confusing referred pain with pain due to nerve root compression, thus leading to the wrong type of surgery.

In the post-laminectomy group, a combined anterior and posterior approach to the previously operated and painful segments provides a very high chance of rehabilitation to a reasonable lifestyle.

References

Burns, B. H. (1933). An operation for spondylolisthesis, *Lancet*, **1**, 1233.

Capener, N. (1932). Spondylolisthesis, *British Journal of Surgery*, **19**, 374.

Fairbank, J. C. T., Couper, J., Davies, J. B. & O'Brien, J. P. (1980). Oswestry Disability Questionnaire, *Physiotherapy*, **66**, 271–3.

Farfan, H. F. & Kirkaldy-Willis, W. H. (1981). The present status of spinal fusion in the treatment of lumbar intervertebral disorders, *Clinical Orthopaedics*, 158, 198.

Frymoyer, J. W. (1981). The role of spine fusion: Question 3, *Spine*, **6**, 284–9.

Holt, E. P., Jr. (1968). The question of lumbar discography, *Journal of Bone and Joint Surgery*, **50A**, 720.

Kane, W. J. (1980). The incidence rate of laminectomy in the USA, Abstract of International Society for the Study of the Lumbar Spine Meeting.

Kellgren, J. H. (1977). The anatomical source of back pain, *Rheumatology and Rehabilitation*, **16**, 3–12.

Kozak, J. A. & O'Brien, J. P. (1989). Simultaneous combined anterior and posterior fusion: an independent analysis of treatment for the disabled low back pain patient, Spine. (In press)

Lehmann, T. R., Spratt, K. F., Tozzi, J. E., Weinstein, J. N., Reinarz, S. J., El-Khoury, G. Y. & Colby, H. (1987). Long-term follow-up of lower lumbar fusion patients, *Spine*, **12**, 97–104.

Mercer, W. (1936). Spondylolisthesis, *Edinburgh Medical Journal*, NS **43**, 545.

Nachemson, A. (1982). The national course of low back pain. In: *Symposium on Idiopathic Low Back Pain*, eds. A. A. White & S. L. Gardon, pp. 46–51. C. V. Mosby, St Louis.

O'Brien, J. P. (1984). Mechanisms of spinal pain. In: *Textbook of Pain*, eds. P. D. Wall & R. Melzack, pp. 240–51. Churchill Livingstone, Edinburgh.

O'Brien, J. P., Dawson, M. H. O., Heard, C. W. *et al.* (1986). Simultaneous combined anterior and posterior fusion, *Clinical Orthopaedics*, **203**, 191–5.

Park, W. M., McCall, I. W., O'Brien, J. P. & Webb, J. K. (1979). Fissuring of the posterior annulus fibrosus in the lumbar spine, *British Journal of Radiology*, **52**, 382–7.

Weber, H. (1983). Lumbar disc herniation: A controlled, prospective study with ten years of observation, *Spine*, **8**, 131–40.

Wiltse, L. (1977). Surgery for intervertebral disc disease of the lumbar spine, *Clinical Orthopaedics*, **129**, 22.

Wright, A. (1981). The role of spine fusion: Question 5, *Spine*, **6**, 292.

Yoshizawa, H., O'Brien, J. P., Smith, W. T. *et al.* (1980). The neuropathology of intervertebral disc removed for low back pain, *Journal of Pathology*, **132**, 95–103.

Young, H. H., Love, J. G., Svien, H. J., Price, R. D. & Kroll, H. G. (1955). Low back and sciatic pain: Long-term results after removal of protruded intervertebral disk with or without fusion, *Clinical Orthopaedics*, **5**, 128–37.

Index